A Colour Atlas of
MULTIPLE SCLEROSIS
& OTHER MYELIN DISORDERS

C W M Adams
MA, MD, DSc, FRCP, FRCPath

*Sir William Dunn Professor of Pathology,
United Medical Schools of Guy's and
St. Thomas's Hospitals, London
University, London SE1 9RT and
Department of Neuropathology,
Runwell Hospital,
Wickford, Essex, SS11 7QE*

Wolfe Medical Publications Ltd

Published by Wolfe Medical Publications Ltd, 1989
Printed by W. S. Cowell, Ipswich, Suffolk, United Kingdom
ISBN 0 7234 0952 8

For a full list of other titles published by Wolfe Medical Publications Ltd, please write to the publishers at Brook House, 2-16 Torrington Place, London WC1E 7LT, England.

A CIP catalogue record for this book is available from the British Library, 2 Sheraton Street, London W1A 6JZ.

Contents

Acknowledgements

I am most grateful to the following for use of illustrations, as further mentioned in the text:

Addis Press Ltd., Professor R M Barlow, Dr K D Barron, Dr Amico Bignami, Professor A C Bird, Dr A P Boon, Messrs Chapman & Hall, the late Professor J N Cumings, Dr J T Done, Professor L Duchen, Messrs Elsevier/North Holland Publishers, Dr Margaret Esiri, Dr Elena Gabrielescu, Dr A L Ganser, Dr N A Gregson, Dr J F Hallpike, Dr B Harding, Professor J McC Howell, Professor R A C Hughes, Professor M Z M Ibrahim, Dr I Janota, Dr D A Kirschner, Dr R L Knobler, Dr J R Kurtzke, Professor S Leibowitz, Dr S Lightman, Dr S K Ludwin, Professor W I Mcdonald, Dr Jia Newcombe, Dr G Petierson, Dr A Petrescu, Dr R N Poston, Dr C S Raine, Professor M C Raff, Dr M Rodriguez, Dr Barbara Smith, Messrs C C Thomas Publishers, Professor H E Webb and Professor R O Weller.

I am much indebted to Mrs Rosemary Brown, Mr S J Buk, Miss Valerie Gray and Dr Olga High for help with the histological preparations. The following provided material for which I am most grateful: Dr David Haler, Professor Keith Mant, the late Professor C K Simpson, Dr William Brander, Dr R Doshi, Dr M O Skelton and other pathologists in the S-E Thames Region, my colleagues at Guy's Hospital, Dr Louise Cuzner, Dr Margaret Esiri, the Department of Morbid Anatomy, Addenbrooke's Hospital, Cambridge and the Department of Neuropathology, Runwell Hospital, Wickford. I am further indebted to the Department of Medical Illustration, UMDS, Guy's Hospital and the Department of Neuropathology, Runwell Hospital, for help with many of the illustrations. Last but not least, I particularly wish to thank Miss Beryl Hilliard for typing the text and bibliography.

Abbreviations

ACAT – acyl-cholesterol: acyltransferase

ASA – arylsulphatase-A

CJ (disease) – Creutzfeldt – Jakob disease

CNS – central nervous system

CPM – central pontine myelinoclasis

CREAE – chronic relapsing experimental allergic encephalomyelitis

CSF – cerebrospinal fluid

CSPE – chronic sclerosing panencephalitis

EAE – experimental allergic encephalomyelitis

EAN – experimental allergic neuritis

GAG – glycosaminoglycan

GFAP – glial fibrillary acidic protein

MAG – myelin associated glycoprotein

MBP – myelin basic protein

MCB – metachromatic bodies

ME – measles encephalitis

MLD – myelin deficient

MRI – magnetic resonance imaging

MS – multiple sclerosis

OTAN – osmium tetroxide – α naphthylamine

PAN – perchloric acid-naphthoquinone

PLP – proteolipid protein

PML – progressive multifocal lencoencephalopathy

PNS – peripheral nervous system

PTAH – phosphotungstic acid haematoxylin

PUFA – polyunsaturated fatty acids

RF – Rosenthal fibres

SACD – subacute combined degeneration

SLE – systemic lupus erythematosus

SSPE – subacute sclerosing panencephalitis

VEP – visually evoked potential

Preface

Multiple sclerosis may present to a doctor or medical scientist as a patient with a clinical problem or as an abstract report from a chemical-immunological laboratory. Hence, it seemed appropriate to a pathologist to assemble an atlas of the tissue changes in MS to provide a fundamental and visible background to the clinical and molecular aspects of the myelin diseases.

The illustrations in this Atlas have been collected over the last 30 years during work in the myelin/MS field. This, together with current difficulties in obtaining autopsy tissue, seemed to make it particularly worthwhile to put our illustrations on record, together with a short explanatory text which also aims to be a concise review of myelin diseases. The original intention was to assemble an Atlas on MS only, but recent developments have widened our interest in myelin disorders. To name but a few instances, demyelination has become of particular relevance to AIDS, oncology and to electrolyte disturbances (central pontine myelinoclasis). Genetic, immune and infective factors are now seen to be of major importance in a range of demyelinating and dysmyelinating diseases, in both human and veterinary medicine.

It is very pleasing to record the great help that I have received from many colleagues in lending illustrations of the experimental, comparative and human aspects of myelin diseases. Their contribution is formally acknowledged in the following pages, but here I wish to add a further deeply felt 'thank you' to them for their generous and invaluable help.

C W M Adams
1989

1 Myelin and demyelinating diseases: introduction and general principles

Before discussing and illustrating the lesions of multiple sclerosis and other myelin diseases, it is necessary to consider the principles relating to the composition, formation, degeneration and repair of myelin.

A major problem is that myelin with its compact membranous composition is a unique structure. It has no immediate comparable in human pathology and its relation to any experimental disease is tenuous or at best inconclusive. There is no great difficulty in understanding the overall pathogenesis of a frank viral or autoimmune disease, but the typical episodic and relapsing course of multiple sclerosis adds another dimension to the problem.

Myelin structure and components

It is well established that myelin is a complex membranous structure laid down around the axon by oligodendroglia in the central nervous system (CNS) and by Schwann cells in the peripheral nervous system (PNS). Its essential molecular structure is a lipid bilayer with connecting struts between the protein layers, known as the intermediate and period dense lines, as seen by electronmicroscopy (**1**) and by Xray diffraction. Interest in the precise molecular topography of the lipid components has probably waned since the earlier studies based on graphic molecular models (Finean, 1957; Vandenheuvel, 1965). More interest is now attached to the functions of the myelin proteins, the ionic and electrostatic forces binding the surface membranes together, and the state of compaction of the myelin lamellae (Kirschner and Ganser, 1984).

The paranodal region of the myelin sheath, next to the node of Ranvier, shows complex interdigitations in electronmicrographs, and is thought to form a centre for metabolic and perhaps electrical activity. The Schmitt-Lantermann cleft, which dips deeply into the myelin sheath and was first recognised in the last century, has now been shown to contain Schwann cell cytoplasm and, in the peripheral nerve, acts as a conduit across the width of the sheath (Hall and Williams, 1970).

The myelin lipids are major components of the myelin sheath: they may be detected by biochemical or histochemical means. Recently a start has been made towards detecting these lipids by immunocytochemical means (Dupouey *et al.*, 1979; Itoyama *et al.*, 1980; Gregson and Leibowitz, 1985). The localisation of free cholesterol, cerebroside, sphingomyelin, sulphatide and phosphoglycerides in myelin by the relevant histochemical methods (Adams and Bayliss, 1975) is shown in **2** to **18**. Esterified cholesterol is essentially absent from adult myelin, but is transiently present during development (Adams and Davison, 1959; Barlow, 1969; **19**; Table 1) and is the major lipid of the myelin breakdown products (Cumings, 1955). This esterified cholesterol is the essential lipid that is 'sudanophilic' (stains with the red Sudan dyes and Oil red O), is coloured pink with Nile Blue sulphate and reacts with the Marchi reagents (**20**; Adams, 1958, 1959). Cholesterol ester synthetase and hydrolase activities have been detected in MS plaques and correlate with the amount of ester in the plaque (Shah and Johnson, 1980). Although the presence of cholesterol ester is the hallmark of a demyelinating disease, it essentially only indicates that the myelin sheath has been irreversibly degraded.

Table 1 Esterified cholesterol in developing human nervous system (Adams & Davison, 1959, 1960)

		% of cholesterol as ester	
		Spinal cord	Corpus callosum
Foetus	17 weeks	5.8	6.60
Foetus	28 weeks	18.8	—
Foetus	33 weeks	20.8	3.1
Foetus	34 weeks	49.0	—
Newborn		7.6	13.4
Infant	7 weeks	0	17.8
Child	5 years	2.8	5.0
Adults	(5 cases)	0	0*

*1.4% in one case only

An important component of both CNS and PNS myelin is myelin basic protein (MBP). PNS myelin contains less MBP than does the CNS but, in addition to P_1, contains P_2, which is not a constituent of CNS myelin (Norton, 1982). MBP can be demonstrated histologically by both immunocytochemical and histochemical methods, the latter using staining methods for basic protein (**21** and **22**). Encephalitogenic activity (the antigen that evokes experimental allergic encephalomyelitis) is mainly located in MBP.

The most abundant myelin protein of the CNS is proteolipid protein (PLP); this lipoprotein behaves as a lipid in that it can be extracted by certain lipid solvents. However, some lipid material remains in histological paraffin sections and such myelin PLP can be stained by the Heidenhain (**23**), Weigert-Pal, Loyez, Solochrome cyanin (**24**) and Luxol fast blue (**24**) methods.

Myelin PLP was originally characterised by Jordi Folch as a trypsin-resistant protein, but it is now known that it is sensitive to trypsin in the presence of detergent (Lees and Chan, 1975). Proteolipid and CNS-MBP can be demonstrated immunohistologically in oligodendroglia during myelination and, susbsequently, in the myelin sheath (Hartmann *et al.*, 1979).

Neurokeratin in the peripheral nerve is shown in **25** and **26**. This is a solvent-resistant and trypsin resistant protein (**27** and **28**), which is probably mainly derived from the myelin protein P_o. It appears in paraffin and cryostat sections in the form of a network (**26** and **29**), but this artefactual distribution is not seen after fixation in buffered osmium tetroxide (**29**). The relationship of neurokeratin to other myelin constituents in histological terms is shown in **30**.

Glycoproteins are represented in myelin by a myelin-associated glycoprotein (MAG; **31**), which is involved in some immune reactions in the human peripheral nerve. MAG can be demonstrated immunocytochemically with anti-MAG and anti-IgM antibodies (Gregson and Leibowitz, 1985); it seems to be associated in the PNS more with the Schwann cell and outer myelin membranes than with the inner compact myelin (Trapp and Quarles, 1984). In the CNS, MAG is located in the periaxonal region and in oligodendroglia during myelination (Itoyama *et al.*, 1980).

Glycosaminoglycan (GAG), in the form of hyaluronic acid, is seen at the node of Ranvier (**32**), endoneurium and axon (**33** to **36**; see Adams, 1965; Langley and Landon, 1968). Conventional staining methods for glycosaminoglycans are hampered in myelin by the presence of sulphatide, which competes with acid GAGs for dye cations (**14**). However, such staining of sulphatide is abolished by the relevant lipid solvents or by trypsinisation to reveal the axonal distribution of acid GAGs (**33** to **36**). Axonal protein is demonstrated by the coupled tetrazonium method (**37**).

The metabolic stability (speed of turnover) of myelin was studied in depth three decades ago (Dawson and Richter, 1950; Davison *et al.*, 1959; Payling Wright, 1961). The results showed that myelin lipids have a rather slow turnover consistent with marked metabolic stability. Later work largely confirmed this view, but certain constituents, such as phosphatidyl-choline and phosphatidyl-inositide turn over much faster. However, the typical myelin lipids cholesterol and cerebroside are confirmed as slow-turnover constituents (Norton, 1982; Benjamins and Smith, 1984). The proteins of myelin appear to turn over much more rapidly (20-40 days) than the 'slow turnover' myelin lipids (Smith and Hasinoff, 1971).

Apart from 2′, 3′-cyclic nucleotide-3′-phosphoesterase activity, myelin membranes show little evidence of respiratory and general metabolic enzyme activity. Figures **38** and **39** show histochemical evidence of respiratory activity in Schwann cell and axon, but none in compact myelin. However, a range of enzymes concerned with lipid and protein synthesis are present in myelin (see Norton, 1982). Earlier work had shown that some neutral catheptic and peptidase activities are located in myelin (**40**; Adams and Bayliss, 1961): neural L-leucyl-β-naphthylamidase activity can be detected biochemically in myelin, but not histochemically because the simultaneous coupling salt inhibits the enzyme in the incubating medium (Adams and Glenner, 1962).

Myelination and myelin control

The oliodendrocyte is responsible for myelination in the CNS (Peters and Vaughan, 1970), whereas the Schwann cell subserves this function in the PNS (Bunge, 1968). The PNS is largely myelinated by birth in most species, whereas the brain is slowly myelinated in the months and years following birth (Yakovlev and Lecours, 1967; reviewed by Einstein and Adams, 1988; Hartmann *et al.*, 1979). Kinney *et al.* (1988) have plotted out the time taken to achieve 50 per cent myelination at various sites in the human brain; it varied between 44 weeks for the internal capsule and 139 weeks for the anterior commissure.

The human cord is myelinated between mid-late term and the third month of life after which further myelin may be laid down within the sheath (Niebroj-Dubosz *et al.*, 1980). It has been suggested that tracts are myelinated when physiological needs first require conduction through them. This delayed myelination in the CNS accounts for the jelly-like nature and vulnerability of the newborn human brain.

Evidence is mounting that thyroxine controls myelination (Dalal *et al.*, 1971; Anderson *et al.*, 1987; Shanker *et al.*, 1987). This accords with the hypomyelinogenesis in border disease of sheep, where the thyroid is damaged in-utero by a toga-virus (*see* Chapter 3).

An oliogodendrocyte is thought to myelinate about 30-40 CNS internodes by a complex series of extrusions around the axon (Bunge *et al.*, 1962). The Schwann cell adopts the simpler manoeuvre of rotating around the outside of a single axon, forming the myelin sheath from extruded mesaxon material (Peters and Vaughan, 1970).

The mature myelin sheath is maintained by these two formative cells: damage to them causes myelin degeneration, as seen after administration of cuprizone (**41** and **42**; Ludwin, 1981, Blakemore *et al.*, 1983), diphtheria intoxication (**194** and **195**) and in diabetic neuropathy (**43**).

Myelination is disturbed in a number of conditions, notably the various leucodystrophies in man (*see* Chapter 2), similar disorders in mutant mice, hypomyelinogenisis congenita and swayback disease of sheep (*see* Chapter 3). Myelin development is at risk when malnutrition occurs in early life (Dobbing, 1968); myelin defects may persist even though brain weight catches up better than bodyweight when alimentation improves. Such early malnutrition may result in irreversible damage to glial cells and subsequent defective myelin formation (Bass *et al.*, 1970).

Characteristics of demyelination

Demyelinating diseases are conditions where the brunt of the disease is born by the myelin sheath – oligodendroglia/Schwann cell system. The axon and nerve cell remain intact (**44** and **45**), although the axon may be damaged at a later stage. (This is discussed further at the beginning of Chapter 2 and in Chapter 7.) Conversely, Wallerian or axonal degeneration involves the whole neurone distal to the seat of damage, for example, the nerve cell of the anterior horn in poliomyelitis (**46** and **47**) or the peripheral part of the nerve after trauma or in intoxication. Rows of hypertrophied Schwann cells (the bands of Büngner) are seen in the peripheral nerve undergoing Wallerian degeneration. At first, these are concerned with myelin digestion, but they persist until the nerve is reinnervated by axonal sprouting. However, only one or two of these sprouts then proceed to be myelinated.

Demyelinating neuropathy in the peripheral nerve is not accepted as a common feature of multiple sclerosis (*see* Chapter 2), but the nerve may be involved in tract (Wallerian) degeneration as a result of damage by a plaque in the cord. True demyelinating disease in the peripheral nerve, as in diabetic neuropathy or Guillain-Barré syndrome, is typically characterised by segmental demyelination, where one complete internodal segment is damaged following death or impairment of the nutritive Schwann cell for that internode (**43** and **48**).

In the CNS, segmental or internodal demyelination are seen when oligodendroglia are damaged (Suzuki *et al.*, 1969; Prineas *et al.*, 1984). However, the complex interrelationships of oligodendroglia with many CNS internodes would complicate the recognition of such segmental damage that occurs.

Remyelination

The damaged peripheral nerve in segmental demyelination repairs relatively rapidly in a matter of weeks following recovery of the Schwann cell. By contrast, repair is slow in Wallerian degeneration, when the complete unit of axon, myelin and Schwann cell has been damaged. Here, the nerve can only repair at a slow rate by regenerative sprouting from the central surviving part of the nerve (Lubinska, 1963).

Repair in the central nervous system is a controversial issue and is thought to be impeded by neuroglial overgrowth preventing axonal sprouting (**49**) or, in some circumstances, by inadequate neurotropic stimulation or both. Provided that the axon is intact, CNS myelin may be repaired by oligodendroglia; the extent depends on various circumstances (see below). After lysolecithin-induced and cuprizone-induced demyelination, remyelination starts at 1 to 2 weeks and is nearly complete at 3 months (**41** and **42**; Smith *et al.*, 1981; Ludwin, 1981, 1987). However, repair and remyelination in multiple sclerosis is more controversial (McDonald, 1974; Harrison, 1983). The occasional or rather more frequent presence of thinly myelinated axons provides evidence for remyelination (Prineas and Connell, 1979; Ludwin, 1987). Shadow plaques are thought to be foci of such remyelinating fibres (*see* Chapter 7; Prineas, 1985; Prineas *et al.*, 1984; Raine, 1983). It is likely that some fibres with inappropriately thin sheaths are undergoing remyelination, but it would be unwise to conclude that all such fibres are recovering in the absence of other more direct evidence of remyelination (Ludwin, 1987). Likewise, some shadow plaques may be caused by focal oedema or arrested incomplete demyelination. Remyelination and shadow plaques are discussed further in Chapter 7.

Schwann cells may remyelinate demyelinated areas that are near the exit points of cranial and spinal nerves (Feigin and Popoff, 1966; Ogata and Feigin, 1975; Ghatak *et al.*, 1973; Blakemore, 1977). Peripheral type myelin derived from Schwann cells during CNS remyelination appears considerably thicker and more deeply stained than normal CNS myelin (**50**), and is also endowed with a limiting basement membrane (Harrison, 1983). Itoyama *et al.*, (1985) showed that areas of Schwann-cell-controlled remyelination (shown by anti-P_0 peroxidase) in the cord are deficient in astrocyte fibres (GFAP-peroxidase). This suggests that astrocytes may inhibit Schwann cell remyelination in the CNS.

Oligodendroglia are at some disadvantage in comparison with Schwann cells as remyelinating cells. Ludwin (1982) points out that at least 20 internodes would have to be remyelinated by one oligodendrocyte and that the membranes concerned would get twisted up in the great complexity of the process. There is also a shortage of oligodendroglia in the brain, so that even satellite oligodendroglia may be recruited for this purpose (Ludwin, 1979). Furthermore, recruitment of macrophages into the damaged peripheral nerve is rapid, but is slow in the CNS (Perry *et al.*, 1987).

Clinical recovery is not necessarily an index of remyelination, as nerve conduction can improve after even the formation of only a few new myelin lamellae. Conduction may also be assumed to improve as a result of subsidence of the oedema that accompanies acute lesions (**51**) and the resulting reduction in tissue pressure. Moreover, there still remains the question whether part of the defect in nerve conduction MS is caused by an IgG synaptic neuroelectric blocking factor, as found in serum from MS patients (Schauf *et al.*, 1978).

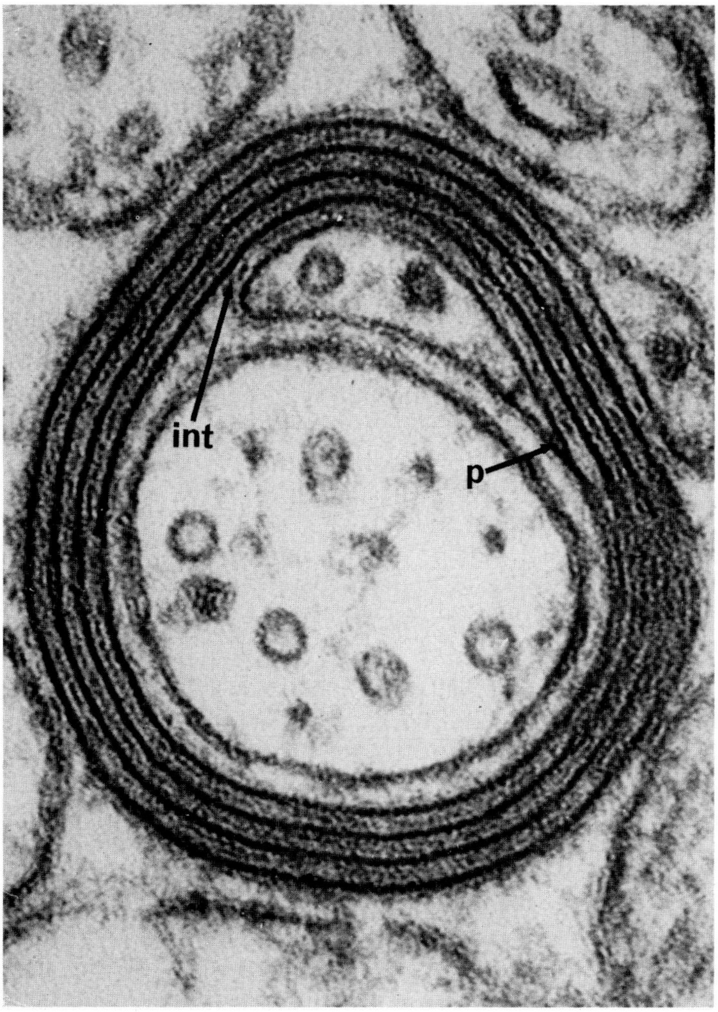

1

1 Electronmicrograph of small axon in rat CNS. The major dense or period line is formed by fusion of the inner aspects of oligodendroglial cell membrane (P), whereas the interperiod line (int) is formed by fusion of the outer aspects of this cell membrane, × 256,000. *(Courtesy of Professor R.O. Weller)*

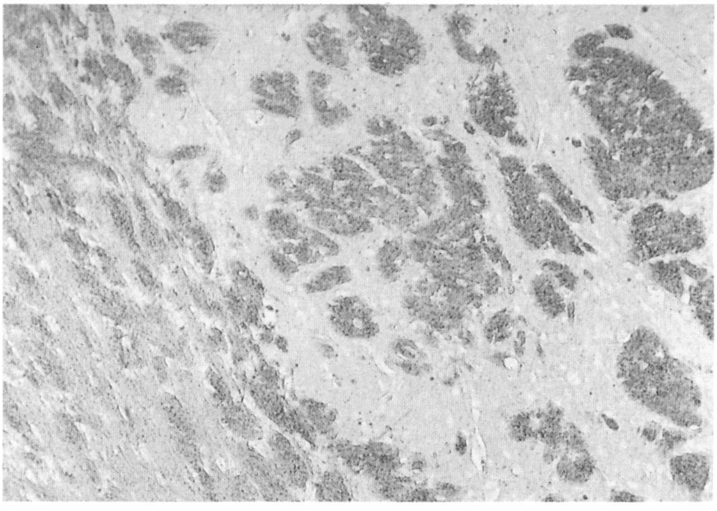

2

2 Cholesterol in callosal radiation of human brain, perchloric acid-naphthoquinone (PAN), × 80.

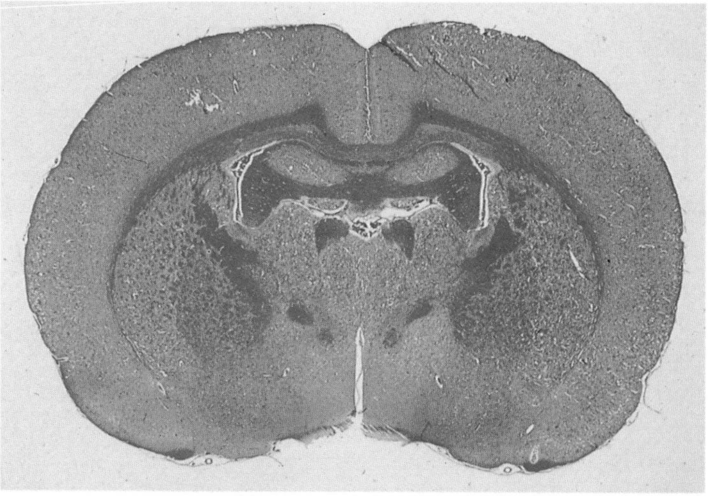

3

3 Cerebroside in corpus callosum of rat brain, modified PAS method, × 5.

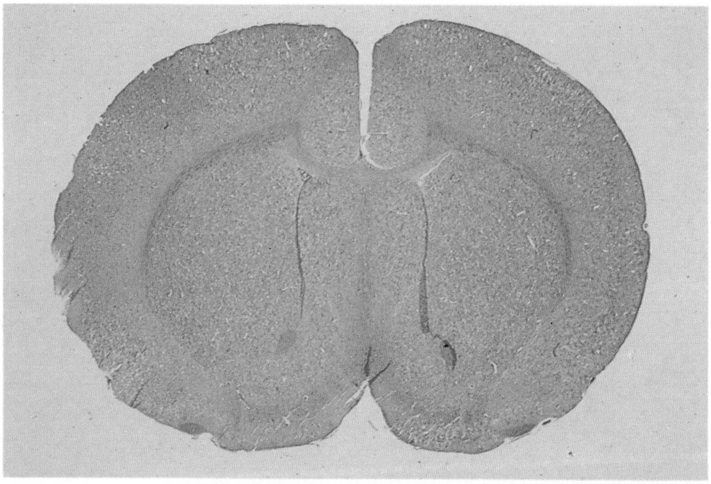

4

4 Negative reaction for cerebroside (see **3**) after extraction with chloroform-methanol (2:1 v/v).

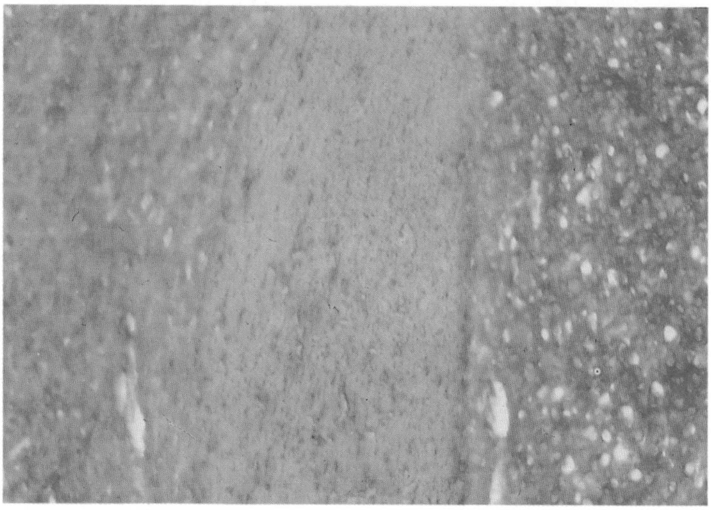

5

5 Sulphatide revealed as brown metachromasia in rat callosal radiation. Cresyl violet, × 150.

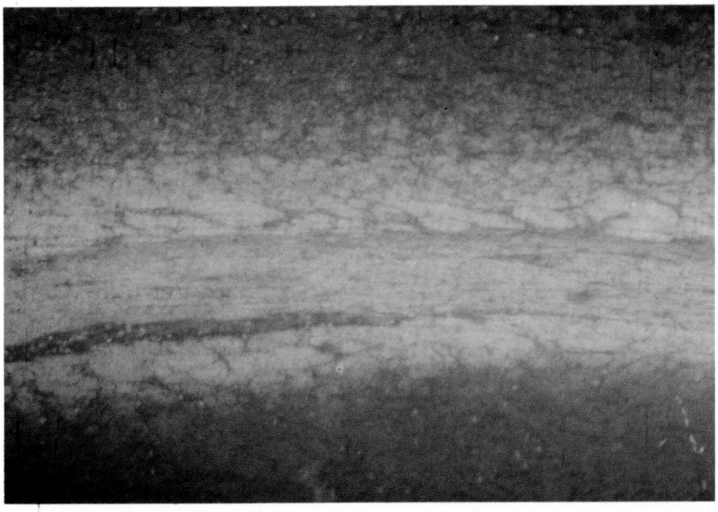

6

6 Sulphatide in rat callosal radiation. Frozen section, acridine orange in 0.3M NaCl, × 150.

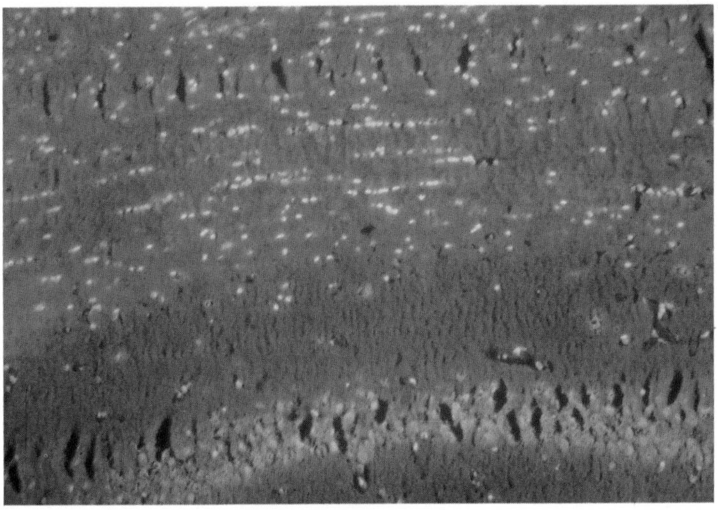

7

7 Negative reaction for sulphatide with acridine orange (see **6**) after chloroform-methanol extraction.

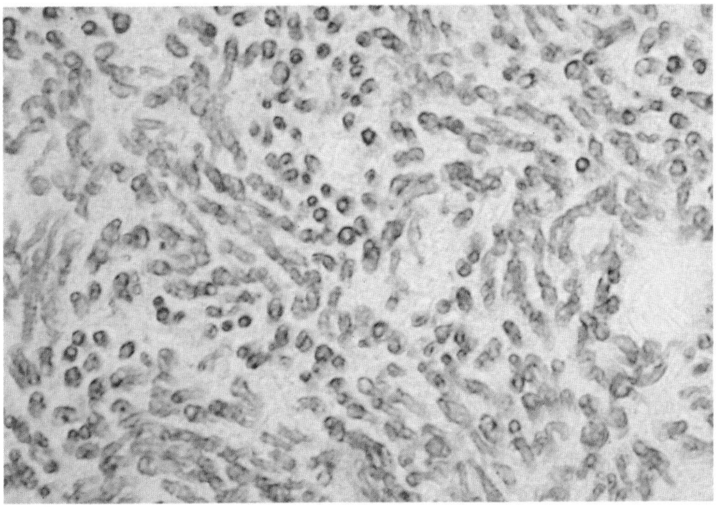

8

8 Myelinated tract in human cord. Gold hydroxamic acid method for phospholipids, × 150.

9

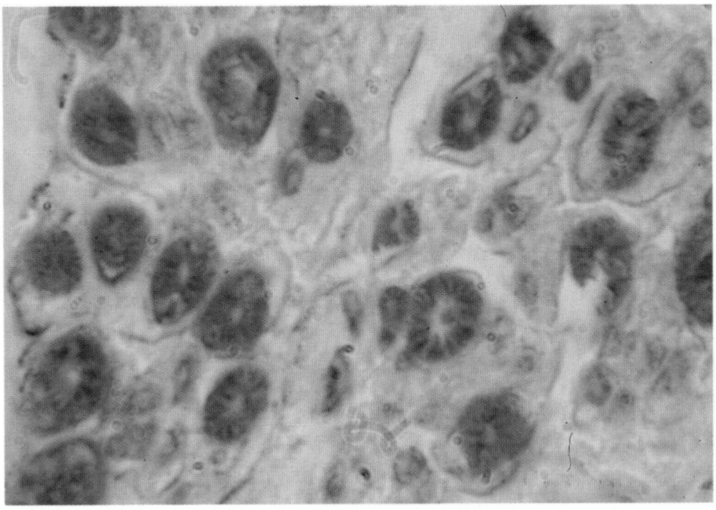

9 Myelin phospholipids. Human cord, gold hydroxamic acid method, × 400.

10

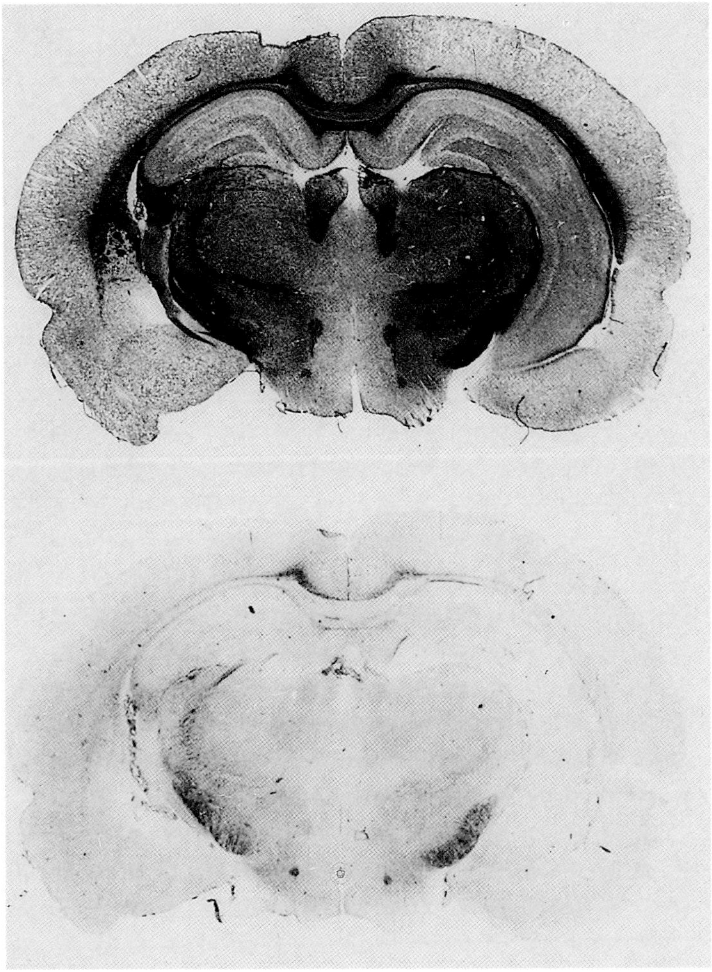

10 Rat cerebral cortex. Plasmal reaction for plasmalogen phospholipids. Chloroform methanol extraction below. Schiff, × 4.

11

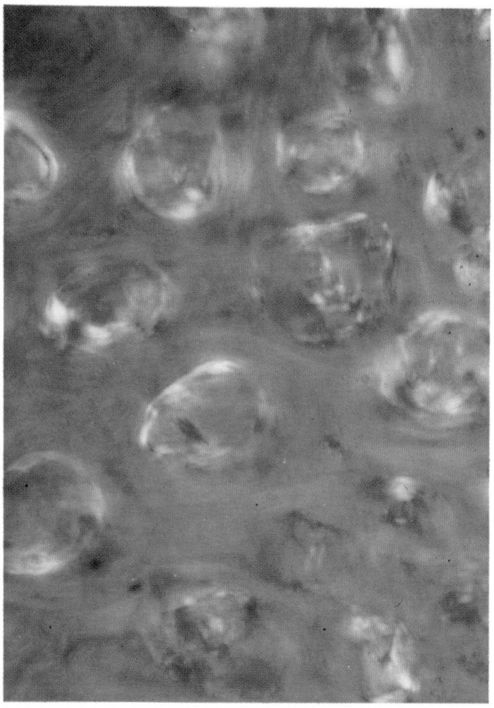

11 Human spinal cord viewed in polarised light. Note birefringent myelin sheaths, × 400.

12

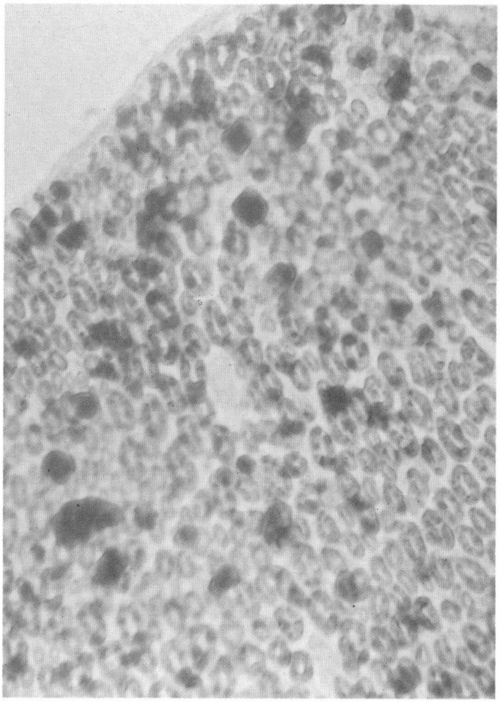

12 Rat sciatic nerve, perchloric acid-naphthoquinone (PAN) to show cholesterol, × 100.

13

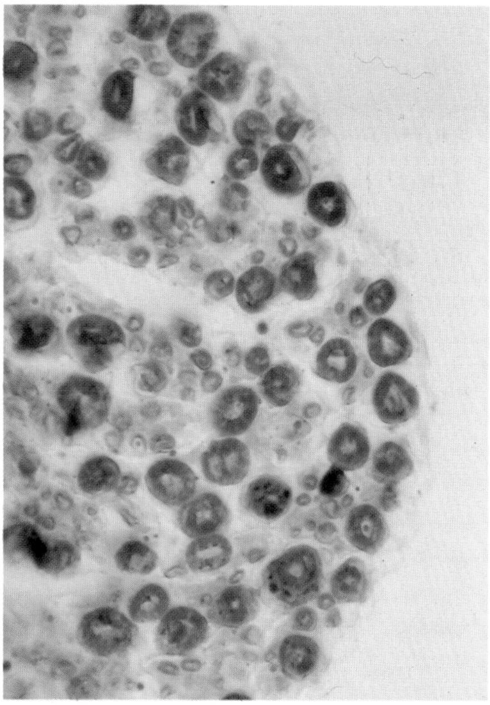

13 As for 12, final black reaction for cholesterol, PAN × 200.

14

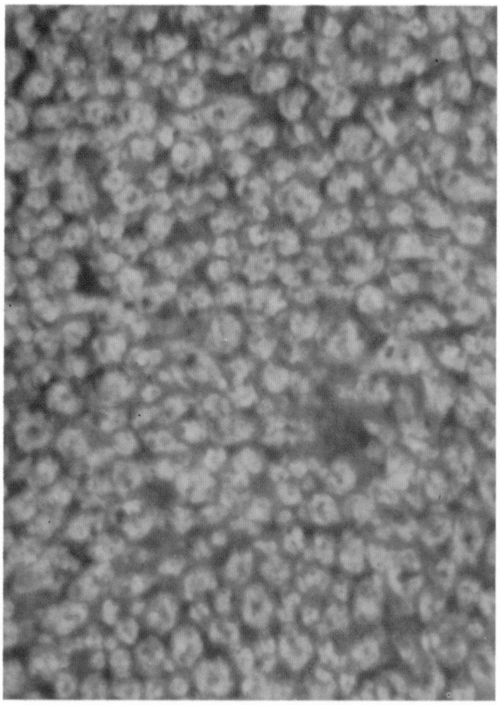

14 Rat peripheral nerve. Acridine orange in 0.3M NaCl to show sulphatide, × 200.

15

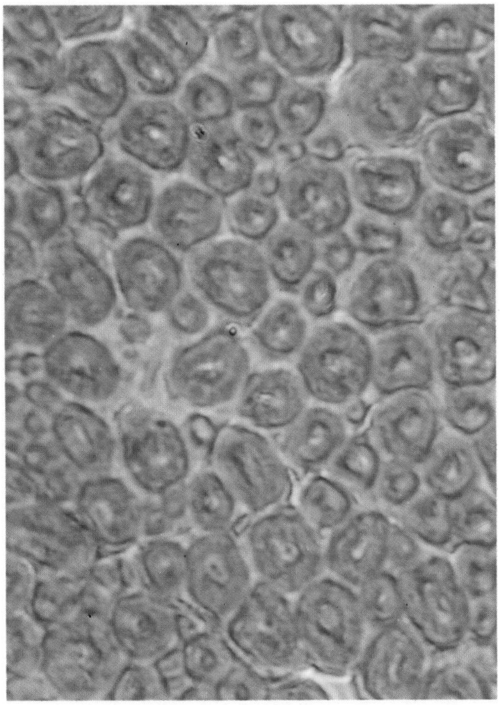

15 Rat peripheral nerve. Acetone – Hale's colloidal iron to show sulphatide, × 300.

16

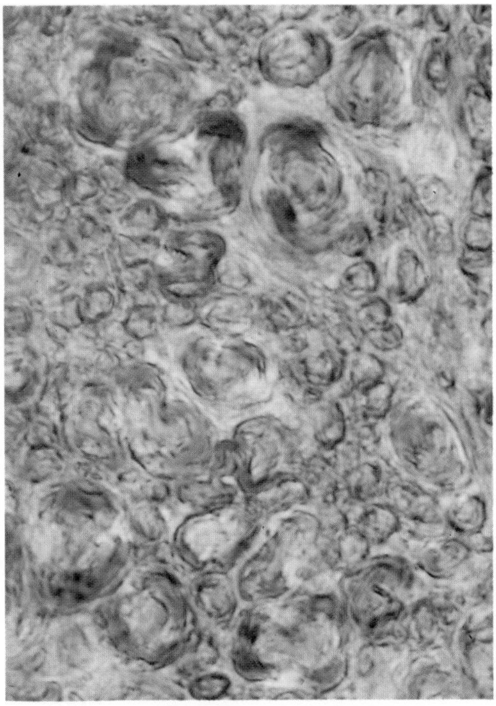

16 Human peripheral nerve. Osmium tetroxide-αnaphthylamine (OTAN) to show phospholipids (orange-red), × 300.

17

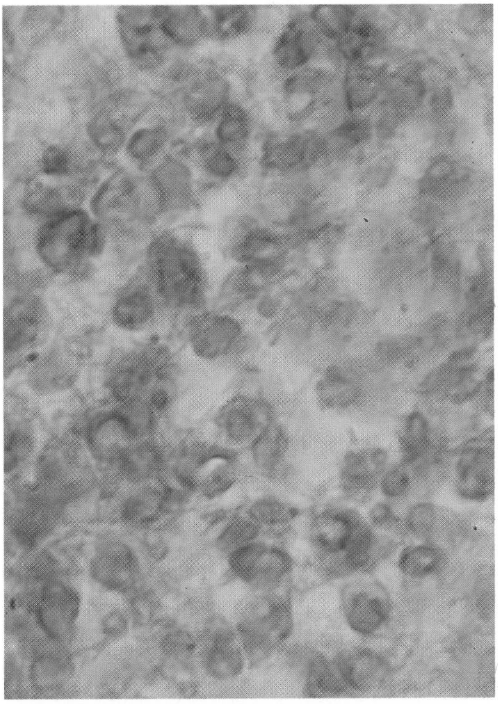

17 Human peripheral nerve. Alkaline hydrolysis to show sphingomyelin (sphingolipids are alkali-stable), NaOH-OTAN, × 300.

18

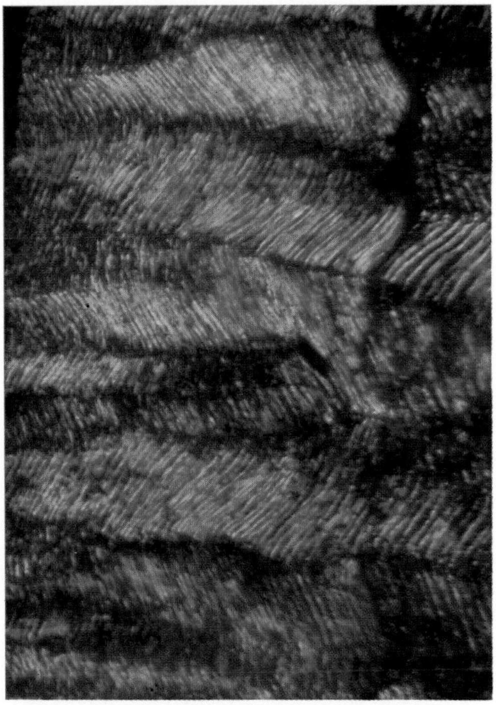

18 Rat peripheral nerve, stained with Sudan black B and viewed in polarised light. The red dichroic colour indicates phospholipids, longitudinal section, × 60.

19

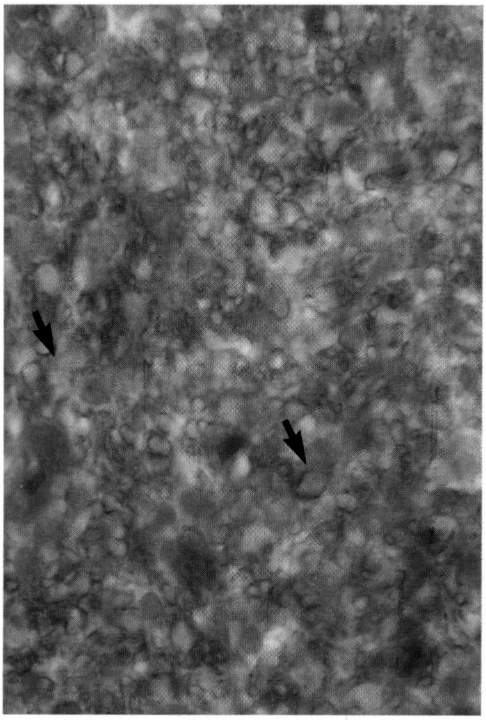

19 Developing chick spinal cord (at hatching). The slight black reaction (arrows) is caused by the transient presence of esterified cholesterol within oligodendroglia and/or early myelin. OTAN, × 100.

20

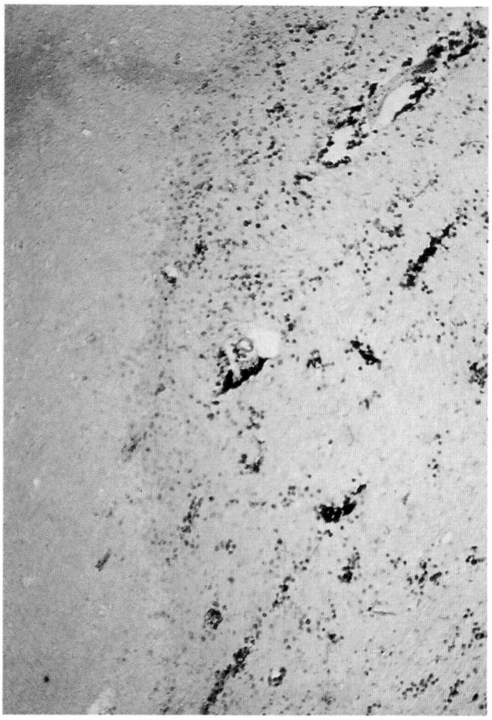

20 Active multiple sclerosis plaque. Black osmiophilic lipid (esterified cholesterol) within macrophages. Osmium tetroxide-α naphthylamine (OTAN), × 30.

21

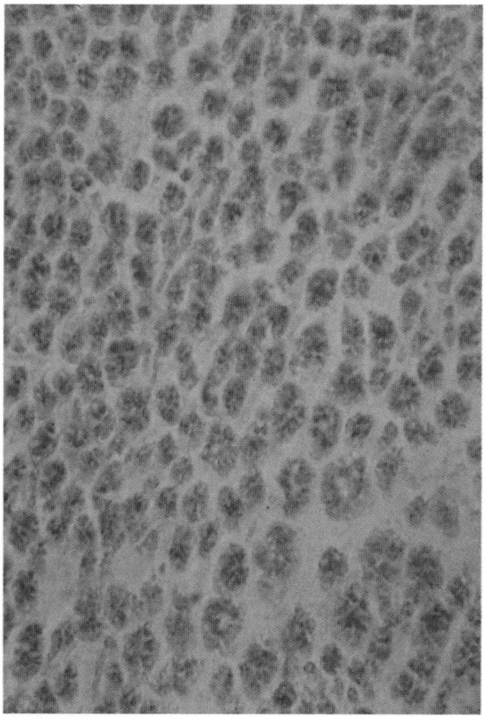

21 Basic myelin protein in human cord. Trypan blue, × 100.

22

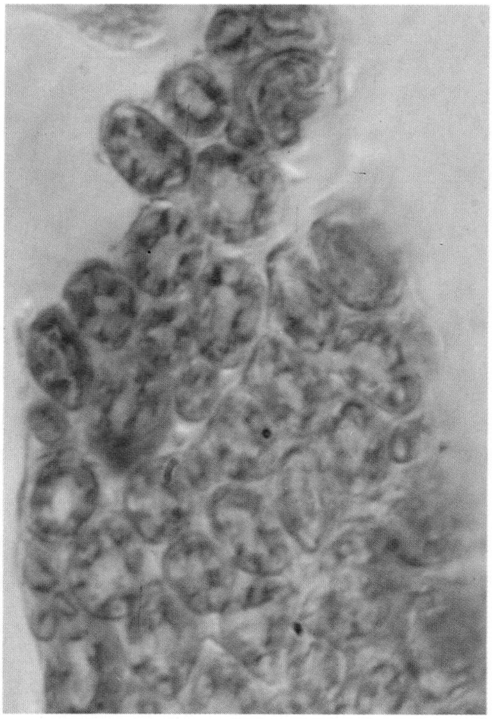

22 Basic myelin protein in rat sciatic nerve. Trypan blue, × 300.

23

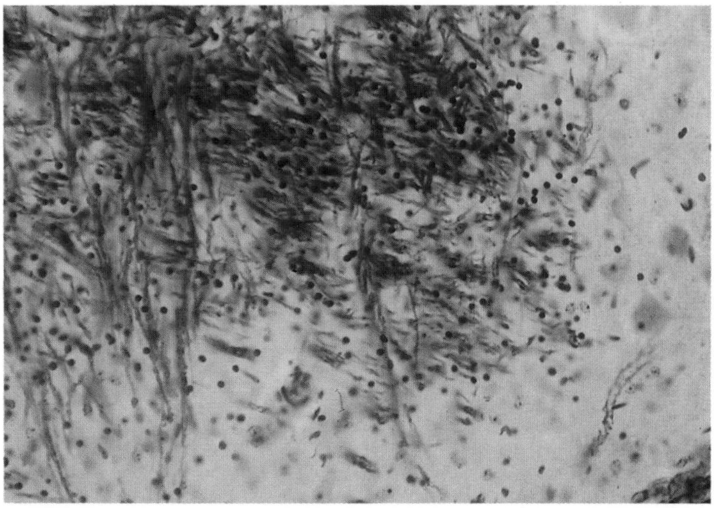

23 Myelinated fibres at edge of MS plaque. Heidenhain, × 80.

24

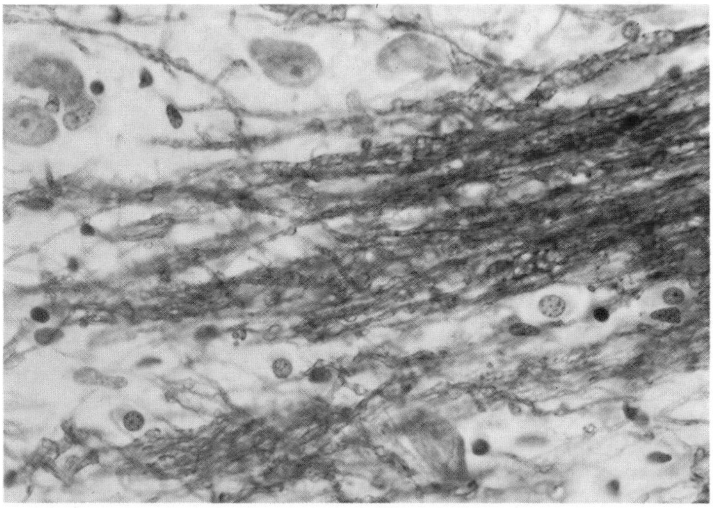

24 Myelinated fibres at edge of MS plaque. Luxol fast blue, × 300.

25

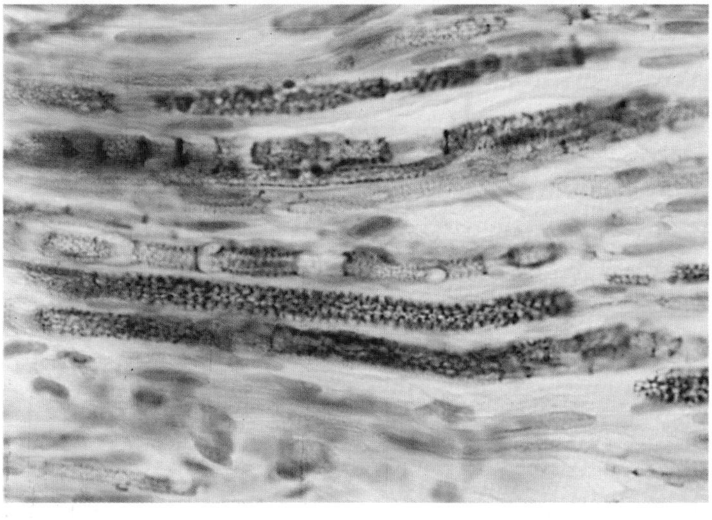

25 Peripheral nerve myelin, showing neurokeratin artefact. Solochrome cyanin, × 150.

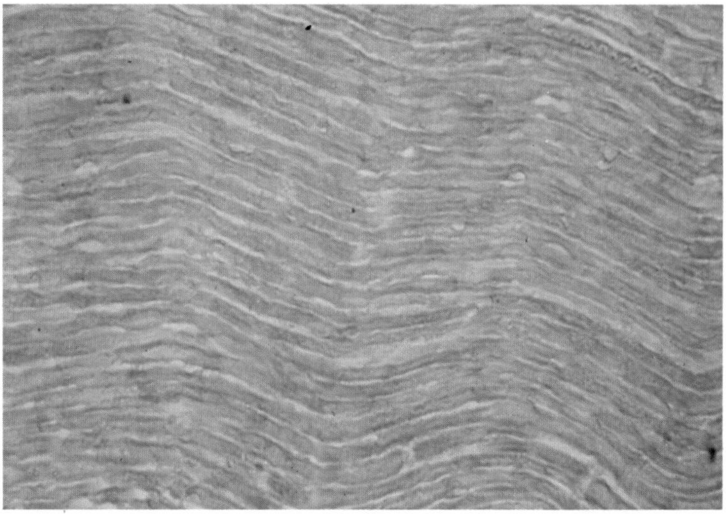
26

26 Neurokeratin in rat sciatic nerve stained by the p-dimethylamino benzaldehyde (DMAB) method for tryptophan, × 80.

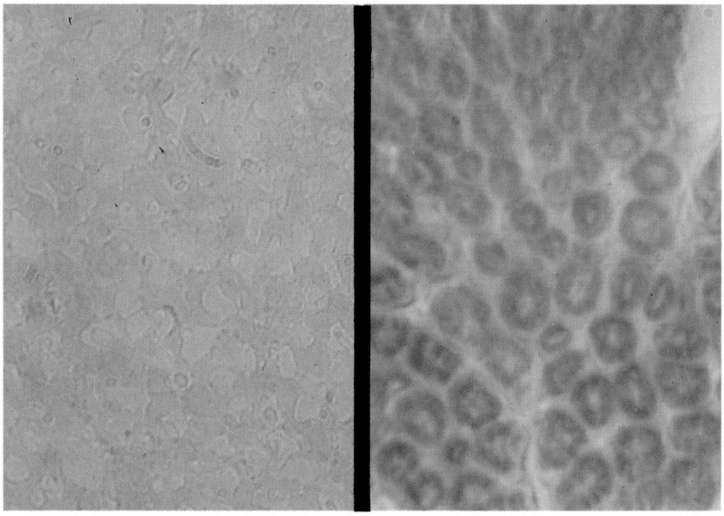
27

27 Rat sciatic nerve subjected to trypsin. Left: trypan blue stain for basic protein (nearly completely digested). Right: DMAB method stains neurokeratin (Po; resistant to digestion), × 300.

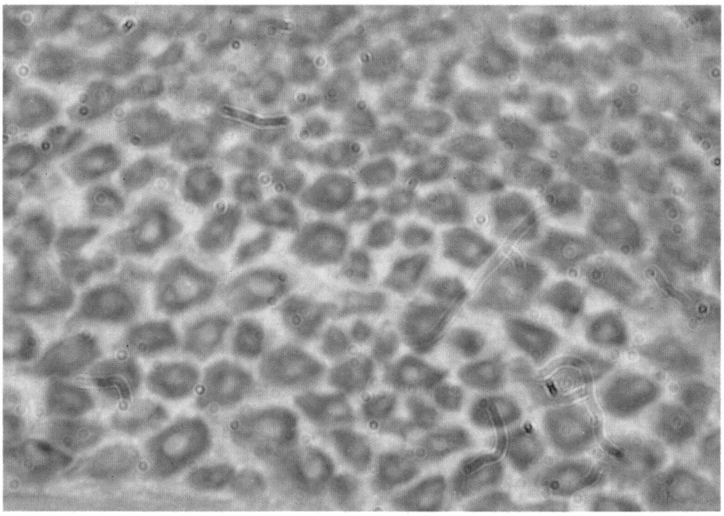
28

28 Neurokeratin (Po) in rat sciatic nerve. DMAB, × 300.

29

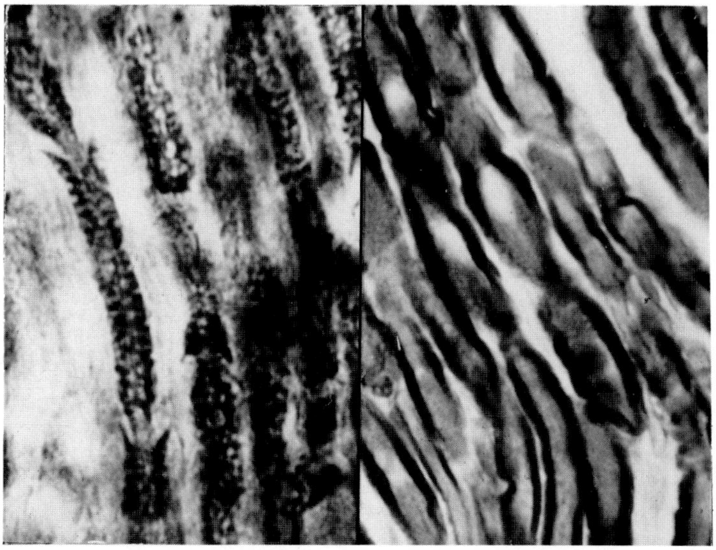

29 Left: neurokeratin network in peripheral nerve fixed in formalin. Right: absence of neurokeratin network in peripheral nerve fixed in buffered osmium tetroxide, × 400.

30

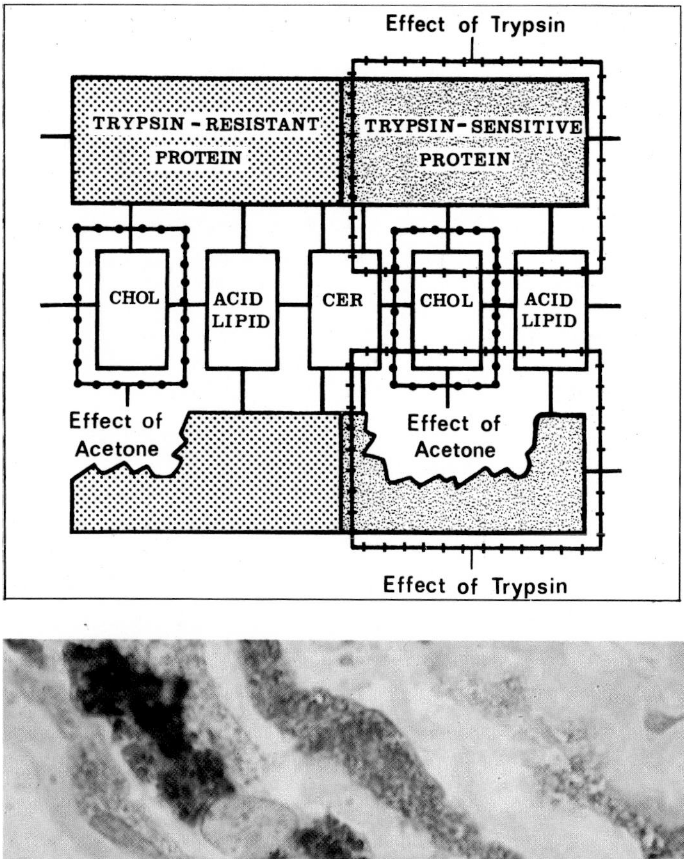

30 Diagram to show effects of trypsin and acetone on subsequent staining of myelin in histological sections. Anhydrous acetone removes only cholesterol. Trypsin removes basic myelin protein and some attached lipids. In histological sections, trypsin does not remove neurokeratin (Po) or proteolipid (trypsin-resistant proteins).

31

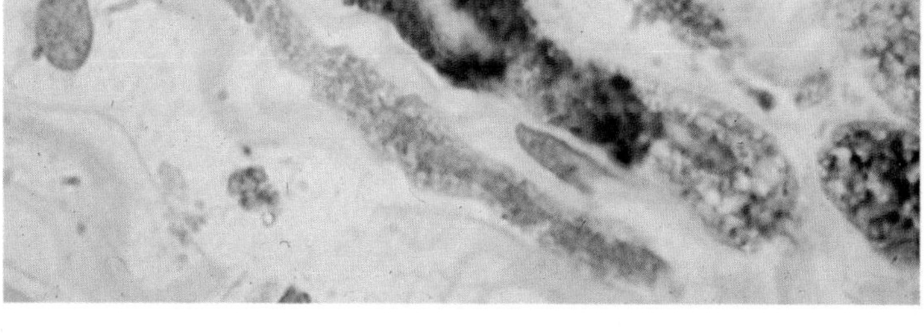

31 Myelin-associated glycoprotein (MAG) stained by anti-IgM-peroxidase in human sural nerve. Positive reaction in myelin and pi-granules in Schwann cell, × 400.

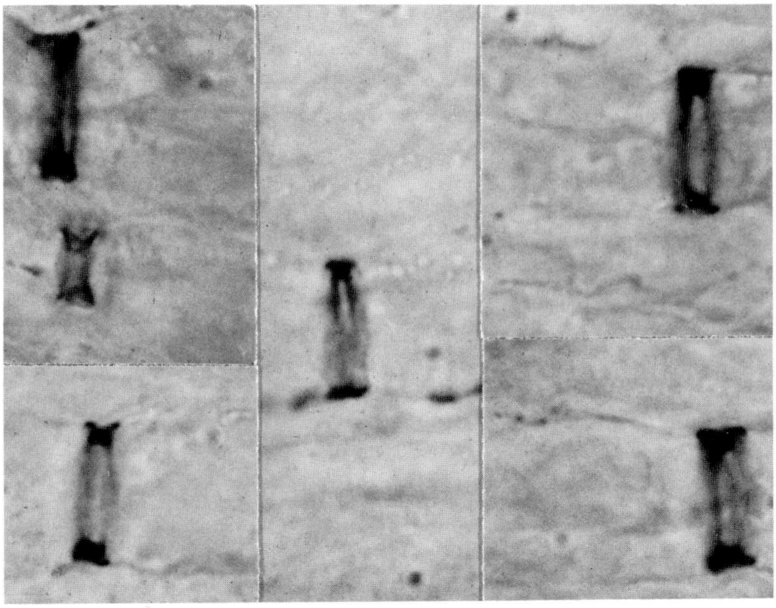

32 Copper-binding by acidic glycosaminoglycans in gap-substance at node of Ranvier in rat nerve, × 700.

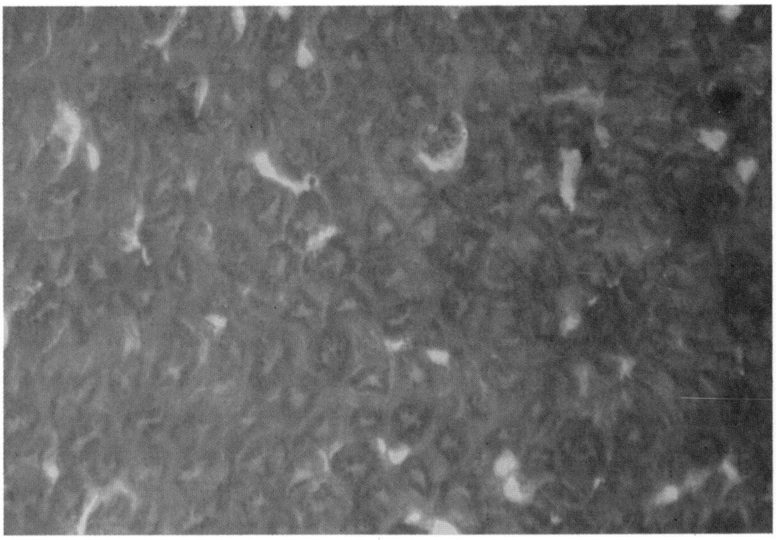

33 Acidic glycosaminoglycans in axon and Schwann cell in rat sciatic nerve. Extracted in chloroform-methanol (2:1 v/v) to remove sulphatide, then stained in acridine orange at pH 7.2, × 150.

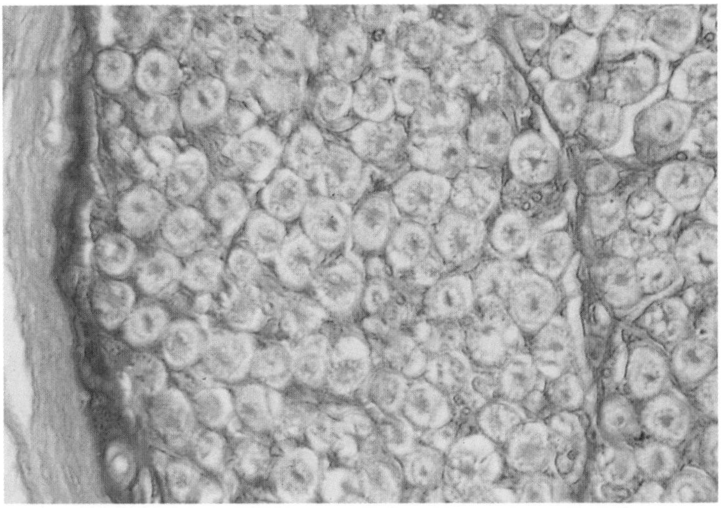

34

34 Acid glycosaminoglycans (GAGS) staining weakly in axon, myelin and endoneurium. Hale's colloidal iron, × 300.

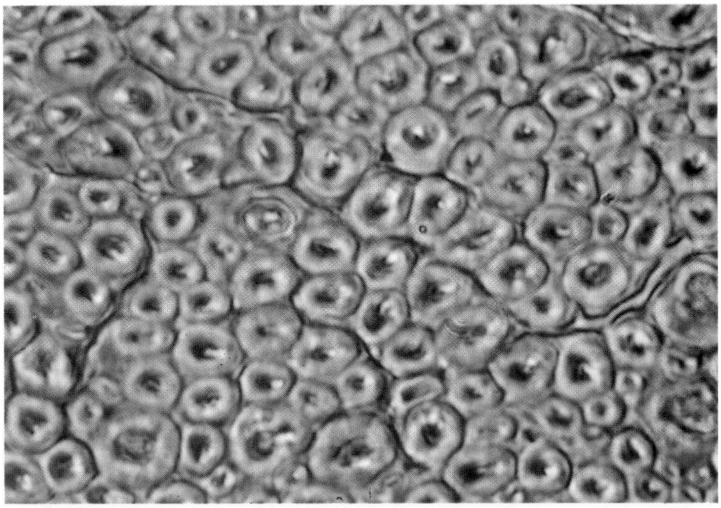

35

35 Acidic glycosaminoglycans in axon and endoneurium. Trypsin, Hale's colloidal iron, × 300.

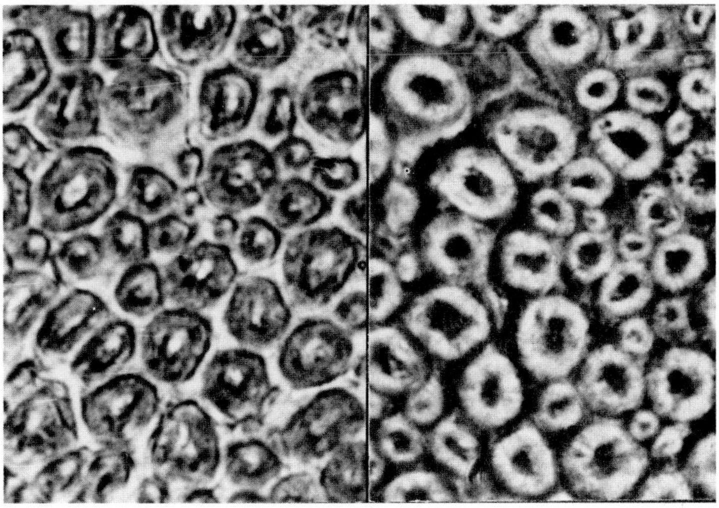

36

36 Rat sciatic nerve. Left: Hale's colloidal iron on frozen section stains myelin sulphatide. Right: Hale's colloidal iron after lipid extraction stains acidic glycosaminoglycans in axon and endoneurium, × 300.

37

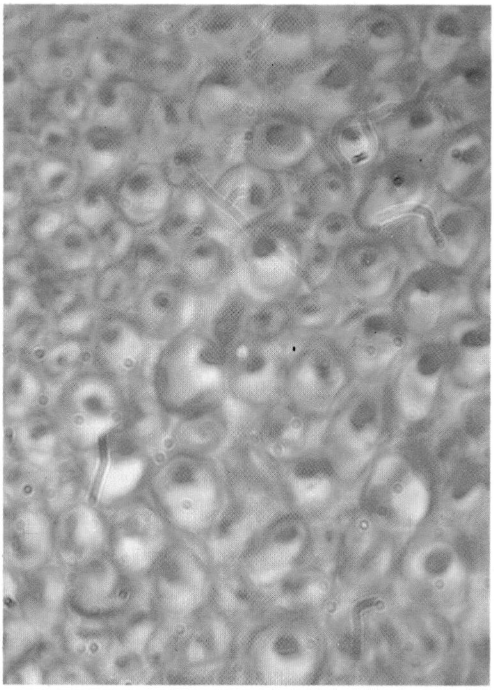

37 Staining of axonal protein in human cord. Danielli's coupled tetrazonium method, × 250.

38

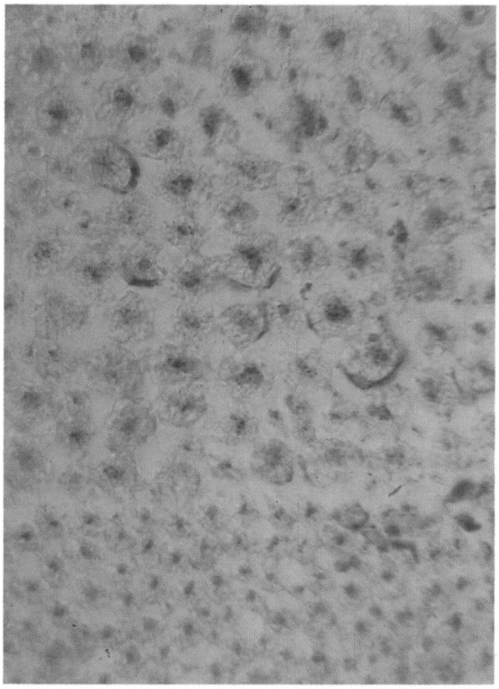

38 Lactic dehydrogenase activity in axon and Schwann cell, but not in myelin in rat sciatic nerve. Lactate: tetrazolium reductase, × 200.

39

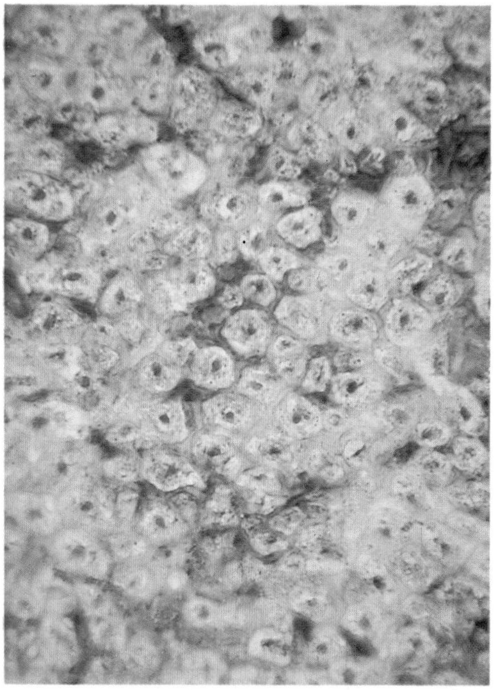

39 ATPase activity in axon and endoneurium in rat sciatic nerve. Padykula-Hermann method, × 200.

40

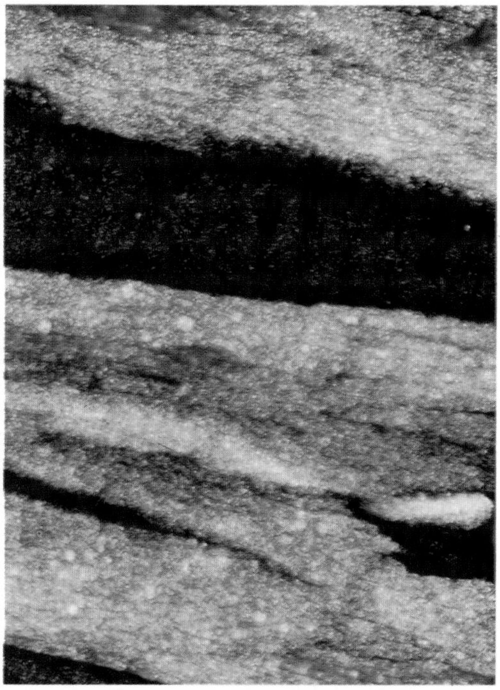

40 Neutral protease activity in rat sciatic nerve. The section is mounted on blackened photographic plate, comprising silver granules embedded in gelatin. Activity is revealed as translucent areas of gelatin digestion. Gelatin-silver film method, pH 7.6, × 30.

41

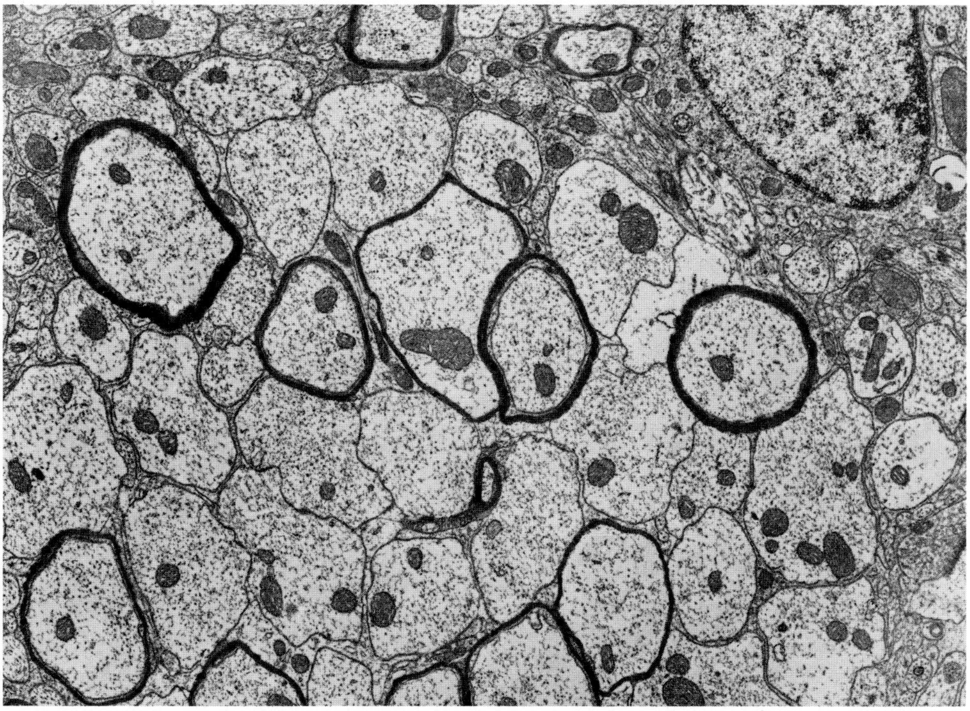

41 Cuprizone intoxication in young mouse. Note demyelinated axons and inappropriately thinly myelinated fibres in superior cerebellar peduncle. These fibres represent early remyelination, × 8,500. *(Courtesy of Dr S.K. Ludwin)*

42

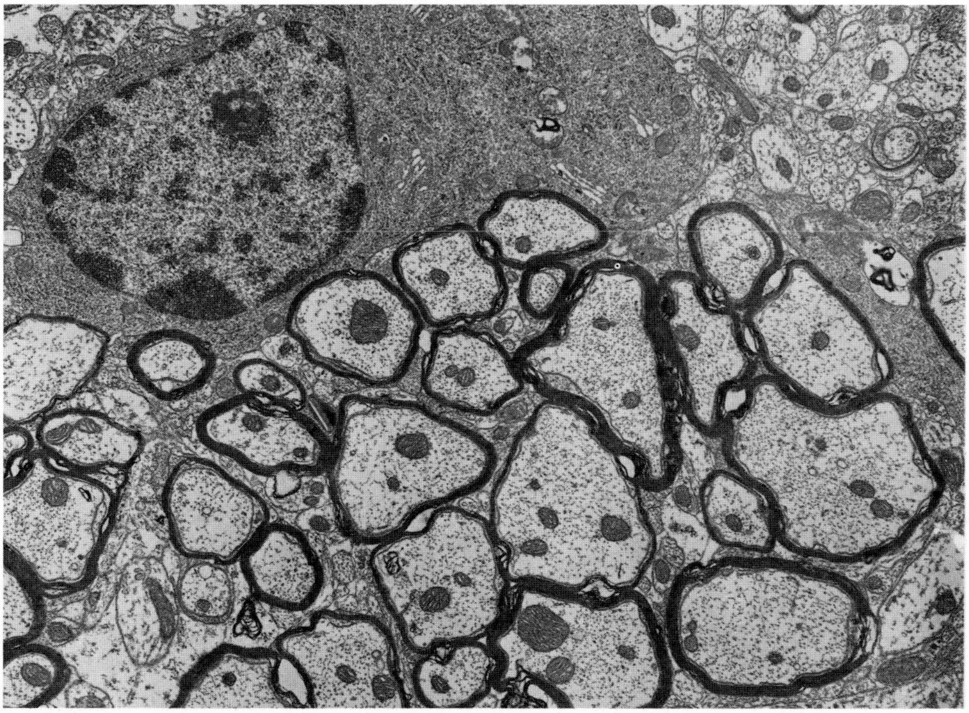

42 Cuprizone intoxication in young mouse. A later stage of remyelination (thinly myelinated fibres). Note one oligodendrocyte (top) remyelinating all these axons × 8,500. *(Courtesy of Dr S.K. Ludwin)*

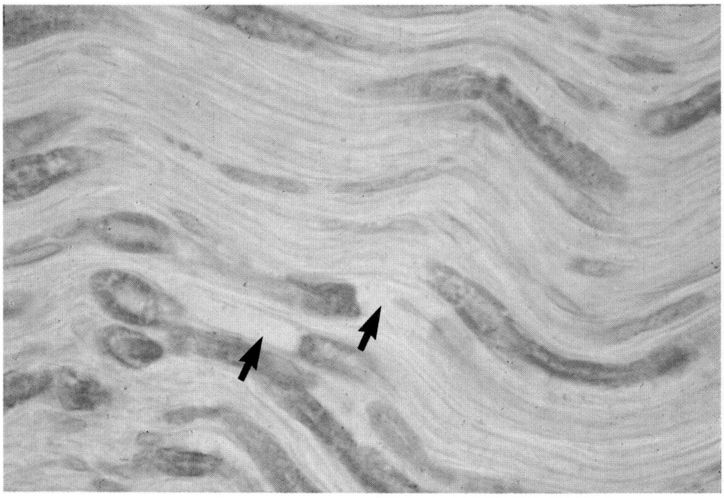

43

43 Diabetic neuropathy. Segmental demyelination. Note abrupt loss of myelin at paranodal region (arrows), gold hydroxamic acid, for phosphoglycerides × 200.

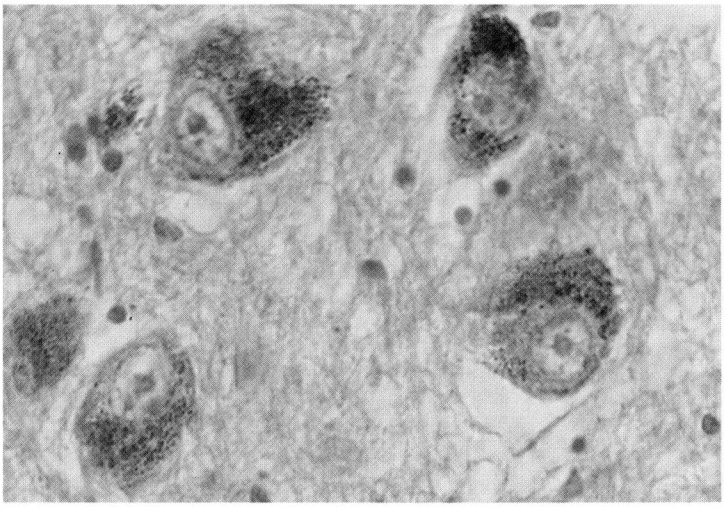

44

44 Persistence of pigmented neuronal cell bodies in substantia nigra within a plaque of MS. Haematoxylin-eosin, × 400.

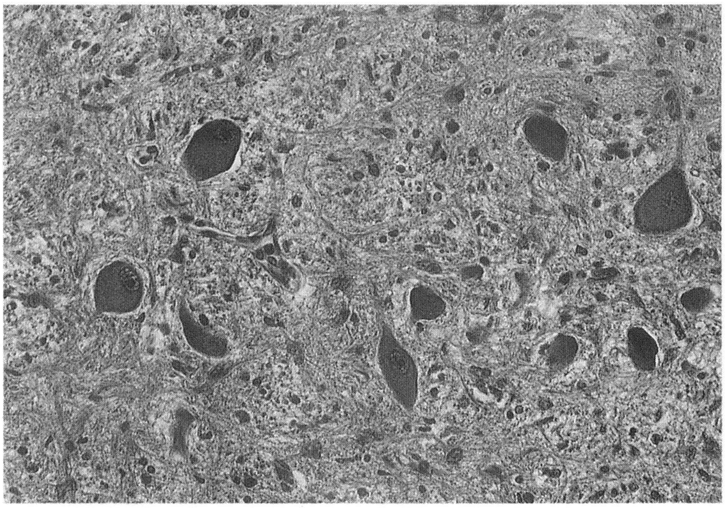

45

45 Persistence of neuronal cell bodies in olivary nuclei within a MS plaque. Phosphotungstic acid-haematoxylin, × 200.

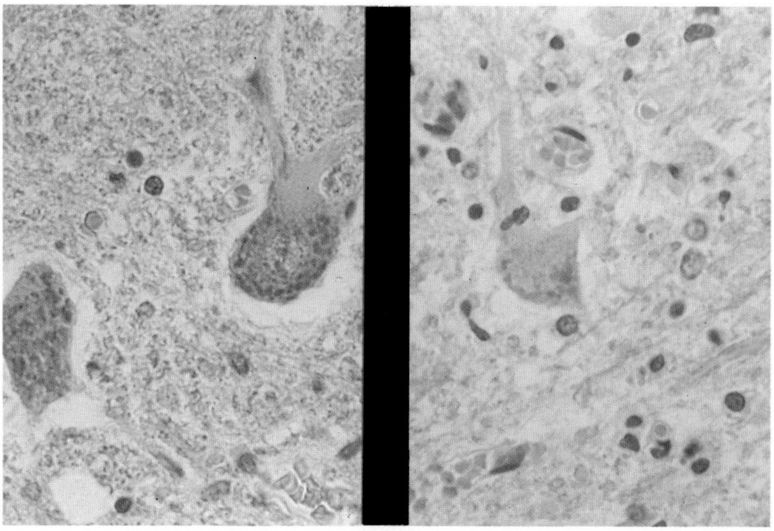

46

46 Anterior poliomyelitis in human cord. Left: normal anterior horn cells. Right: chromatolysis of Nissl substance (RNA) in damaged anterior horn cell. Haematoxylin-eosin, × 400.

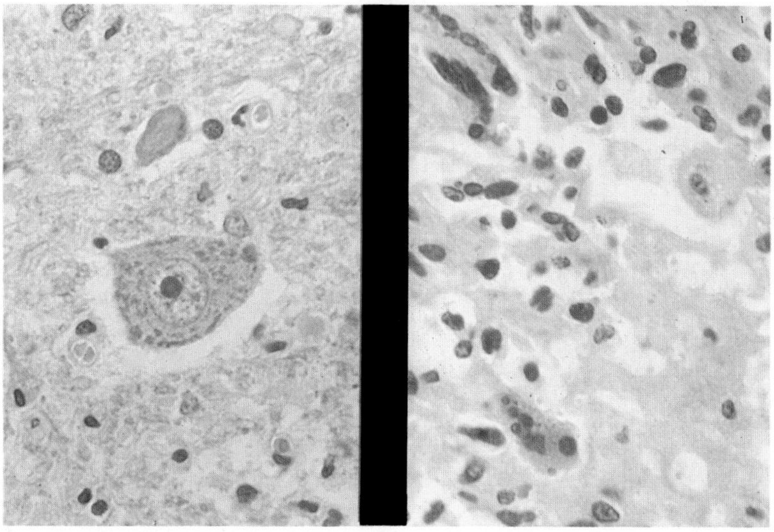

47

47 Anterior poliomyelitis. Normal anterior horn cell on left; neuronophagia (digested dead neurone) on right. Haematoxylin-eosin, × 400.

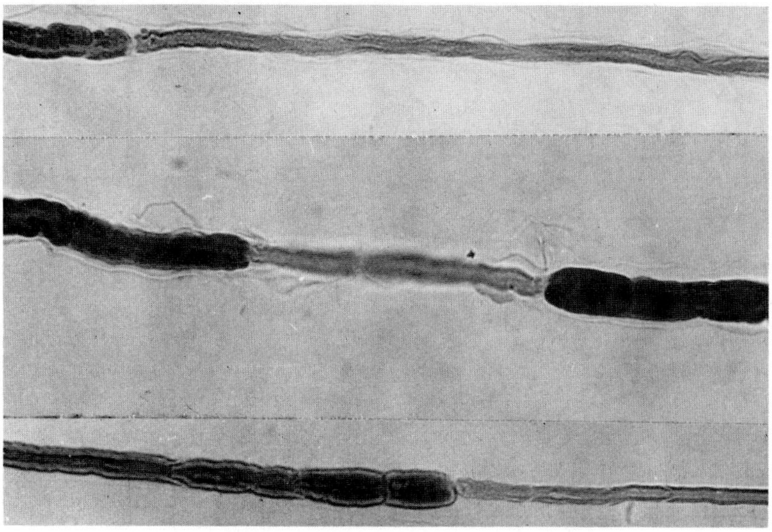

48

48 Segmental demyelination in mouse sciatic nerve, 40 days after intraneural administration of lysolecithin. Note short internodal segment of demyelination. Teased fibres, × 30. *(Courtesy of Dr Susan Hall)*

49

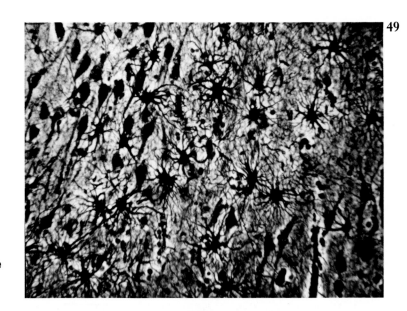

49 Astrocytic proliferation (spider cells) at edge of MS plaque. These spider cells secrete a dense network of glial fibres. Cajal's gold sublimate, × 250.

50

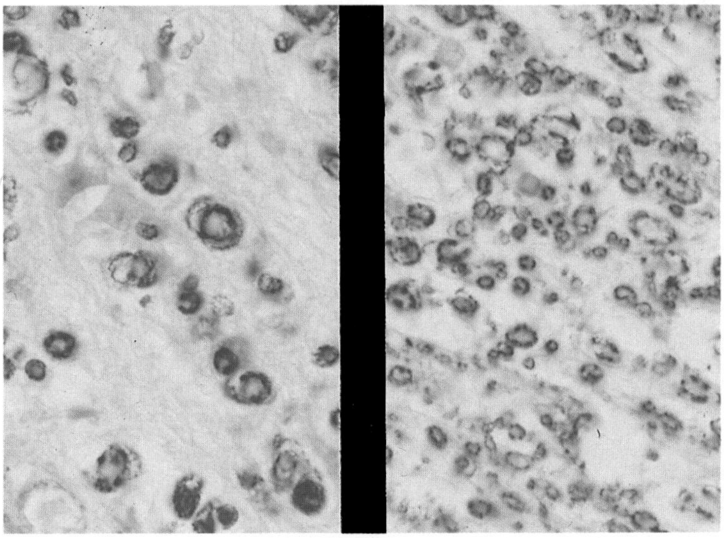

50 Left: remyelination by Schwann cells at edge of plaque of MS near ventral root in human cord. **Right: distant normal CNS myelin in the same section.** Note thicker and darker staining of Schwann-cell myelin. Luxol fast blue, × 200.

51

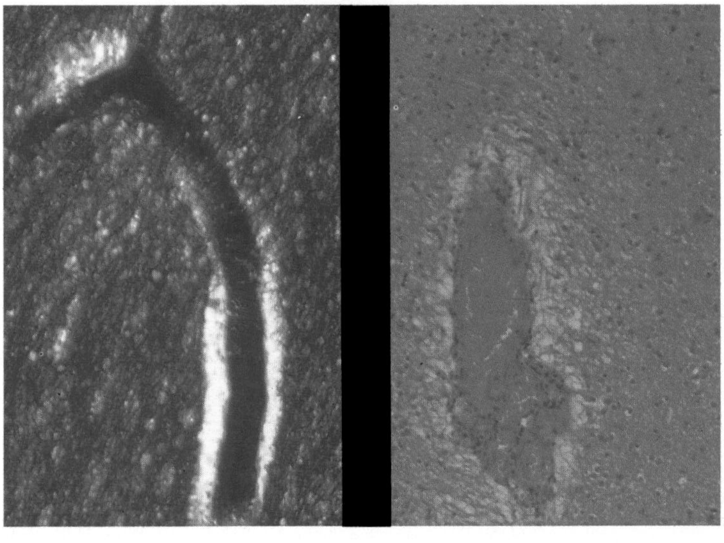

51 Left and right. Oedema around venules near MS plaque. H & E and Luxol fast blue, × 150.

2 Demyelinating and other myelin diseases in man

Although a disease resembling multiple sclerosis (MS) was described in the Low Countries in the Middle Ages (St Ludwina van Schiedam, 1380-1433), the disease was not formally recognised until the 19th century following descriptions by Carswell and Cruveilhier in the 1830s (Medaer, 1979). The subsequent definition of a demyelinating disease that it initially selectively damages the myelin sheath (Charcot, 1868, 1877) was a crucial advance in knowledge about MS.

A little earlier in 1863, it had been recognised that MS (grey degeneration) is closely related to veins (see Rindfleisch, 1863, 1873). As the disease develops and, particularly, with more aggressive progress, axons are damaged and lost (also see Madrid and Wisniewski, 1977). Acetylcholinesterase activity is at first retained but subsequently falls in advanced MS plaques (Lumsden, 1957). This loss of cholinesterase activity is matched by a corresponding loss of axons. Figures **52** to **54** show loss of myelin but good preservation of axons in an early plaque, while **55** to **57** show substantial loss of axons in the chronic plaque. Torpedoes and retraction bulbs may sometimes be seen in such areas of axonal damage (**56**). Loss of silver staining in the chronic plaque – assessed by scanning microdensitometry – represents a substantial loss of axons (*see* Table 2). This selective destruction of myelin in the early stages of multiple sclerosis will be considered further in Chapter 4 in relation to myelin vulnerability.

Multiple sclerosis is by far the commonest human demyelinating disease with a general prevalence rate in northern Anglo-Saxon communities of about 50-100 per 100,000 population, and is discussed and illustrated in detail in Chapters 5 to 10. Rarer variants of MS include (a) Balo's disease, characterised by concentric rings of demyelination in rapidly advancing disease (Balo, 1928; Courville, 1970; **58** and **59**), and (b) a form of Devic's disease where a characteristic solitary inflammatory or necrotic lesion in the cervical cord is accompanied by a lesion in the optic pathway only (**60** and **61**). Devic's disease is not confined to MS but may develop in pulmonary tuberculosis (Hughes and Mair, 1977) and other inflammatory diseases. These two variants of MS (Balo's and Devic's diseases) are further discussed in Chapters 6 and 7. Schilder's disease or diffuse sclerosis (which is akin to sudanophilic leucodystrophy) can be regarded as another variant of MS, but this disease usually involves younger persons, is monophasic and rapidly progressive. Large areas of white matter are affected by demyelination (**62**) or dysmyelination, with accompanying cavitation and massive accumulation of myelin breakdown products within microglia and other phagocytic cells (**63**; Suzuki and Grover, 1970a; Lhermitte *et al.*, 1981).

Table 2 Scanning microdensitometry of axonal and myelin staining in multiple sclerosis plaques (% of staining in surrounding brain)

	Axon (Palmgren)	*Myelin (luxol)*
Acute plaques (n = 14)	92.7 (±14.5)	32.5 (±1.4)
Chronic plaques (n = 12)	51.7 (±3.2)	31.6 (±.6)

S.E. in parenthesis. Silver staining of acute and chronic plaques is significantly different $P < 0.001$. Luxol staining is not statistically different between acute and chronic plaques.

A not uncommon form of demyelinating disease is acute disseminated encephalomyelitis (post-infectious encephalomyelitis). The pathogenic mechanism of most of these postviral encephalomyelitides must be autoimmune disease, of which post-rabies-vaccination encephalomyelitis in Japan (Uchimura and Shiraki, 1957) and post-vaccinial encephalomyelitis (Turnbull and McIntosh, 1926) are well-known examples. (*Professor H.M. Turnbull was actively discouraged from publishing his results because of the effect they were expected to have on the smallpox vaccination programme in the early 1920s.*)

These postviral encephalomyelitides are characterised by marked perivenular lymphocytic infiltration, with a surrounding narrow zone of perivenular demyelination (**64**). A similar encephalomyelitis accompanied by perivascular infiltration, demyelination and focal necroses may also be seen in Behcet's disease (**65**; Alema and Bignami, 1966; Hayashi *et al.*, 1982). Occasionally, these diseases may be more haemorrhagic (**66** to **68**), which may be an expression of the generalised Schwartzman reaction (Graham *et al.*, 1979) and a reflection of inflammatory damage to the vein wall (*see* Chapter 8). These postviral encephalomyelitides never produce massive confluent demyelination but, nevertheless, might represent an early pre-confluent stage of the disease process in MS. Possibly, demyelination in postviral encephalomyelitis is caused by lysosomal enzymes in the inflammatory infiltrate locally digesting the myelin sheath (*see* Chapter 4).

More intense damage to the white matter leads to a necrotic lesion, such as is seen in subacute necrotising leucoencephalitis (**69** and **70**), leading on to the gross necrotising lesion encountered in an acute encephalomyelitis, such as that caused by the herpes simplex virus (**71**). However, even the more virulent organism may only cause demyelination as, for example, sometimes occurs with herpes simplex (Ludwin, 1987).

Infection of the neurone with an incomplete form of measles virus in childhood results in the disease, known as subacute sclerosing panencephalitis (SSPE; Dayan, 1969). This slow virus disease results in progressive neuronal destruction and gliosis (**72** to **76**). The neurones display a variable number of inclusion bodies, containing the incomplete measles virus (**76**). This is why the disease was originally termed 'subacute inclusion encephalitis' by Van Bogaert. The oligodendroglia are also infected in the chronic form of sclerosing panencephalitis (CSPE), leading to demyelination in addition to the neuronal damage (**72**).

Opportunistic infection complicating immune deficiency is the underlying mechanism of progressive multifocal leucoencephalopathy (PML). Immune deficiency accompanying Hodgkin's lymphoma, other lymphomas, other neoplasms or AIDS allows the oligodendroglia to become infected with a polyoma (papova) virus. Damage to the oligodendroglia results in multifocal and later confluent demyelinating lesions (**77** and **78**). Rounded intranuclear inclusion bodies are seen in the oligodendroglia, while the astrocytes are hypertrophied and assume bizarre shapes (**79** and **80**; Waksman and Adams, 1962).

The nervous system is involved in about 70-80 per cent of cases of acquired immuno-deficiency syndrome (AIDS), as reported by Moskowitz *et al.*, (1984) and Lehmann *et al.*, (1985). Indeed AIDS seems to have taken over from syphilis in more ways than one, particularly in the clinical role of the Great Imitator. The involvement of the CNS in AIDS is often a result of opportunistic infection, such as cerebral toxoplasmosis, candida and cryptococcal abscesses, cytomegalovirus infection, herpes simplex encephalitis or PML. These often result in necrotic or microgranulomatous subacute encephalitis with giant cells (Kato, 1987; Rhodes, 1987) but sometimes a microvascular response occurs, which is a cause of focal necrotic lesions. Occasionally, focal or diffuse cerebral intravascular coagulation is encountered (**81** and **82**; Moskowitz *et al.*, 1984; Anders *et al.*, 1986). Intracranial lymphomas occur in about 13 per cent of cases. Non-vascular necrotic lesions may be seen (**83** and **84**; Vinters *et al.*, 1987), as well as demyelinating lesions in the spinal cord, pons, brainstem (**85**) and elsewhere (Anders *et al.*, 1986; Rhodes, 1987). Parkinsonism, Shy-Drager syndrome (autonomic central neuropathy), multisystem disease (Miller and Semple, 1987) and peripheral neuropathy may all be features of neuro-AIDS.

A vacuolar myelopathy is common in AIDS (*see* Chapter 7, oedema). This myelinopathy of the spinal cord resembles subacute combined degeneration (SACD; Goldstick *et al.*, 1985; Lehmann *et al.*, 1985; Petito *et al.*, 1985, 1986; Rhodes, 1987), but some patients show a similar myelinopathy in cerebral and cerebellar white matter (Petito *et al.*, 1985). This vacuolar myelopathy in AIDS might be caused by folate deficiency. Thus, two children with congenital AIDS were found to have very low folate levels (Smith *et al.*, 1987), similar to those found in SACD (Clayton *et al.*, 1986). Pteridine metabolism is linked with folate metabolism, and patients with dihydropteridine and 5, 10-methylene tetrahydrofolate reductase deficiencies both develop demyelinating disease (Smith *et al.*, 1986). In parenthesis, it is of interest that CSF neopterin levels are increased in active MS (Frederikson *et al.*, 1987).

Apart from HTLV-3 (HIV), other retroviruses have been linked with demyelinating disease. HTLV-1 seems to be an important cause of tropical spastic paraparesis, and magnetic resonance imaging reveals a high signal in the periventricular region in such patients, similar to that seen with the periventricular lesions of MS (see Chapter 6; Rodgers-Johnson *et al.*, 1985; Roman *et al.*, 1897; Tournier-Lasserve *et al.*, 1987). It has been shown that HTLV-1 can both incorporate host antigen into its envelope and 'transactivate' expression of Class II antigen (Ia) in certain cells, such as astrocytes and macrophages. After incorporating newly-formed Ia antigen into its own envelope, HTLV-1 then masquerades as an antigen-presenting-cell, presenting host antigen as foreign and thus promoting an autoimmune disease (Dalgliesh *et al.*, 1987). However, a search for HTLV-1 and HTLV-3 (HIV) antigens in 32 MS patients (paired serum and CSF samples) was essentially negative (De Rossi *et al.*, 1986). A further study confirmed this negative finding in both MS patients and their close relatives (Swingler *et al.*, 1987).

Non-inflammatory demyelinating diseases

Adams and Richardson (1961) pointed out that central pontine myelinoclasis, Marchiafava-Bignami disease and subacute combined degeneration are non-inflammatory demyelinating conditions, all of which probably result from a metabolic failure (see below). This group contrasts with MS, its variants and encephalomyelitis, which are all inflammatory conditions principally involving white matter.

Central pontine myelinoclasis (CPM) was first described by Adams, Victor and Mancall in 1959 and was thought to be due to chronic malnutrition and alcoholism (see Messert *et al.*, 1987). Minor forms are quite common (**86**; Laureno and Karp 1988; Boon and Potter, 1987) but severe forms are often associated with sudden correction of hyponatraemia (**87** and **88**; Norenberg *et al.*, 1982; Laureno and Karp, 1988). It is now apparent that extrapontine cases of CPM are quite common (10 per cent of cases; Wright *et al.*, 1979; Boon and Potter, 1987) and lesions may be found in the thalamus, internal capsule, and central and cerebellar white matter. The demyelination in CPM is complete with production of sudanophilic lipid (esterified cholesterol; **89**). The oligodendroglia are very sensitive to a rapid change from hyponatraemia to hypernatraemia during correction of an electrolyte disturbance, and become shrunken and pyknotic as a result (Norenberg and Papendick, 1984). The occurrence of CPM in both chronic alcoholism and rapid correction of hyponatraemia could be reconciled by recalling that ethanol has a marked diuretic action. Indeed ethanol and vasopressin are seen to have diametrically opposite effects on cerebral water distribution as shown by magnetic resonance imaging (Besson *et al.*, 1981). An electrolyte-induced demyelinating disorder in the rat can be ameliorated by dexamethasone (Rojiani *et al.*, 1987), which suggests that steroids can protect glial cells against the effects of a sudden increase in $[Na^+]$.

Marchiafava-Bignami disease is a disorder of myelin with predominant involvement of the corpus callosum. However, it can also affect the middle cerebral peduncle (McLardy, 1951). The characteristic changes are loss of myelin, oedema and vascular proliferation. It was first suggested that it results from excessive consumption of the red wines of Tuscany, such as Chianti, but it has now been found in other countries either in alcoholics or associated with Wernicke's encephalopathy (**90** to **93**; USA, UK and Roumania; Ironsides *et al.*, 1961; Petrescu *et al.*, 1975; Koeppen and Barron, 1978).

Creutzfeldt-Jakob (C-J) disease is not a demyelinating disease. It is an infection of grey matter (neuronal cell body) by a primitive viral form, known as a prion, resulting in death of the neurone (revealed as a hole) and astroglial scar formation (**94** to **97**). These holes are separated by glial fibres and, thus, give the generic name of 'spongiform encephalopathy' to the group of diseases of which C-J disease is a member. C-J disease is mentioned here, in the context of MS, because of the previous interest in the spongiform encephalopathy of sheep, known as scrapie, as a possible cause of MS. However, repeat of the original work now shows that MS brain extracts do not cause scrapie in sheep (Dick *et al.*, 1965). The illustrations presented here show that the two diseases are so clearly different (Gadjusek, 1967) that it is difficult to see how the possibility of a common aetiology was ever considered.

Dysmyelinating diseases

The group of human demyelinating diseases discussed above are essentially viral-associated conditions. The next type of myelin disorder to be considered is not demyelinating but dysmyelinating in nature, that is, myelin is not formed properly in the first place. In spite of this distinction, a major element of demyelination may be seen in these diseases, probably because the myelin that is formed is imperfect and soon degenerates. A metabolic abnormality causing dysmyelination would presumably also fail to maintain such myelin as had been formed.

There are in excess of 4,000 known inborn catabolic errors and many of these conditions affect the central nervous system. The basic cause of these metabolic disorders is the absence of the specific enzyme for a particular stage in catabolism so that the catabolic or degradative product accumulates within the tissues. These disorders can thus be distinguished from the anabolic defects discussed in Chapter 3. The most common of these genetic errors is phenylpyruvic aciduria, which results from an absence of phenylalanine hydroxylase. It may cause demyelination in older subjects (Forsmann *et al.*, 1967), but its presenting feature in early life is the accumulation of phenylpyruvic acid in the blood and tissues.

The lipid storage diseases of the nervous system are further well-known examples of these genetic metabolic disorders, and have recently been reviewed in depth by Lake (1984). It is obvious that a congenital defect in lipid metabolism (whether genetically controlled or not) might affect myelin development, in particular where the lipid concerned is an essential part of the myelin lipid-protein molecular structure. The storage cells concerned often show characteristic ballooning or complex ultrastructural storage bodies. Myenteric ganglion cells in the rectum or appendix, lymphocytes in lymphnodes or spleen, peripheral lymphocytes and urine provide easily accessible material from which many of the stored lipids may be identified (see Lake, 1984).

The human dysmyelinating diseases are caused by a defect in the formation of myelin, as a result of genetically controlled metabolic and neuroglial dysfunction. Collectively, they form the group of leucodystrophies:

a) Metachromatic leucodystrophy results from a deficiency of arylsulphatase-A (ASA; sulphatylgalactosylceramidase; Austin *et al.*, 1963; Mehl and Jatzkewitz, 1965). One form of the disease is distinguished by a deficiency of the activator for ASA (Norton and Cammer, 1984). The disease is characterised by the accumulation of sulphatide within the brain (**98** and **99**), peripheral nerve (**100**), kidney (**101**), gall-bladder and bile duct epithelium (**102**). The excess sulphatide overflows into the urine, where it can be detected by a variety of simple diagnostic tests. As sulphatide is an important constituent of myelin, this disorder severely impairs normal development of the sheath: metachromatic material may be seen as deposits in the glia and Schwann cells around the myelinated tracts in central and peripheral nervous systems.

The preparative yield of myelin is low in MLD (Norton and Poduslo, 1982), which confirms that dysmyelination due to sulphatide deficiency is the essential pathology of the disease.

b) Sudanophilic leucodystrophy. This is similar to or identical with Schilder's disease, mentioned above. It is characterised by massive breakdown or defective synthesis of myelin. It is commonly seen in children and can be regarded as equivalent to an acute monophasic form of MS (*see* **62** and **63**). The histology reveals a substantial uptake of sudanophil lipid by microglia and other glial cells (**103**). The lipid is esterified cholesterol formed by the breakdown of myelin. A form of sudanophilic leucodystrophy in older subjects has been identified as hereditary diffuse leucoencephalopathy; it is characterised by demyelination, axonal spheroids and other changes (Axelsson *et al.*, 1984).

c) Adrenoleucodystrophy is a disease closely related to sudanophilic leucodystrophy, but of X-linked recessive inheritance. Demyelinating lesions are seen in the brain (**104** and **105**), together with an inflammatory infiltrate, while there are varying degrees of adrenocortical failure and psychiatric illness (Jablensky *et al.*, 1970). The original cases were described as 'bronzed Schilder's disease' because of the concurrent adrenal failure. Heterozygote females develop minor manifestations of the disease (Powers *et al.*, 1987). A lipid abnormality has recently been detected in this disease, the inability of peroxisomes to β-oxidise C24, C25 and C26 (hexacosanoic acid) unbranched long-chain fatty acids with resulting accumulation of these fatty acids in plasma (Moser *et al.*, 1981; Singh *et al.*, 1981; Norton and Cammer, 1984; Powers *et al.*, 1987).

d) Pelizaeus-Merzbacher disease. The nosology of this disease is complex. There are several different types, which are mainly distinguished by the age of onset. The classic type presents as a leucoencephalopathy with severe demyelination in middle to late childhood. In the congenital form, there is disordered myelinogenesis (**106**) and cavitation in the brain (Seitelberger, 1970), reminiscent of the dysmyelination in swayback (Chapter 3).

Dysmyelination in Pelizaeus-Merzbacher disease is associated with scanty or absent oligodendroglia (**106**), near-absent proteolipid-protein (PLP) and reduced amounts of CNP, MAG and MBP (Koeppen *et al.*, 1988). Similar changes are seen in the Jimpy mouse and the MLD rat (*see* Chapter 3). The major fault in these diseases is in the snythesis of PLP and, in Pelizaeus-Merzbacher disease and the Jimpy mouse, this has been shown to be caused by deletion of DNA transcript (Morello *et al.*, 1986; Koeppen *et al.*, 1987).

e) Krabbe's leucodystrophy (Krabbe, 1916). In this disease of children, accumulation of galactocerebroside (**107**) is caused by deficiency of galacteroceramidase, leading to accumulation of this lipid as characteristically angulated tubular structures in the typical binucleate PAS-positive globoid cells of the disease (**108** and **109**; Suzuki and Grover, 1970b), myelin deficiency (**107**) and impaired CNS function (Suzuki and Suzuki, 1970). In spite of the similarity in enzymatic defects between Krabbe's and Gaucher's diseases, the appearances of the storage cells and inclusions are quite different: Gaucher's disease is characterised by ballooned pear-shaped microglia or macrophages, while the storage macrophages in Krabbe's disease are globoid and sometimes binucleate (**108** and **109**).

Experimentally, globoid cells can be produced by local injection of cerebroside: they seem to be a characteristic macrophage response to accumulation of this lipid (Austin and Lehfeldt, 1965; Olsson *et al.*, 1966).

f) Alexander's disease is a dysmyelinating leucodystrophy of unknown cause (Alexander, 1949; Friede, 1964). There is marked destruction of central white matter (**110**), and perivascular accumulation of lipid and protein debris (**111** and **112**). The debris contains an abundance of Rosenthal fibres (RF), which are thought to represent degraded astrocytes in areas of longstanding reactive gliosis (Herndon *et al.*, 1970). However, RF in Alexander's disease give only a surface reaction with the anti-glial fibrillary acidic protein peroxidase method (GFAP: Towfighi *et al.*, 1983). Smaller RF stain more strongly than larger ones, so their origin in Alexander's disease is not altogether clarified by GFAP; Herndon *et al.*, (1970) considered that RF are derived from hyaline bodies containing degenerate astrocytes (*see* RF in MS in Chapter 7).

g) Niemann-Pick's disease. This disease is characterised by sphingomyelin accumulation within the brain and lymphoreticular tissues. The enzymatic defect in Group I Niemann-Pick's disease is in shingomyelinase activity (review: Brady and Barranger, 1981). There may be defects of myelination in the classic form (Type A) of Niemann-Pick's disease, but the main brunt of the disease is born by neurones, which are distended by sphingomyelin storage (**113**), and by visceral tissues (**114**).

h) The cerebral forms of Gaucher's disease do not result in defects in myelination. The enzyme defect is in glucosylceramidase resulting in accumulation of glucocerebroside in the typical pear-shaped Gaucher cells. Although cerebroside is a major component of myelin, it is galactocerebroside and not glucocerebroside that is located there.

i) Gangliosidoses. The infantile, but not the juvenile, forms of the gangliosidoses GM1 and GM2 may show some defects in myelination, but the main brunt of these diseases is born by neurones, which accumulate gangliosides both in the cerebral cortex and in the peripheral nervous system (**115** and **116**). This is not surprising as gangliosides are essentially neuronal lipids and only minor myelin components, except in birds where the myelin contains considerably more ganglioside (mainly GM1) than in mammals (Norton, 1982).

GM2 was the first gangliosidosis to be chemically characterised; the disorder being previously known as Tay-Sachs' disease (**117**). The accumulation of GM2 is associated with a defect in hexosaminidase activity, whereas the associated defect in GM1 is in β-galactosidase activity. These defects cause gangliosides to accumulate in neurones and the overflow is taken up by the microglia and other glial cells in the affected areas of the nervous system.

i) Fabry's disease (angiokeratoma corporis diffusum) is caused by deficiency of ceramide trihexosidases, which causes accumulation of ceramide trihexosides (Brady *et al.*, 1967). This leads to deposits within skin, small arteries (**118**; Lehner and Adams, 1968), glomerulus, peripheral nerve (**119**) and brain. However, this deposition results in only minor myelin defects.

j) Ceroid-Lipofuscinosis (Batten's disease) is an ill-understood (probably recessive) genetic disorder, causing cerebromacular degeneration and widespread accumulation of lipofuscin (lipos=fat; fuscus=dark) in both central and peripheral nervous systems, in muscle and at other sites. Lipids undergo peroxidation to become insoluble autofluorescent PAS-stainable pigmented granules, particularly within neurones (**120** and **121**) and muscle, but myelin is not seemingly impaired and there is no record of peroxidation of myelin lipids. The metabolic defect is likely to be a genetic disorder in mitochondrial metabolism resulting in peroxidation and polymerisation of lipids. The possible roles of free radicles, antioxidants and superoxide dismutase do not seem to have been explored in Batten's disease. However, experimental vitamin-E deficiency leads to axonal loss and formation of neuronal lipo-pigments in the CNS, while axonal neuropathy and necrotising myopathy are seen in the peripheral nervous system (Nelson *et al.*, 1981). In the peripheral nerve, bands of Büngner are seen which are characteristic of Wallerian degeneration. These observations underline the neuronal/axonal target in vitamin-E deficiency and confirm that the myelin sheath is spared.

A rare pigmented form of orthochromatic leucodystrophy has been described by Gray *et al.*, (1987). Lipofuscins are deposited within macrophages and glial cells in dystrophic cerebral white matter; while parallel lamellated or fingerprinted intracellular inclusions are seen on electronmicroscopy. The distribution of ceroid/lipofuscin is different from that in Batten's disease as white matter is primarily involved, but demyelination is not a feature of the condition.

The spinal cord (myelopathic myelinopathy)

It is confusing that both spinal cord disease (myelopathy) and myelinopathy are derived from the same classical Greek word, muelos = marrow, inner part. The two terms can be easily confused, and even more so with the term myelosclerosis = sclerosis of the bone marrow.

A number of tract degenerations of the spinal cord are characterised by loss of myelin. Subacute combined degeneration presents as a vacuolar myelopathy and myelinopathy of the lateral and posterior columns (**122**). As discussed above (under AIDS), it is due to deficiency of cyanocobalamin (vitamin B_{12}). Other tract degenerations cause secondary loss of myelin (Wallerian degeneration) due to damage to the neurone. These include motor neurone disease (**123** and **124**), tabes dorsalis (**125**) and Friedreich's ataxia (**126**). The near-absolute symmetry of the lesions of these tract degenerations contrasts with the irregularity, geographical outlines and, at best, pseudosymmetry of the MS plaque (**127**). These tract degenerations are clearly confined to specific anatomical tracts, in contrast to MS, where the disease process is based on vascular (venous) territories (Chapter 8) and overlaps neuroanatomical zones.

Peripheral nervous system

Demyelinating disease of the PNS, as distinct from axonal neuropathy (Wallerian degeneration), may be due to:

a) A metabolic, vascular or toxic effect on Schwann cells, for example diabetes mellitus (**43**), and diphtheritic and lead neuropathy. Hexachlorophene and triethyltin have a direct toxic action against water metabolism within myelin.

b) Acute post-infective polyneuropathy or polyradiculitis (Guillain-Barré syndrome), its chronic and relapsing forms and related conditions (**128**; Hughes, 1985). Inflammatory demyelinating neuropathy is also seen in leprosy (**129**).

c) Genetic cyclic demyelinating disorders. These are characterised by hypertrophic neuropathy and onion-bulb formation, which are caused by repeated episodes of demyelination and abortive attempts at remyelination. The less rare forms are demyelinating Charcot-Marie-Tooth disease (**130** and **131**; Dyck *et al.*, 1974; Weller and Cervos-Navarro, 1977), Dejerine-Sottas disease (Weller, 1967; Weller and Cervos-Navarro, 1977; Dyck *et al.*, 1970) and Refsum's disease, which is caused by intraneural accumulation of phytanic acid resulting from a deficiency of phytanic acid-α-hydroxylase (Rake and Saunders, 1966; Asbury and Johnson, 1978).

d) Genetic enzyme disorders. Here lipid may accumulate in the PNS, as well as in the CNS. These conditions include metachromatic neuropathy (**100**), globoid cell neuropathy (Sourander and Olsson, 1968) and Fabry's disease (**119**).

e) Paraproteinaemis. The IgM type, with antibodies directed against myelin-associated glycoprotein (MAG) typically causes disordered compaction of the outermost myelin lamellae (**132**; Hughes, 1985; Gregson and Leibowitz, 1985). IgG types of paraproteinaemia may occasionally show segmental demyelination.

f) Entrapment and compressive neuropathies. Pressure on the nerve produces segmental demyelination. Such disorders include carpal tunnel, cubital tunnel and ulnar nerve syndromes, meralgia paraesthetica and prolapsed intervertebral disc. They cause segmental demyelination, with clinical recovery after abatement of the pressure about 4 to 6 weeks later. These disorders are not caused by the ischaemic effects of pressure, but rather by the direct effect of pressure on the nerve; they can be experimentally produced by use of a sphygmomanometer arm band inflated to 500-1000 mm Hg (Gilliatt, 1975).

g) Certain drug-induced disorders.

h) Remodelling disorders of myelin. Some fibres in giant axonal neuropathy are thickly myelinated. However, the myelin over the typically swollen axons, which are caused by focal accumulation of intermediate filaments, may be very thin as a result of remyelination or degeneration (**133**; Kretzschmar *et al.*, 1987). An axonopathy in Boxer dogs shows similar remodelling changes in the myelin (Griffiths *et al.*, 1987).

i) The PNS in multiple sclerosis. It is customary to regard the PNS as uninvolved in MS. However a recent paper by Thomas *et al.*, (1987) describes 6 cases of clinically definite MS where peripheral nerve biopsy showed short internodes and inappropriately thin myelin sheaths, that is, the typical changes of a demyelinating neuropathy. Further cases of demyelinating neuropathy (including onion-bulb formation), complicating MS, have been recorded by Pollock *et al.*, 1977; Schoene *et al.*, 1977; Forrester and Lascelles, 1979; Lassman *et al.*, 1981; Rubin *et* *al.*, 1987; Sanders and Lee, 1987. Autonomic neuropathy has been described in MS by Sterman *et al.*, (1985), while target fibres in the disease are a clear indication of denervation due to peripheral neuropathy (Riggs *et al.*, 1986).

Wallerian degeneration

Most of the more common diseases of the PNS result in an axonal neuropathy (Wallerian degeneration; **134**). This includes ischaemic neuropathy due to various vasculitides (**135** to **140**) and 'dying-back' neuropathies caused by chronic alcoholism, thiamine and other vitamin deficiencies, various drugs, industrial compounds, plastics, agricultural sprays and other toxic agents acting on the neuronal cell body. The most peripheral parts of the neurone are first affected, hence the term 'dying-back' neuropathy.

Dysmyelinating diseases of the PNS

Occasional dysmyelinating disorders of the peripheral nervous system occur in children, such as the defect in myelination (hypomyelination neuropathy) seen in **141**. Here, there is a nearly complete myelin deficiency, and Schwann cells surround small scanty unmyelinated axons.

Table 3 summarises the various forms of demyelinating and dysmyelinating diseases occurring in man, and those occurring spontaneously in animals and under experimental conditions. In some instances it is not certain whether a disease is primary demyelination or axonal (Wallerian) degeneration. In some instances both processes may operate; the result depends on the local severity of the pathogenic insult.

Table 3 Spontaneous and experimental disorders affecting myelin

A	**Human diseases: CNS**	
1	Multiple sclerosis	Most common human demyelinating disease and most common neurological disorder after brain tumours and cerebrovascular disease.
2	Balo's concentric sclerosis	An acute variant of multiple sclerosis with concentric zones of demyelination.
3	Devic's neuromyelitis optica	A syndrome sometimes caused by multiple sclerosis, sometimes associated with systemic inflammation.
4	Schilder's disease	Acute massive monophasic demyelination in childhood or early adolescence. Some cases are X-linked adrenoleucodystrophy.
5	Hereditary diffuse leucoencephalopathy	May be equivalent of Schilder's disease in older persons.
6	Binswanger's disease	Ischaemic damage to central white matter in hypertension.
7	Acute disseminated encephalomyelitis (post-infectious and para-infectious) leucoencephalomyelitis	Allergic response to viral infections; post-vaccinial; focal perivenular demyelination.
8	Rabies post-vaccinal leucoencephalomyelitis	Vaccine cultivated in rabbit CNS; allergic reaction to encephalitogen as in chronic relapsing EAE.
9	Acute haemorrhagic leuco-encephalomyelitis	Post-influenzal and other. Similar appearances in cerebral malaria.
10	Progressive multifocal leuco-encephalopathy	Associated with lymphomas and ? immune disturbance. Papova virions in oligodendroglial nuclei.
11	Chronic sclerosing panencephalitis	'Slow' measles encephalitis with demyelination.
12	AIDS leucoencephalopathy and myelopathy	Various manifestations of demyelinating disease in AIDS.
13	Tropical spastic paraparesis	Associated with HTLV-1 infection.
14	Subacute combined degeneration	Vitamin B_{12} deficiency: primary demyelination in early stages.

15 Central pontine myelinoclasis	Associated with malnutrition, alcoholism, or with correction of hyponatraemia.
16 Marchiafava-Bignami disease	Associated with alcoholism.
17 Canavan's disease	Dysmyelination in infants: intramyelin oedema comparable to triethyl tin intoxication.
Leucodystrophies	Variable proportions of demyelination and dysmyelination, depending upon age of clinical onset.
18 metachromatic	Accumulation of metachromatic sulphatide due to deficiency of arylsulphatase A.
19 sudanophilic	Dysmyelination with accumulation of sudanopholic lipid.
20 adreno- l/d	Similar to sudanophilic l/d but with adrenal failure. B-oxidation of fatty acids $C_{24} - C_{26}$ impaired. X-linked.
21 globoid cell (Krabbe)	Accumulation of galactosylceramide due to lack of galactosylceramidase.
22 Pelizaeus-Merzbacher	Congenital type is dysmyelination. Classic older type is a leucodystrophy with tigroid pattern of demyelination.
23 Alexander's disease	Dysmyelination: accumulation of peri-vascular lipid and Rosenthal fibres.
24 Phenylpyruvic aciduria	Deficiency of phenylalanine hydroxylase. Demyelination in chronic stage.

B Human Diseases: PNS – demyelinating neuropathy

1 Diphtheritic neuropathy	Segmental demyelination; Schwann cell degeneration. Impaired protein synthesis. Also used as an experimental model.
2 Landry-Guillain-Barré syndrome and related conditions	Segmental demyelination. Auto-immune demyelinating neuropathy. Equivalent to EAN (see Chapter 9).
3 Paraproteinaemia (anti MAG)	IgM antibody (Kappa chain) that reacts with MAG in myelin. Non-compaction of outer myelin lamellae.
4 Paraproteinaemia with multiple myeloma	IgG/IgA antibodies; segmental demyelination.
5 Diabetic neuropathy	Segmental demyelination. Schwann cell degeneration.
6 Lead neuropathy	Segmental demyelination; Schwann cell degeneration.
7 Hypomyelination neuropathy	Defective myelin formation, and may be accompanied by onion bulb formation.
8 Metachromatic neuropathy	Arylsulphatase A deficiency; metachromatic deposits in nerve.
9 Globoid-cell neuropathy	Counterpart to Krabbe's disease in CNS.
10 Drug-induced demyelinating neuropathy	Isoniazid and others.
11 Charcot-Marie-Tooth, Dejerine-Sottas' and Refsum's diseases	Genetic disorders of myelination. Recurrent demyelination; onion bulbs; excess collagen (hypertrophic neuropathy). Accumulation of phytanic acid in Refsum's disease is due to lack of phytanic acid alpha hydroxylase.
12 Trauma	Segmental demyelination with nerve compression.

Animal diseases*

1 Swayback	Copper deficiency in sheep. Dysmyelination in younger animals: demyelination in older animals.
2 Hypomyelinogenesis congenita	Demyelination and dysmyelination in sheep (Border disease). Also in pigs and calves. Viral aetiology.
3 Visna	Slow demyelinating disease in sheep caused by this lentivirus. It may follow the pulmonary disease, maedi.
4 JCM virus disease	Demyelination in mice and rats caused by direct infection of oligodendroglia by this corona virus.
5 Theiler's virus disease	Infection of oligodendroglia in mice by this picovirus causes demyelination and relapsing autoimmune disease.
6 Semliki virus disease	Glial cells are infected in the rat causing necrotic lesions. Subsequent autoimmune disease causes demyelination.
7 Canine distemper virus	This measles-like (morbilliform) virus causes an acute encephalomyelitis in dogs followed by a chronic demyelinating phase.
8 Marek's disease	Herpes-virus-induced lymphoma and peripheral neuropathy in the chicken.
9 Jimpy disease	Recessive sex-linked dysmyelinating disease of mice. Defective oligodendroglia. Hypomyelinogenesis.
10 Quaking disease	Recessive autosomal dysmyelinating disease of mice. Hypomyelinogenesis. Failure of cerebroside synthesis and defective assembly of myelin.
11 Shiverer disease	Recessive autosomal defect in myelin basic protein synthesis in mice.
12 Myelin deficient (MLD) mouse	Recessive sex-linked less-penetrating form of Shiverer disease.
13 Myelin deficient (MD) rat	Genetic disease with defective oligodendroglia and dysmyelination.
14 Twitcher disease	Recessive autosomal globoid cell leucodystrophy of mice. Similar disease in the dog and cat.
15 Trembler disease	Dominant autosomal hypomyelination with Schwann cell defect and onion bulb formation.
16 Murine muscular dystrophy	Recessive autosomal neuropathic muscle disease, with hypomyelination and dystrophic Schwann cells.
17 Dilute lethal and Wobbler lethal diseases	Autosomal recessive neurological diseases in young mice, with doubtful demyelinating pathogenesis.

D Experimental diseases**

1 Experimental allergic encephalomyelitis (EAE)	Demyelinating lesions in larger animals.
2 Chronic relapsing EAE (CREAE)	Causes demyelinating lesions in smaller animals with chronic relapsing course.
3 Experimental allergic neuritis (EAN)	Primary demyelination of peripheral nerves.
4 Antigalactocerebroside antibody	Experimental demyelination (PNS and CNS).
5 Cyanide and azide encephalopathy	Partly necrotic and partly demyelinating lesions.
6 Carbon monoxide encephalopathy.	Partly necrotic and partly demyelinating lesions.

7 Methotrexate toxicity	Demyelination of central white matter, also microangiopathy and necroses. Myocardial necroses.
8 Alkyltin, hexachlorophene and isoniazid toxicity	Triethyltin and hexachlorophene cause intense intra-myelin oedema, while trimethyltin is neurotoxic. Isoniazid causes oedema of cerebellar white matter.
9 Diphtheria toxin injection	Demyelination in both CNS and PNS, caused by reduced protein synthesis.
10 Intraneural lysolecithin or phospholipase A.	Lysophosphatides cause myelin disruption in vivo or in vitro.
11 Inhibition of cholesterol biosynthesis	AY9944 and triparanol cause accumulation of 7-dehydrocholesterol and desmosteriol, respectively. This results in dysmyelination and atheroma.
12 Barbitage	Perturbation of CSF with superficial trauma to cord.
13 Cord or nerve compression	Moderate trauma causes segmental demyelination in PNS.
14 Wallerian degeneration	Secondary demyelination with simultaneous degeneration of the axon.

* See Chapter 3.
** See Chapter 4

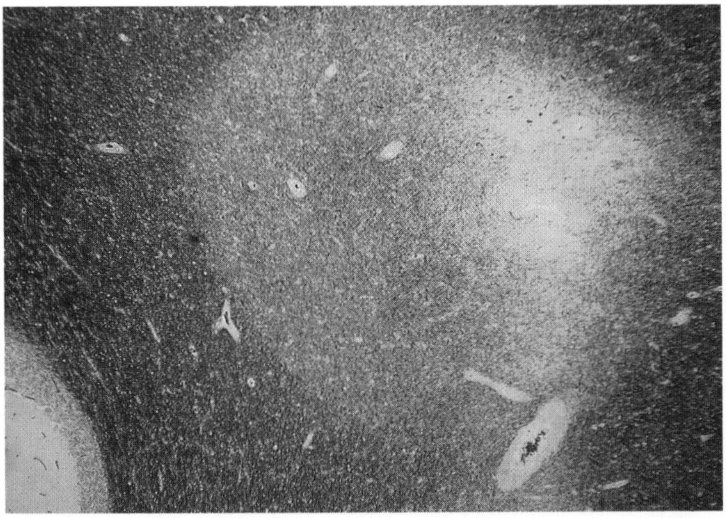

52

52 Shadow plaque in active MS. Luxol fast blue, × 10.

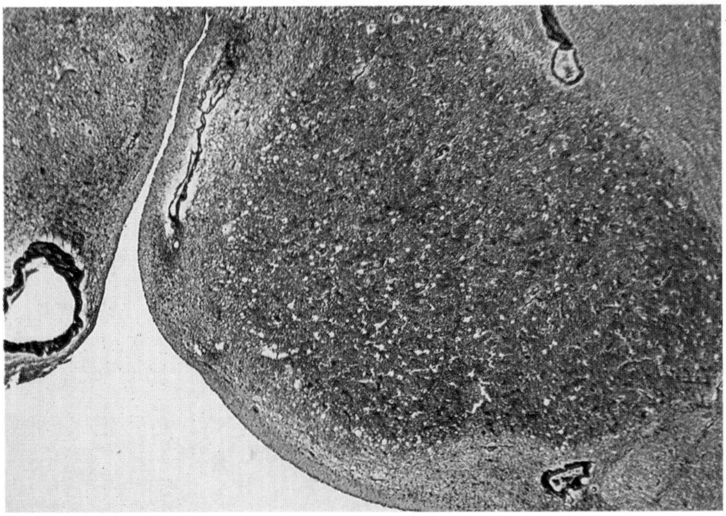

53

53 No loss of axons from same area as **52.** Palmgren silver, × 10.

54

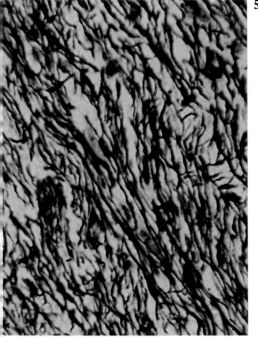

54 Intact axons in acute MS plaque. Palmgren silver, × 200.

55

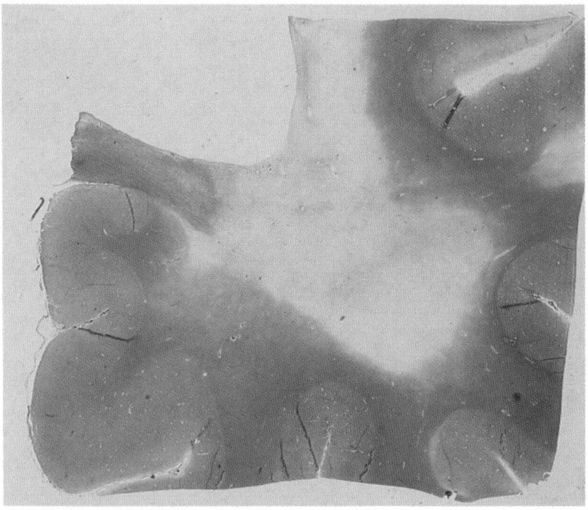

55 Loss of silver staining from chronic plaque. Palmgren silver, × 2.

56

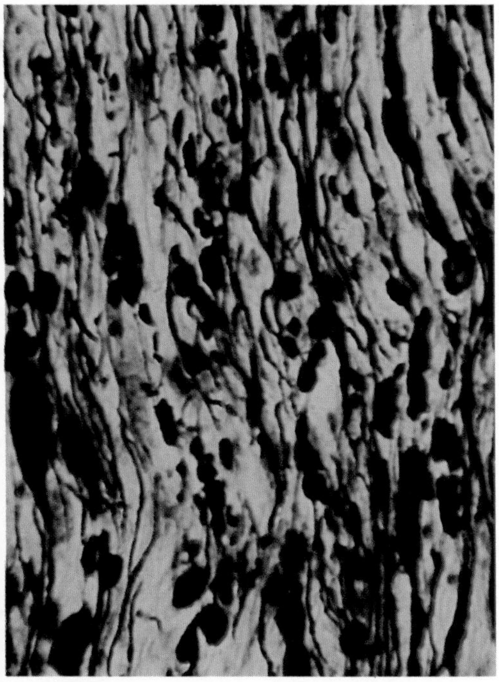

56 Moderate loss of axons, frequent torpedoes and retraction bulbs in chronic MS plaque. Palmgren silver, × 200.

57

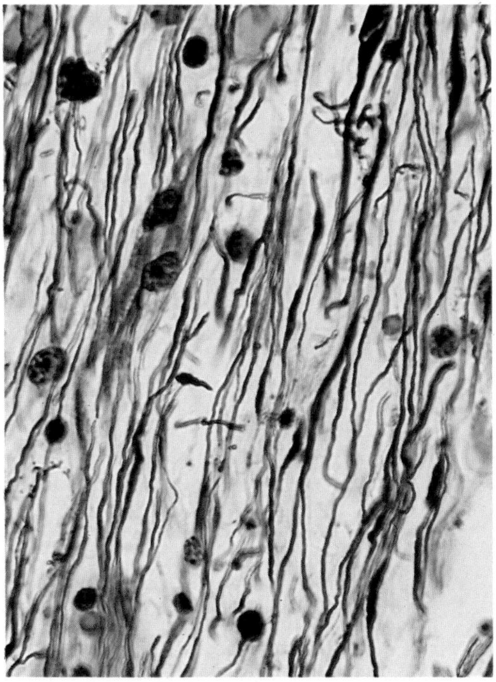

57 Severe loss of axons from chronic burnt-out MS plaque. Palmgren silver, × 200.

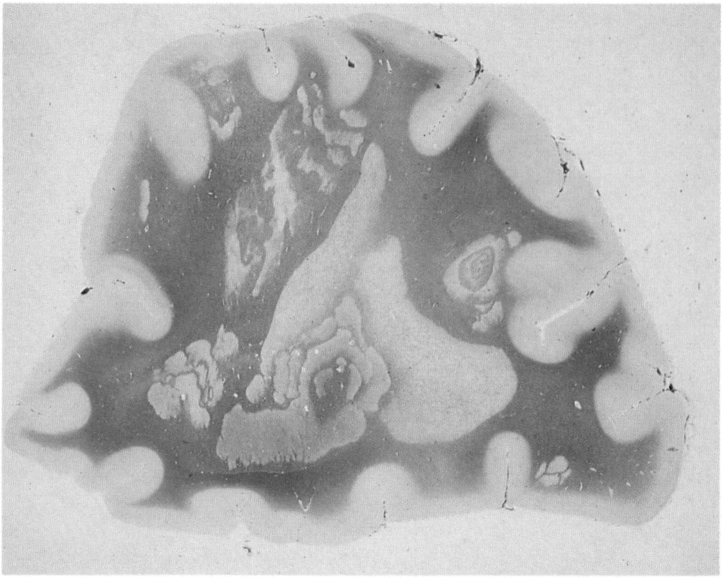

58

58 Balo's concentric sclerosis. Note ripples of concentric demyelination in cortical white matter. Heidenhain, × 1.

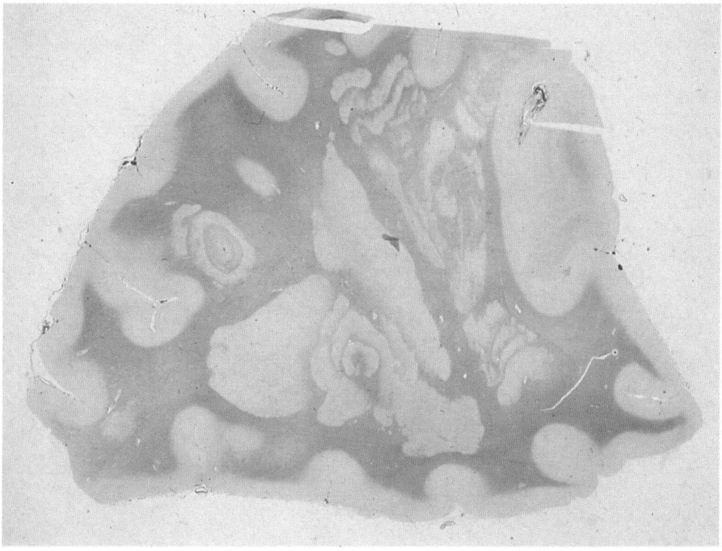

59

59 Balo's concentric sclerosis. Phosphotungstic acid-haematoxylin, × 1.

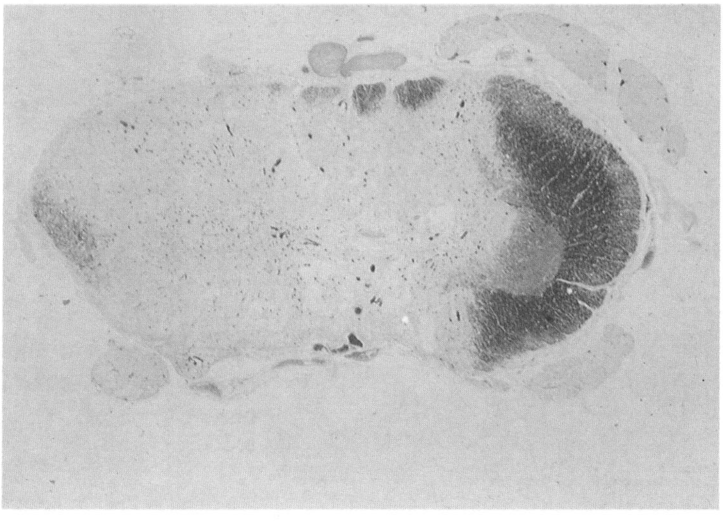

60

60 Devic's disease (neuromyelitis optica). Necrotic lesion in cervical cord (C8), accompanied by optic neuritis in a case of pulmonary tuberculosis. Haematoxylin-eosin, × 6. *(Courtesy of Professor R.A.C. Hughes)*

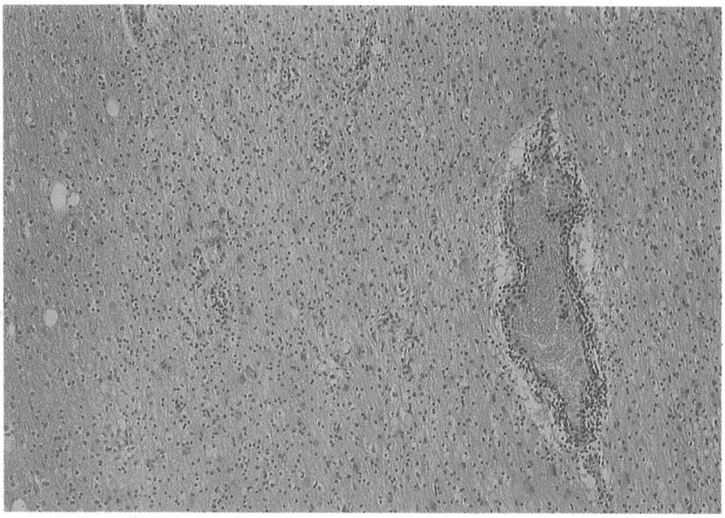

61

61 Devic's disease (neuromyelitis optica). Acute myelitis in the cervical cord. Haematoxylin-eosin, × 25. *(Courtesy of Dr Barbara Smith)*

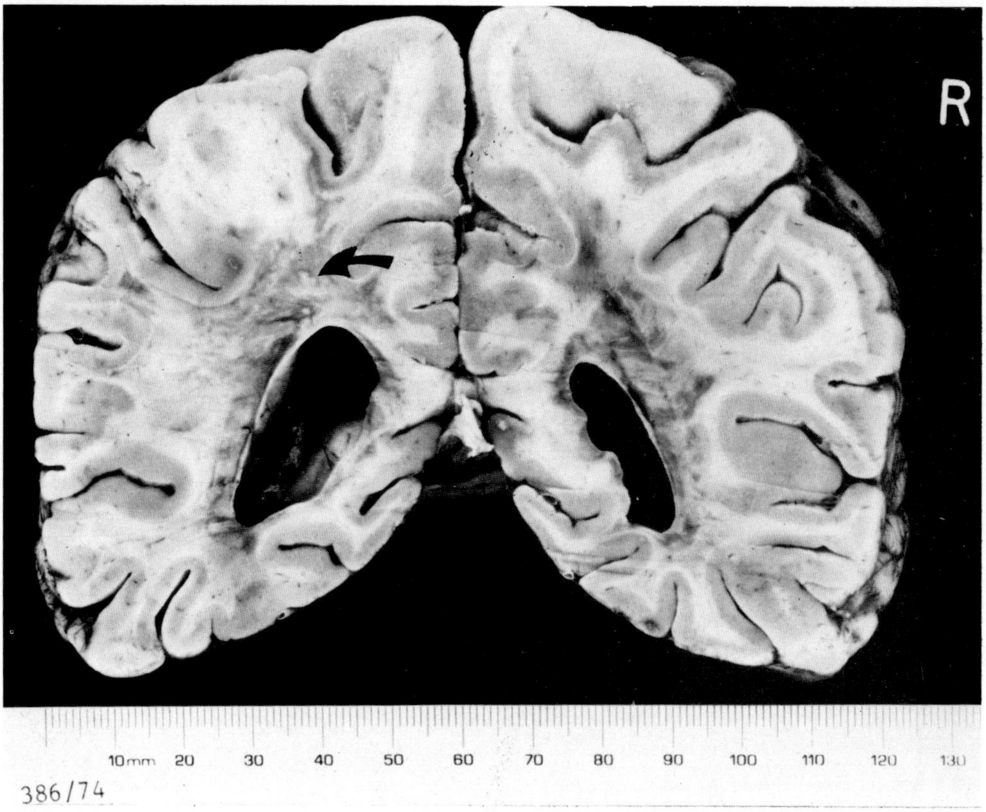

62

62 Diffuse sclerosis or Schilder's disease in a young woman. Note widespread sclerosis of central white matter and periventricular regions. This can be regarded as a severe rapidly progressive form of multiple sclerosis with gross confluent lesions × 1.

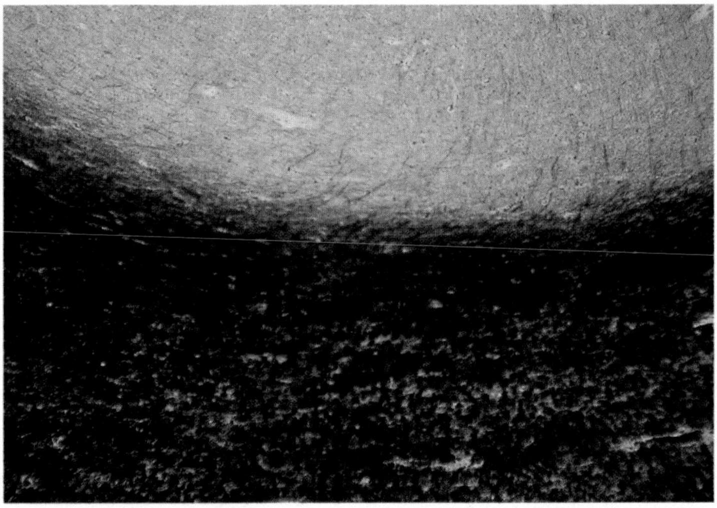

63

63 Demyelination in callosal radiation in Schilder's disease. Much of the lipid lies within macrophages. Sudan black, × 100.

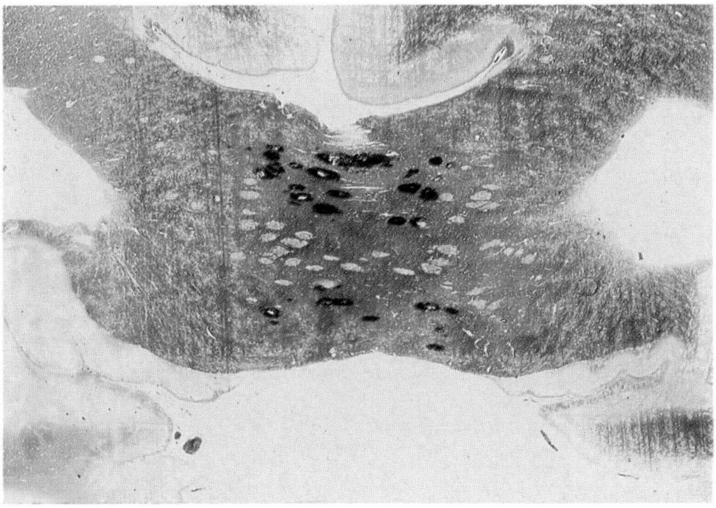

64

64 Perivenular demyelination (partly haemorrhagic) in anterior pillar of fornix in postviral allergic encephalomyelitis. Loyez, × 2.

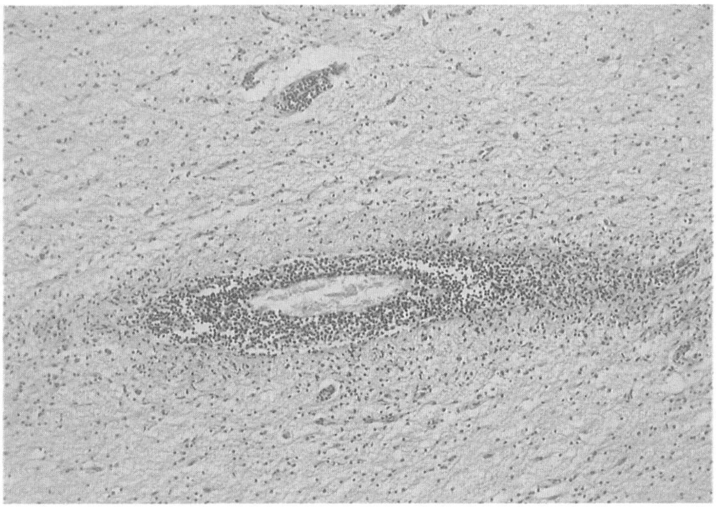

65

65 Leucoencephalomyelitis with marked perivascular infiltration in Behcet's disease. Haematoxylin-eosin, × 25.

66

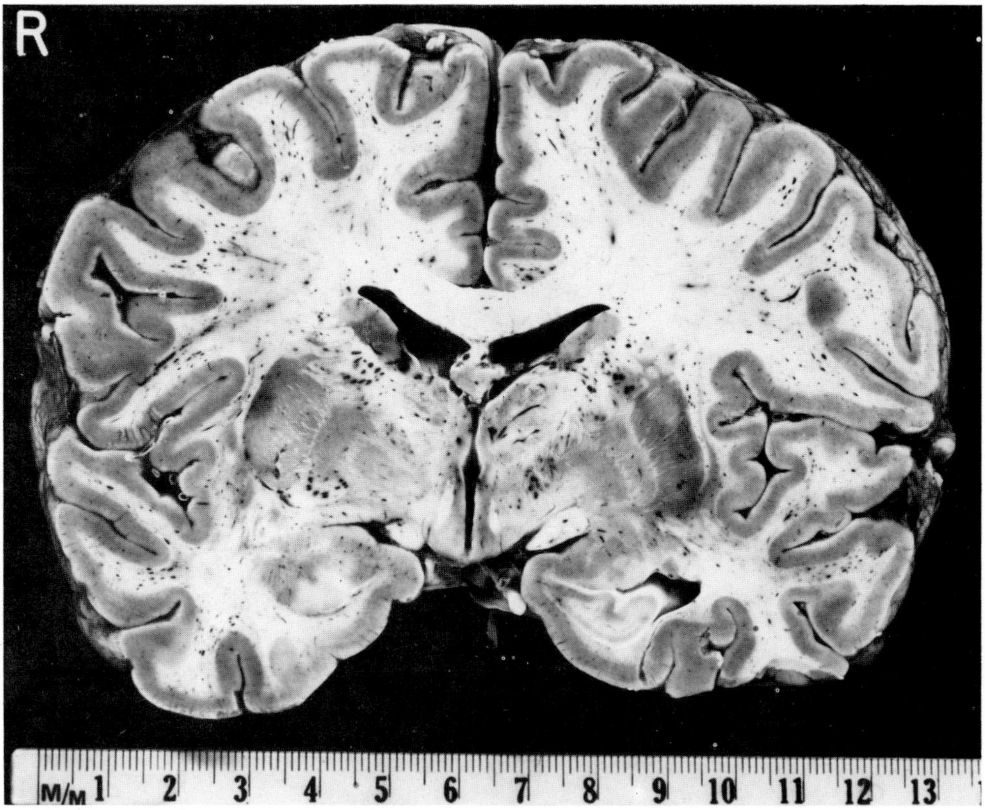

66 Acute haemorrhagic leucoencephalitis. Typical severe haemorrhagic lesions, × 1.

67

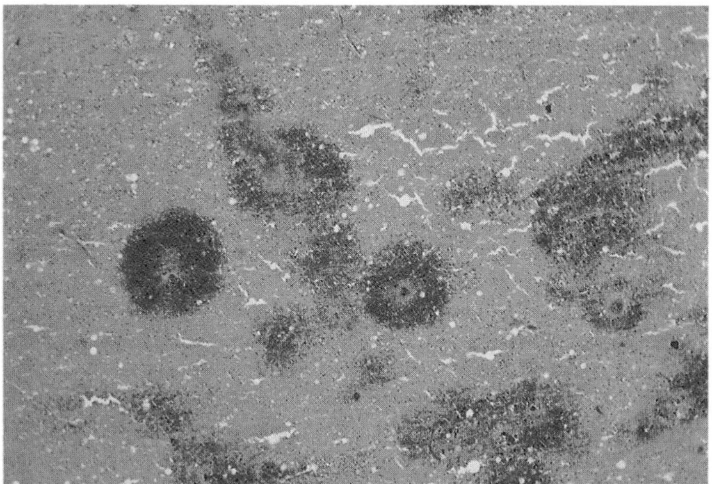

67 Ring haemorrhages in acute haemorrhagic leucoencephalitis. Haematoxylin-eosin, × 40.

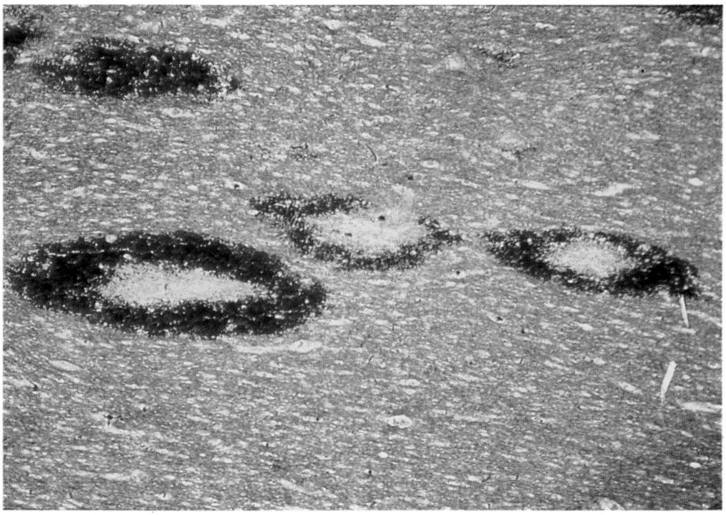

68

68 Ring haemorrhages in acute haemorrhagic leucoencephalitis. Phosphotungstic acid-haematoxylin, × 40.

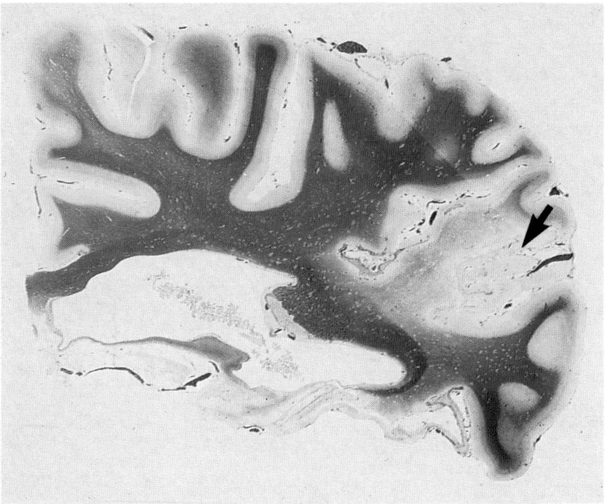

69

69 Subacute necrotising leucoencephalitis. Note necrotic focus in subcortical white matter (arrow). Heidenhain, × 1.

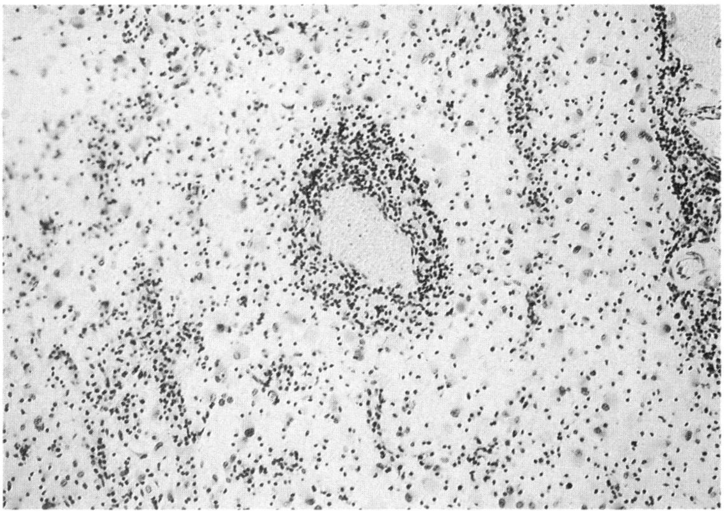

70

70 Subacute necrotising leucoencephalitis. Note severe inflammation and necrosis with loss of structure. Crystal violet, × 40.

71

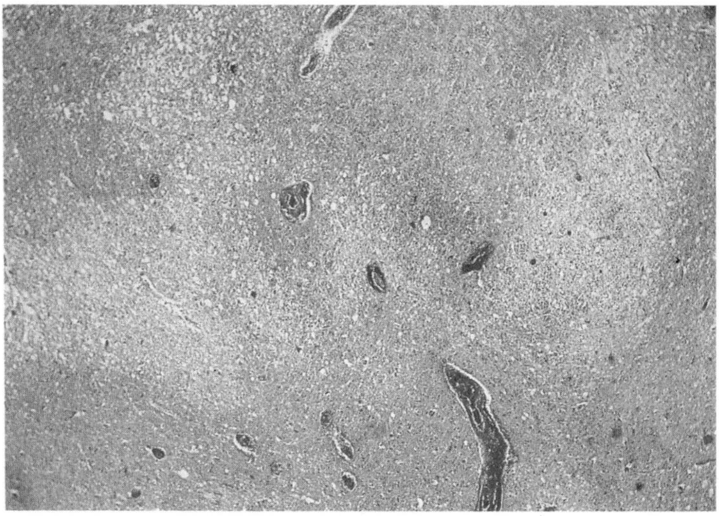

71 Herpes simplex encephalitis. Note multiple focal necrotic lesions and resulting thrombosed vessels. Phosphotungstic acid haematoxylin, × 50.

72

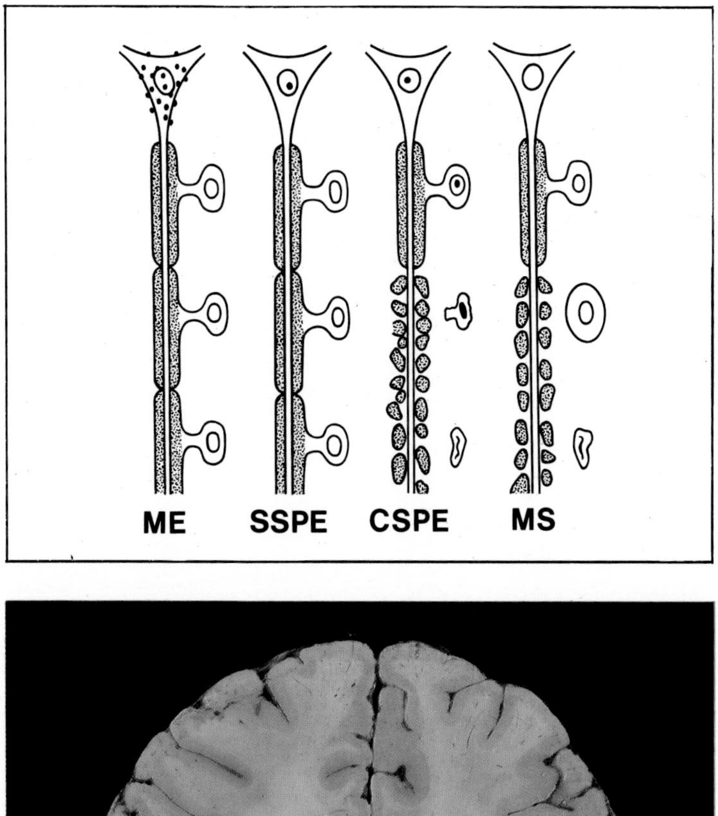

72 Measles infections of the nervous system compared with multiple sclerosis. Neuronal damage is caused by viral infection of the neuronal cell body in acute measles encephalitis (ME). Incomplete slow virus is present in the neuronal nucleus in subacute sclerosing panencephalitis (SSPE) causing Wallerian degeneration. Incomplete virus is present in both neurone and oligodendrocyte in chronic sclerosing panencephalitis (CSPE) causing demyelination. These are contrasted with MS, where the neurone is not involved and the initial change in the oligodendroglia is hypertrophy and hyperplasia, to be followed by loss of oligodendroglia. *(Reproduced from Adams, 1972, 'Research on Multiple Sclerosis', by courtesy of C.C. Thomas, Springfield)*

73

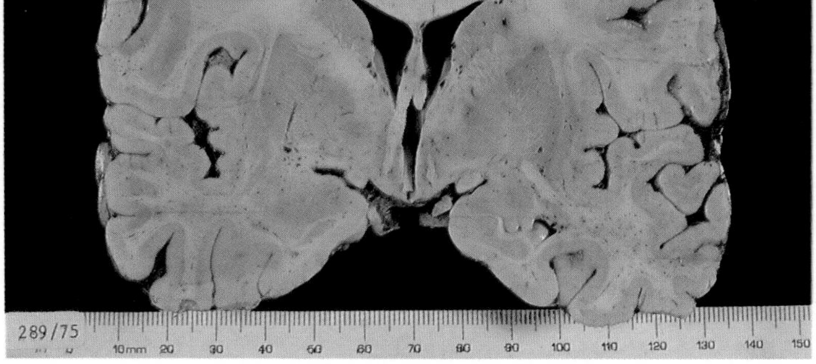

73 Subacute sclerosing panencephalitis (SSPE). Ill-defined sclerosis of subcortical white matter and cortex, particularly in the temporal lobes, × ½.

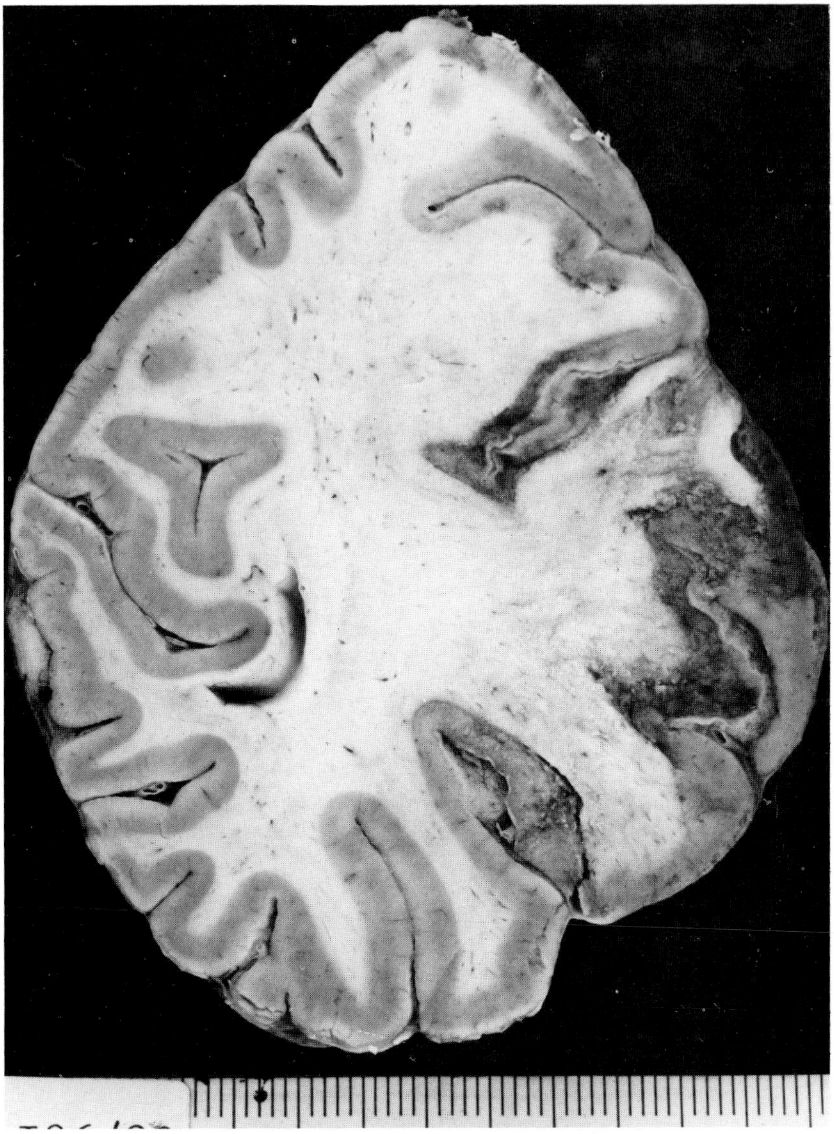

74 SSPE. Focal necrosis in cortex and adjacent white matter.

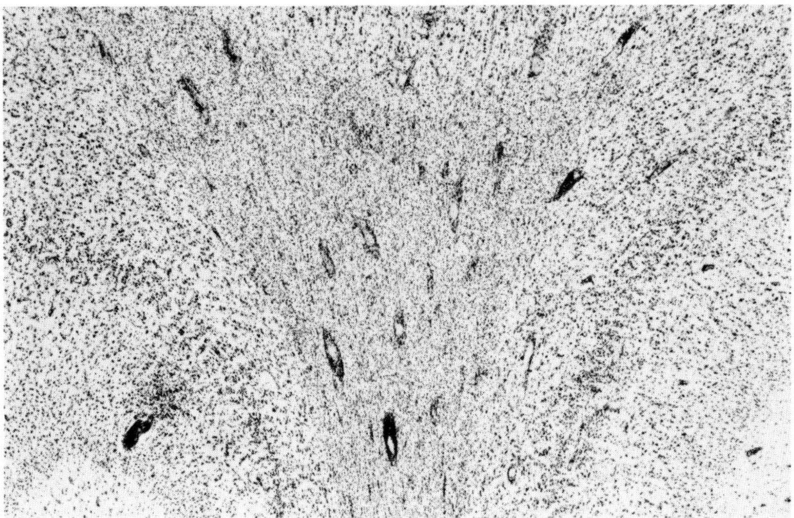

75 SSPE. Astrocytic proliferation, scanty Punkinje cells and neuronal loss in the cerebellum, together with moderate perivascular infiltration. Cresyl violet, × 30.

76

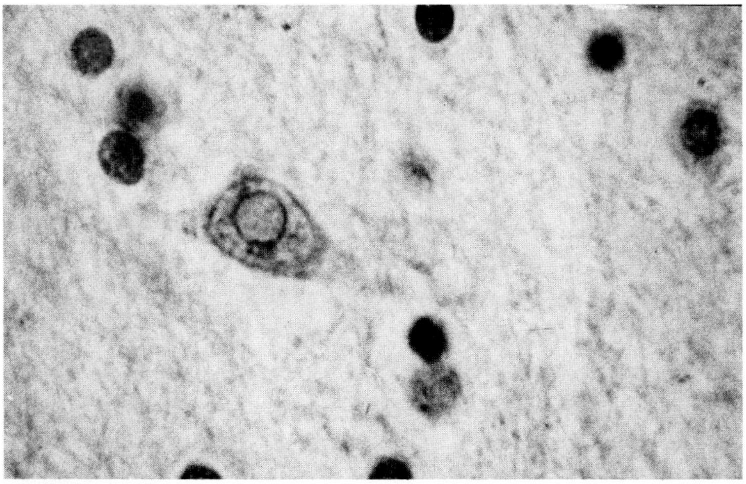

76 SSPE. Intranuclear inclusion in cortical neurone. Haematoxylin-eosin, × 500.

77

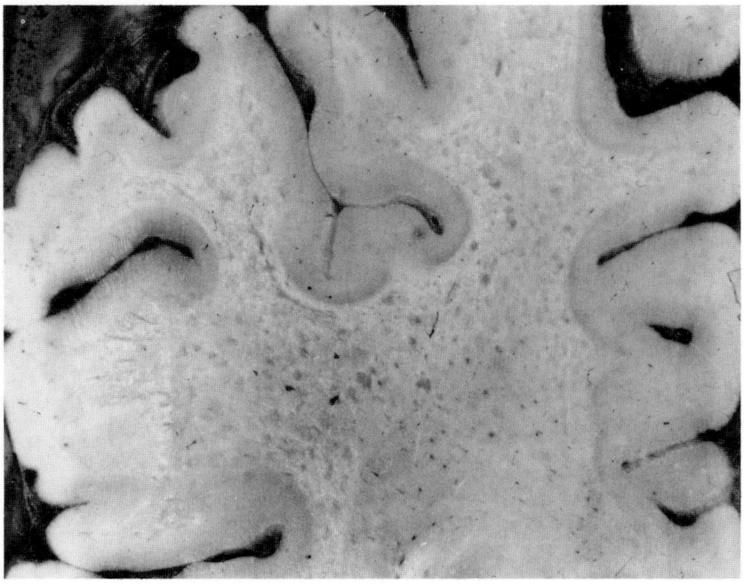

77 Progressive multifocal leucoencephalopathy (PML). Gross appearance of multifocal demyelinating lesions, × 2.

78

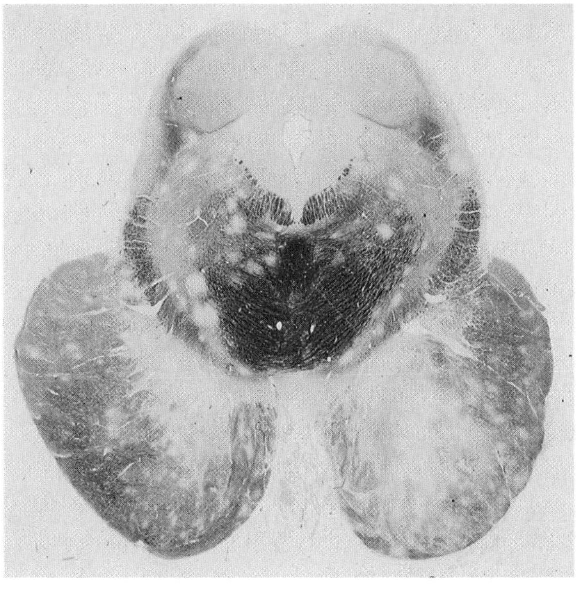

78 PML. A severe chronic case showing multifocal demyelinating lesions in tegmentum and basis pedunculi of brainstem. Heidenhain, × 2.

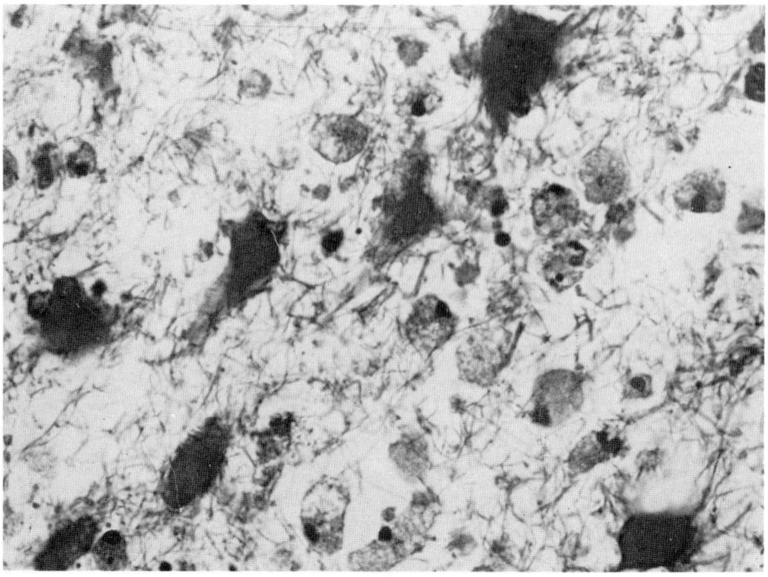

79 PML. Characteristic enlarged bizarre multiangulated fibrillary astrocytes. Haematoxylin-eosin, × 250.

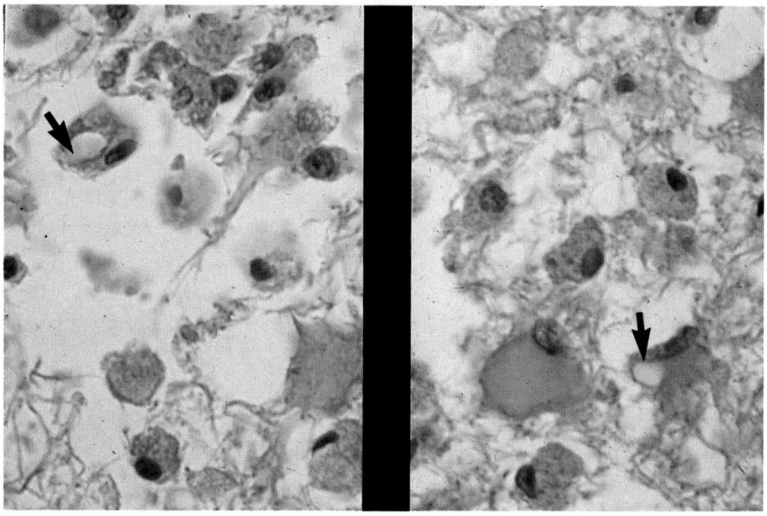

80 PML. Enlarged oligodendroglia with cytoplasmic inclusion bodies (upper left and lower right, arrows). Haematoxylin-eosin, × 300.

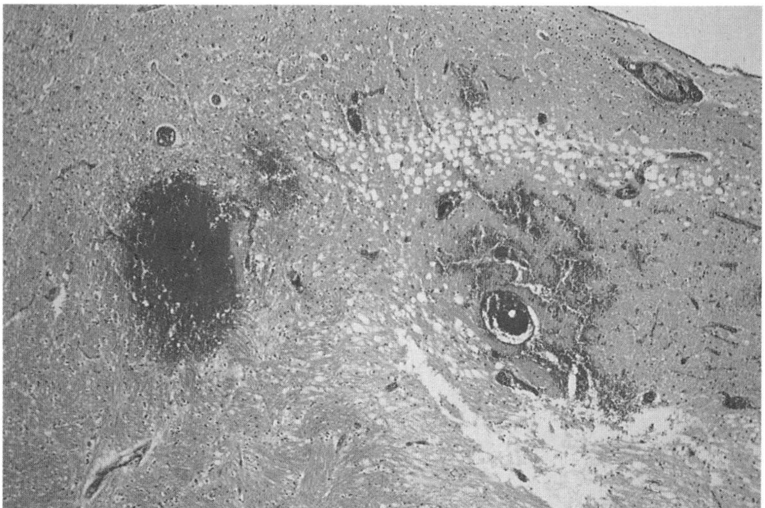

81 AIDS. Intravascular coagulation and focal cerebral infarction in a case of acquired immunodeficiency syndrome. Haematoxylin-eosin, × 80.

82

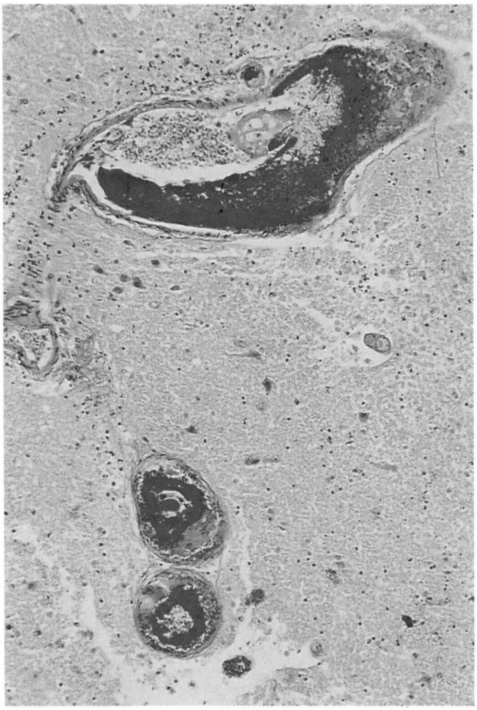

83

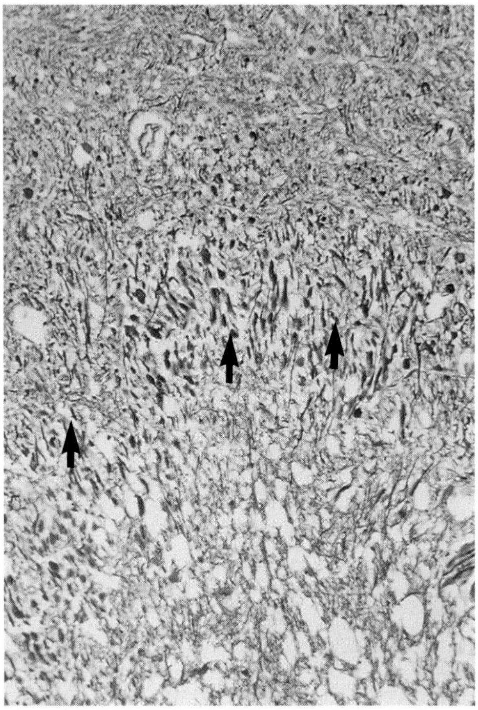

82 AIDS. Intravascular coagulation (fibrin deposition) as a localised form of diffuse intravascular coagulation, confined to the CNS. Same case as **81**. Mallory trichrome-MSB, × 120.

83 AIDS. Edge of necrotic lesion with axons ending in retraction balls at edge of lesion (arrow). Palmgren's silver stain, × 80.

84

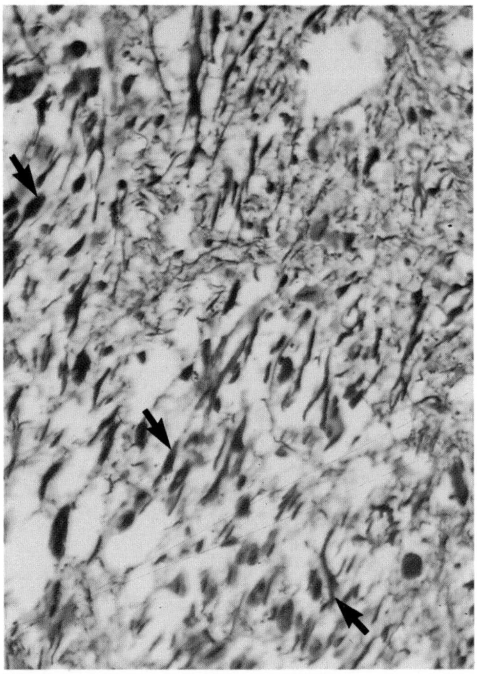

85

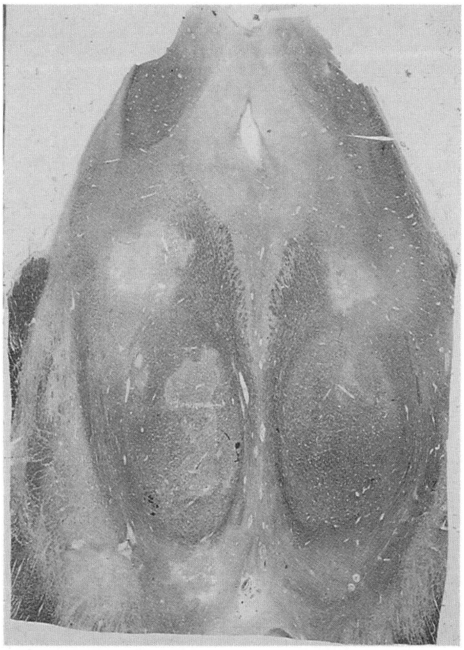

84 AIDS. Higher power view of **83** to show retraction balls (arrow). Palmgren silver, × 200.

85 AIDS. Group of four demyelinating lesions in midbrain in and around the red nucleus. Luxol fast blue, × 2.

86 Central pontine myelinoclasis. Minor form in a terminal patient. *(Courtesy of Dr Barbara Smith)*

87 Central pontine myelinoclasis in a rehydrated-dehydrated patient. Pons at level of middle cerebellar peduncle. Luxol fast blue, × 2. *(Courtesy of Dr A.P. Boon)*

88 Central pontine myelinoclasis; same patient as **87**. Posterior midbrain. Luxol fast blue, × 2. *(Courtesy of Dr A.P. Boon)*

86

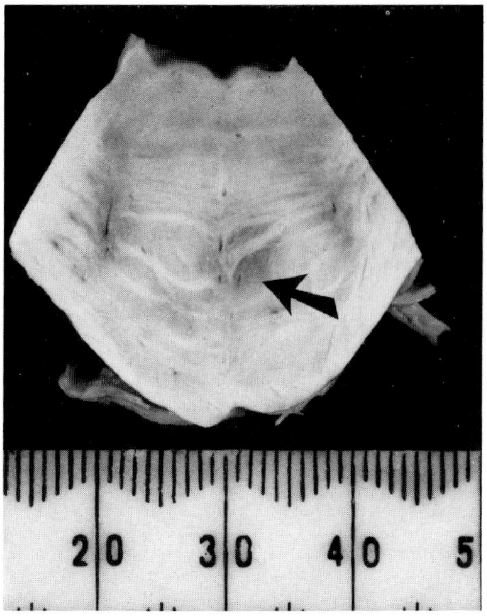

87

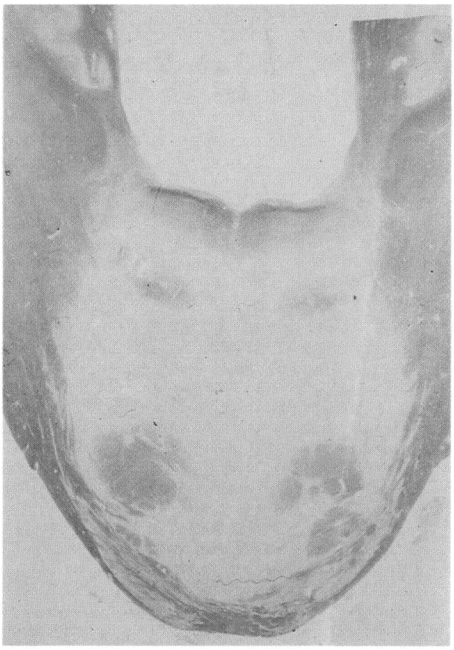

88

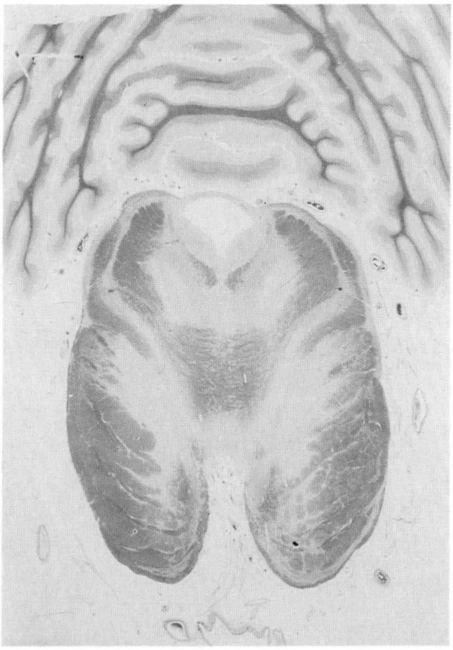

89

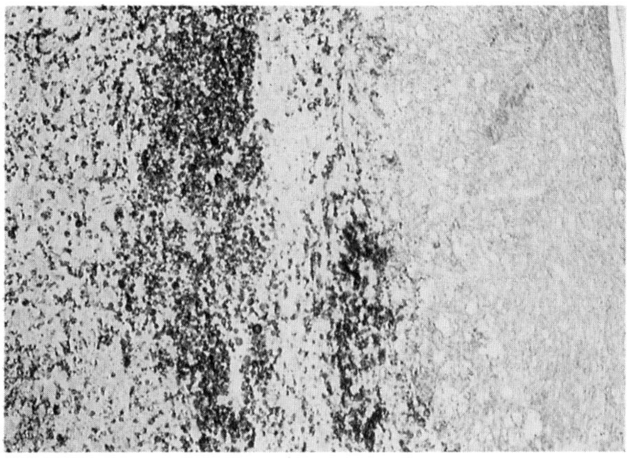

89 Central pontine myelinoclasis. Sudanophilic myelin breakdown products (esterified cholesterol) within macrophages in an active case of CPM. Oil Red O, × 80. *(Courtesy of Dr A.P. Boon)*

90 Marchiafava-Bignami disease. Demyelination of central corpus callosum (D) with sparing of margins. C = caudate nucleus; G = cingular gyrus; O = orbital gyri; V = lateral ventricle. Spielmeyer stain, × 1. *(Courtesy of Dr A. Petrescu)*

91 Marchiafava-Bignami disease. Demyelinating lesions in corpus callosum, subcortical white matter and middle cerebellar peduncle (arrows). Photograph of drawings in Marchiafava and Bignami (1903). *(Courtesy of Dr Amico Bignami)*

90

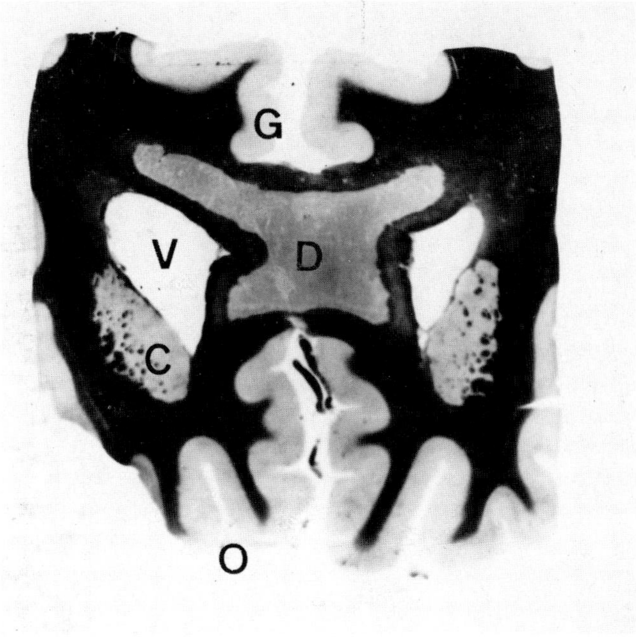

91

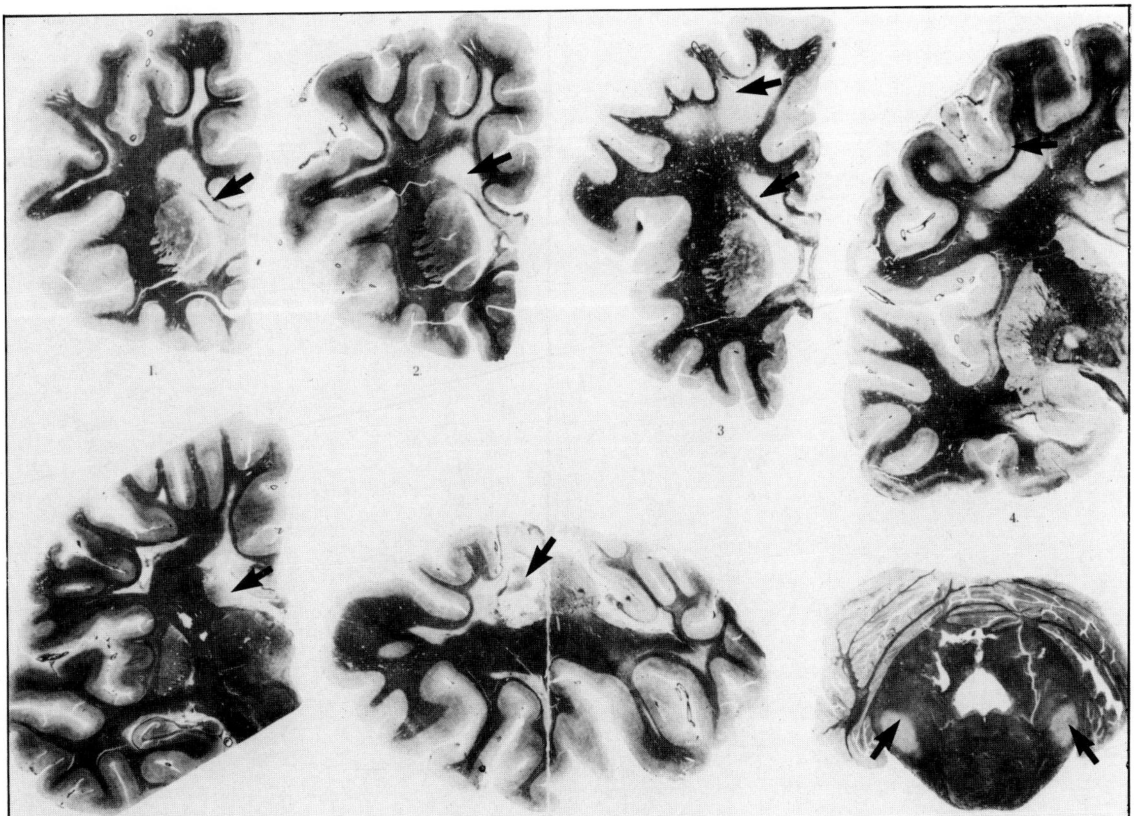

92
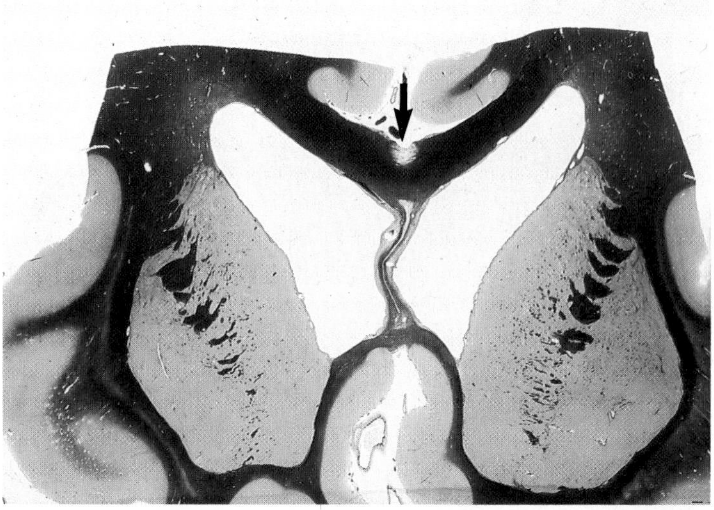

92 Marchiafava-Bignami disease. A patient with Wernicke's encephalopathy, Korsakow's psychosis and peripheral neuropathy showed this small central demyelinating lesion in the corpus callosum at the level of the anterior pillars of the fornix. This minor demyelinating lesion is not located in the middle layers of the corpus callosum, which is the characteristic position in Marchiafava-Bignami disease. Heidenhain, × 1/2, × 1.

93
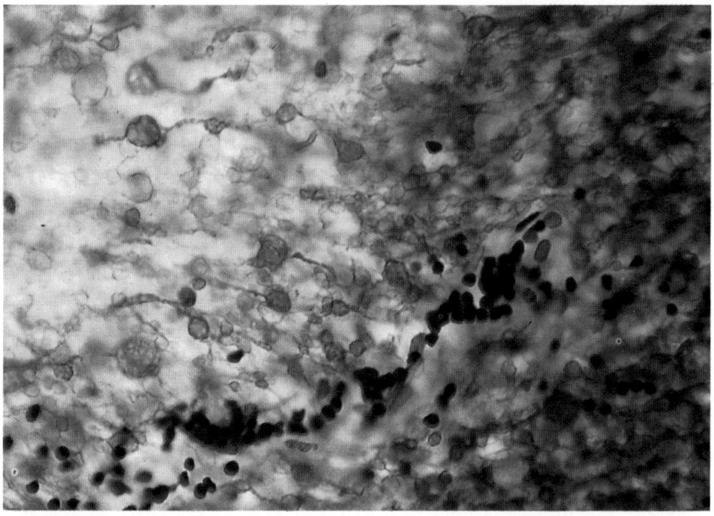

93 Same case as 92 to show loss of myelin and oligodendroglia, myelin balls, oedematous swelling and vascularity. Heidenhain, × 200.

94
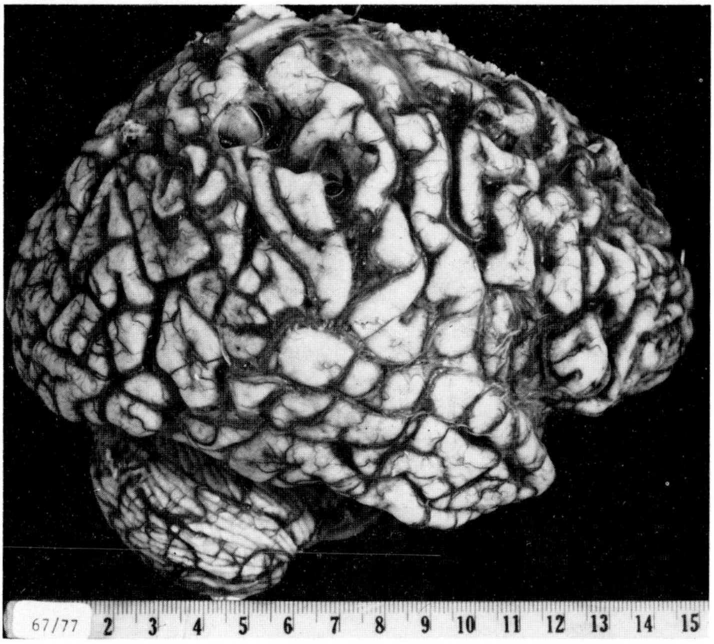

94 Creutzfeldt-Jakob (CJ) disease. Marked atrophy of cerebral gyri with widening of sulci, particularly over the frontal and temporal lobes, × ½.

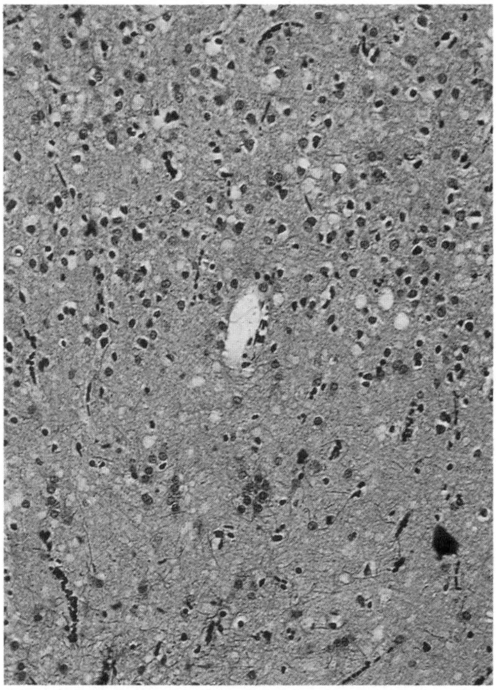

95

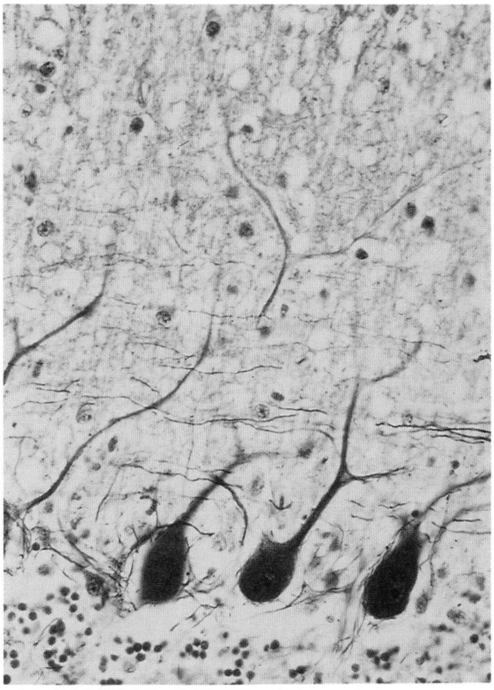

96

95 Creutzfeldt-Jakob disease. Loss of neurones in cerebral cortex with proliferation of astrocytes. Lost neurones are represented by vacuoles, hence the term spongiform encephalopathy. Heidenhain, × 100.

96 Creutzfeldt-Jakob disease. Loss of neurones from granular layer (left) and replacement by spongiform structure. Gros-Bielschowsky, × 250.

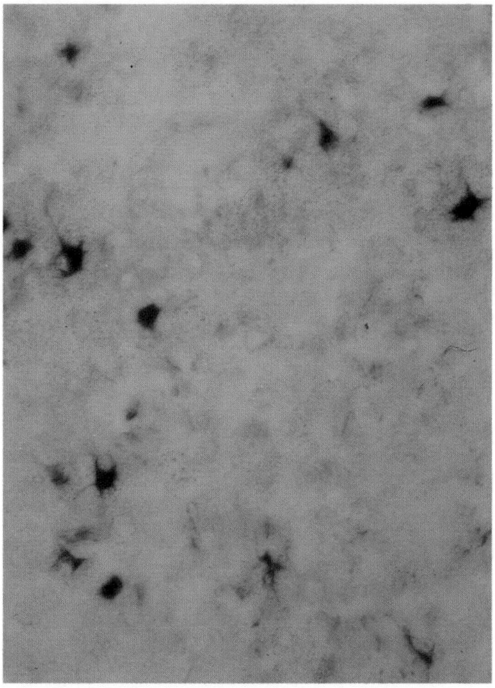

97

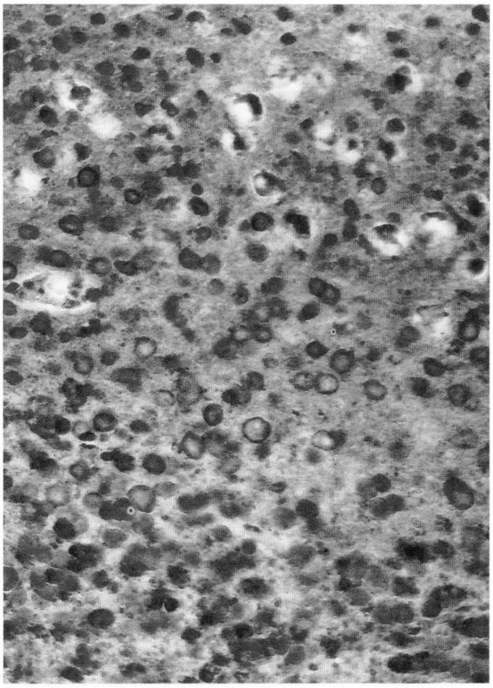

98

97 Creutzfeldt-Jakob disease. Activated astrocytes within cerebral cortex. NADH-tetrazolium reductase, × 200.

98 Metachromatic leucodystrophy (MLD). The stored sulphatide within microglia is stained metachromatically brown. Cerebral biopsy, cresyl violet, × 120. *(Tissue by courtesy of the late Professor J. Cumings)*

99

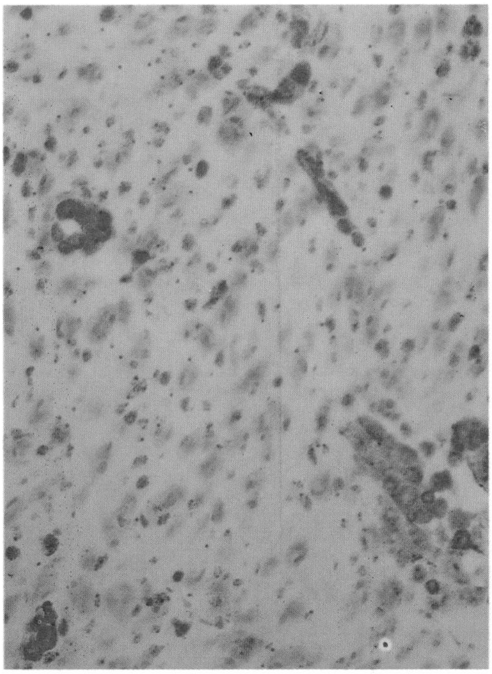

99 MLD, same case as **98**. Sulphatide stained by Hollander's acridine-DMAB method, × 120.

100

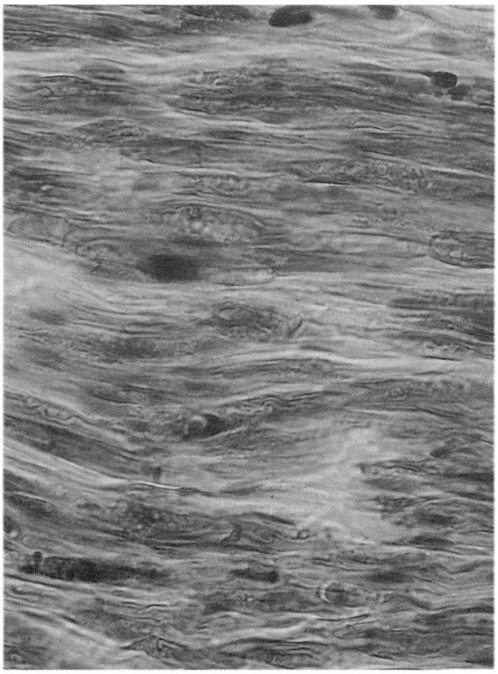

100 MLD. Sulphatide deposits in peripheral nerve stained metachromatically purple. Sural nerve biopsy, thionin, × 200.

101

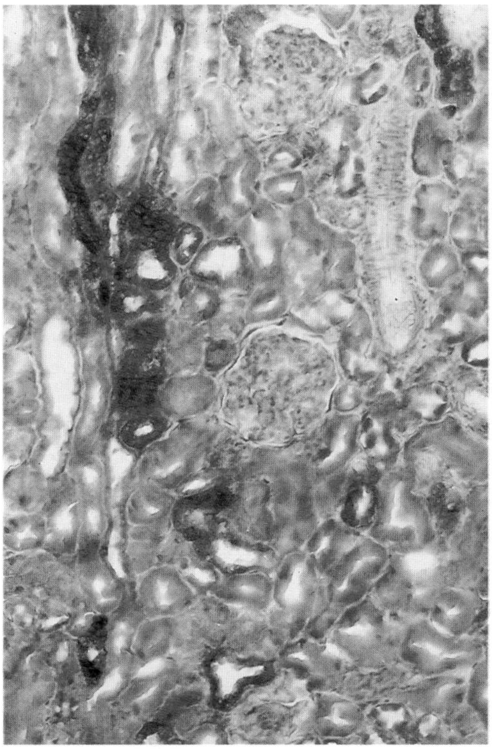

101 MLD. Sulphatide deposits in convoluted and collecting tubular epithelium in the kidney. Autopsy case, cresyl violet, × 150.

102

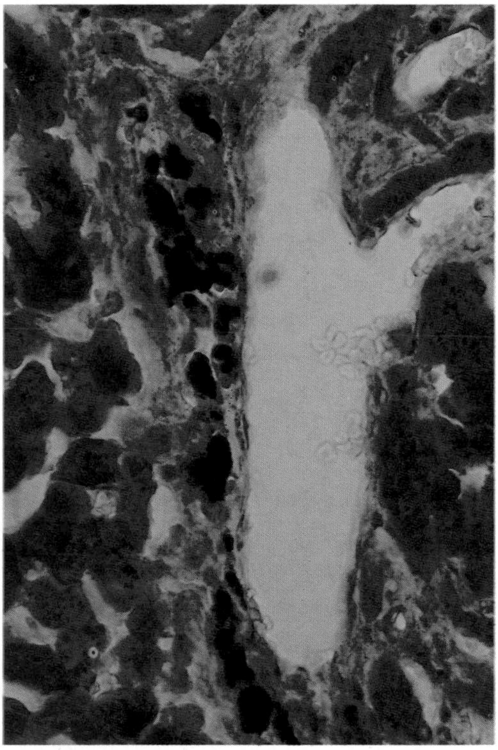

102 MLD. Sulphatide deposits in bile-duct epithelium. Cresyl violet, × 300.

103

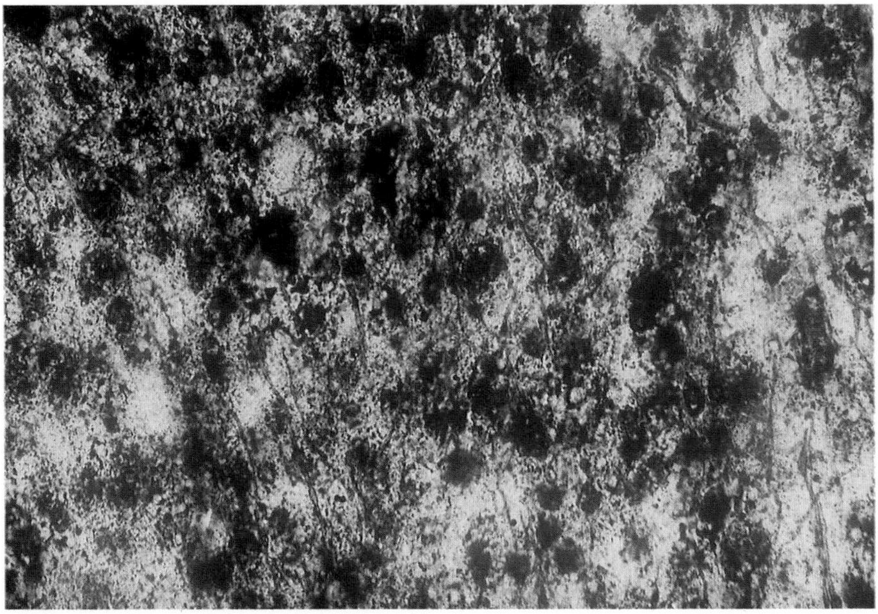

103 Sudanophilic leucodystrophy. Note massive accumulation of sudanophilic lipid (esterified cholesterol). Sudan black, × 200.

104

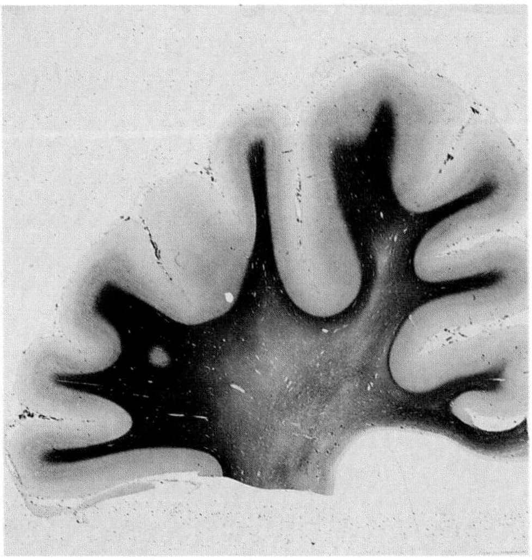

104 Adrenoleucodystrophy. Massive demyelinated area in central white matter of frontal cortex. Loyez's myelin stain, × 1. *(Courtesy of Dr Ivan Janota)*

105

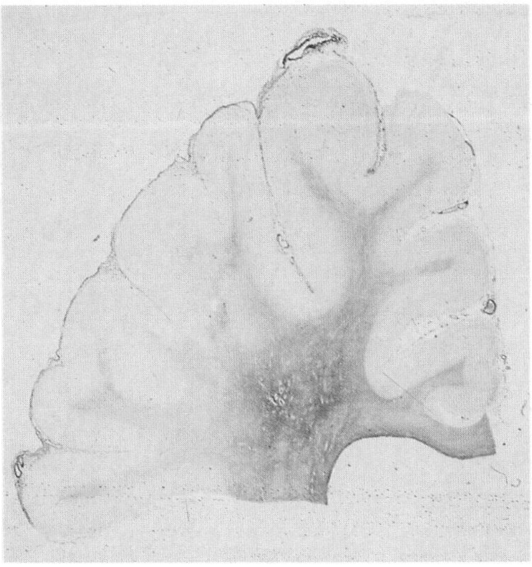

105 Adrenoleucodystrophy. Gliosis in demyelinated area. Holzer's stain, × 1. *(Courtesy of Dr Ivan Janota)*

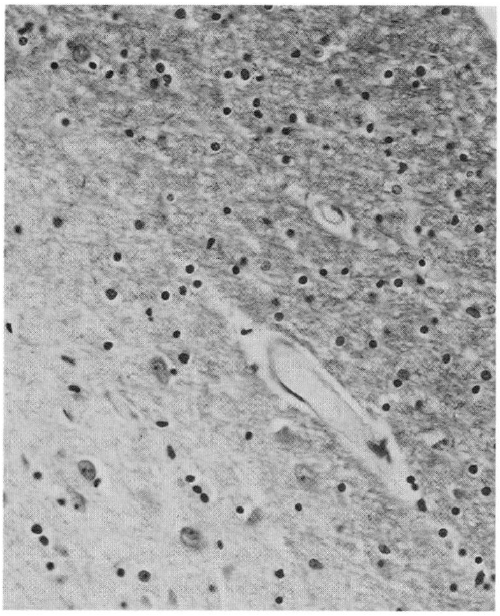

106

106 Pelizaeus-Merzbacher disease (infantile or congenital form). Note gross dysmyelination in white matter of callosal radiation and only scanty oligodendroglia. This dysmyelinating disease results from defective synthesis of proteolipid protein by oligodendroglia (see text). Luxol fast blue-cresyl violet, × 150. *(Courtesy of Professor Daria Haust)*

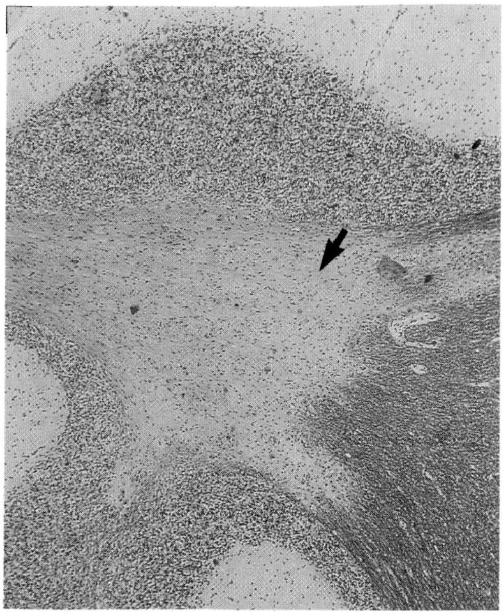

107

107 Krabbe's leucodystrophy. Demyelination and dysmyelination at root of cerebellar medullary lamina (arrow). Luxol fast blue-cresyl violet, × 32.

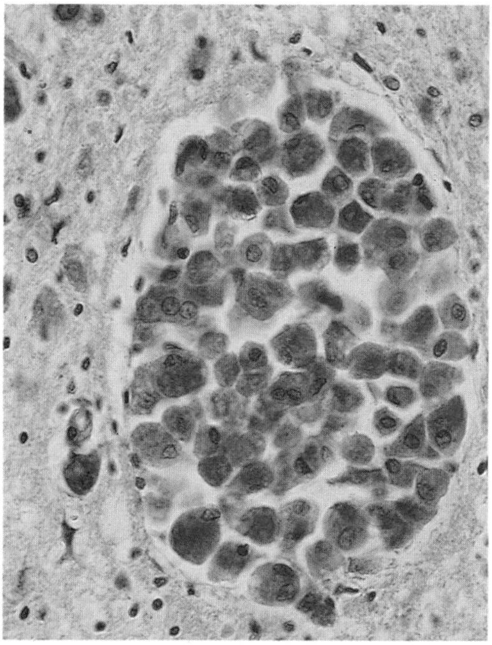

108

108 Krabbe's leucodystrophy. These globoid cells give immunocytochemical reactions for macrophages and store galactosyl cerebroside. Typically, the globoid cells form clumps and a proportion are binucleate. Haematoxylin-eosin, × 200.

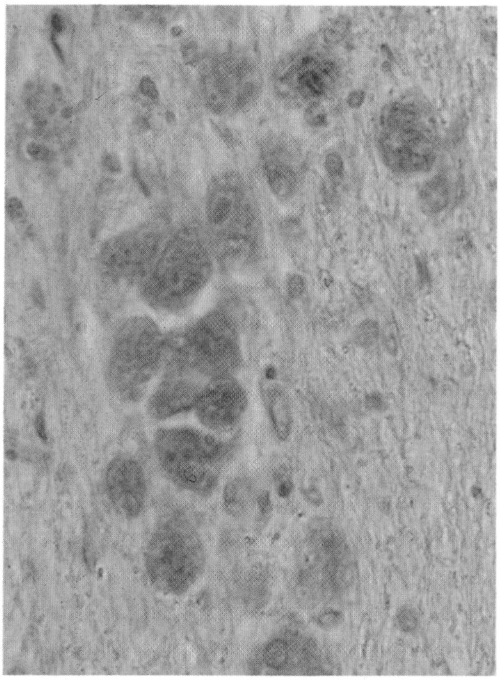

109

109 Krabbe's leucodystrophy. Galactosyl cerebroside is stained by PAS. Periodic acid-Schiff, × 200.

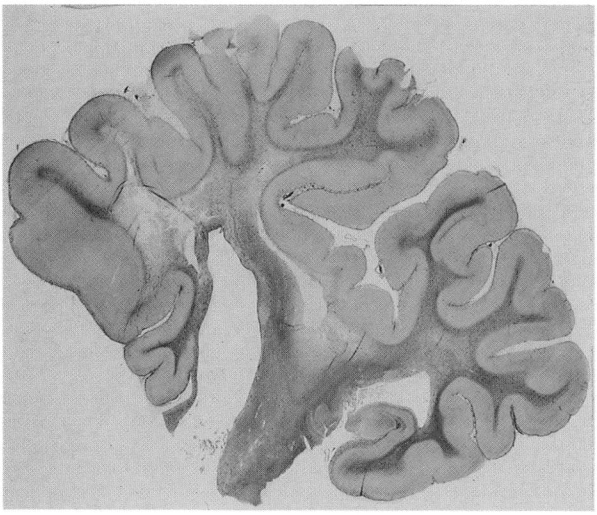

110

10 Alexander's disease. Cortical .trophy, and demyelination, 'ysmyelination and sclerosis of central vhite matter. Phosphotungstic acid- aematoxylin, × 1.

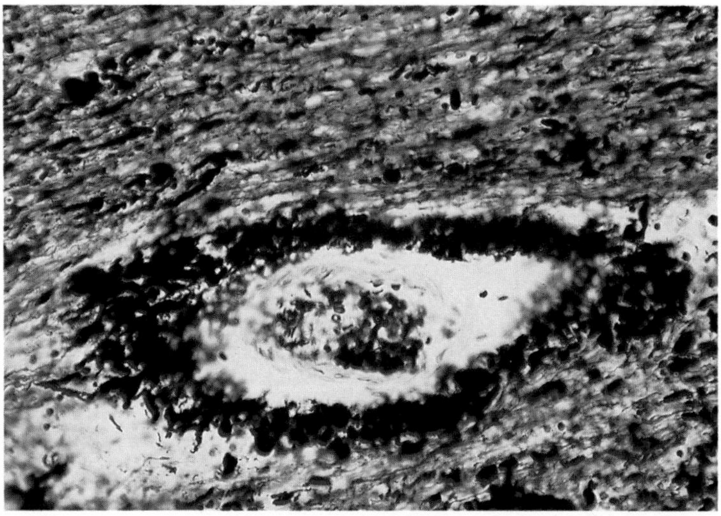

111

11 Alexander's disease. ›emyelination, and perivascular ccumulation of lipid material and Rosenthal fibres. Heidenhain, × 100.

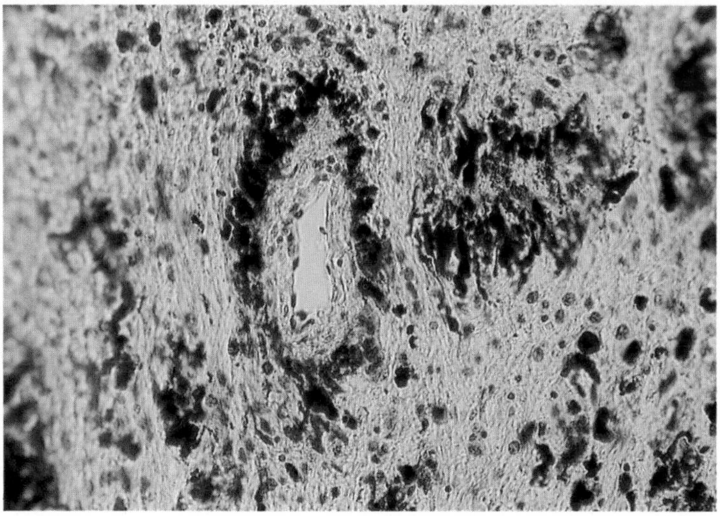

112

12 Alexander's disease. Rosenthal bres stained blue by phospho- ungstic acid-haematoxylin, × 100.

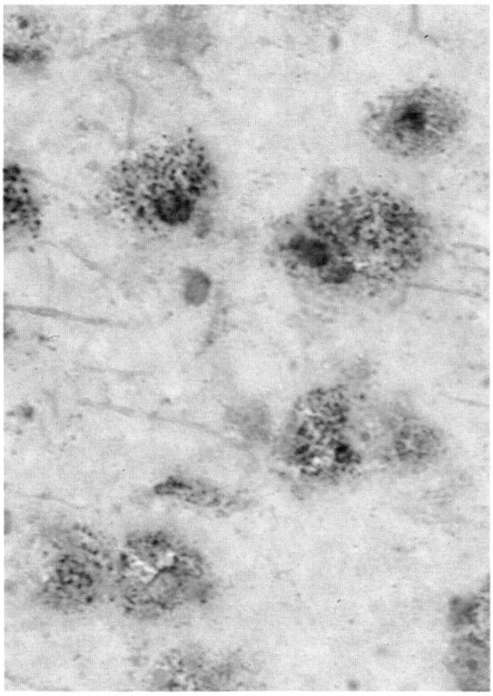

113

113 Niemann-Pick's disease. Accumulation of sphingomyelin in cerebral neurones. Alkali-stable lipid. Baker's acid haematein, × 300.

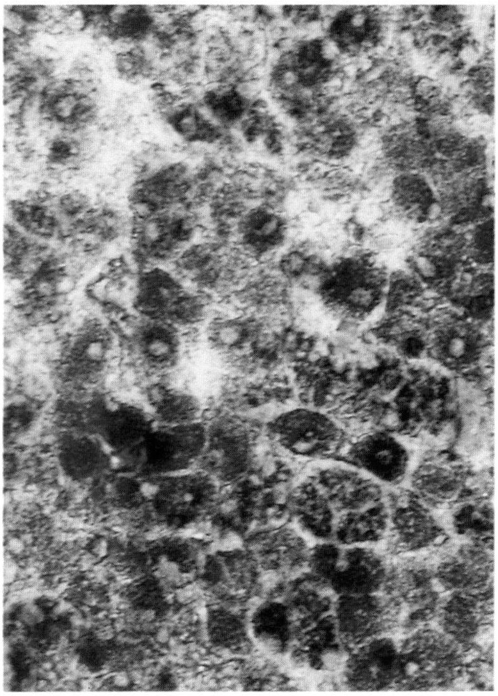

114

114 Visceral Niemann-Pick's disease. Sphingomyelin in liver; in Kupffer and parenchymal cells. Baker's acid haematein, × 300.

115

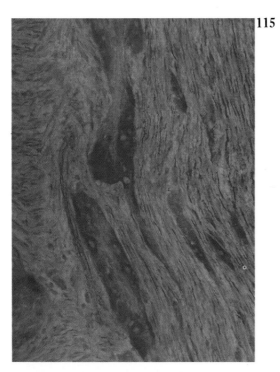

115 GM1 gangliosidosis. Ganglioside in myenteric ganglion cells. Appendix biopsy, periodic acid-Schiff, × 300.

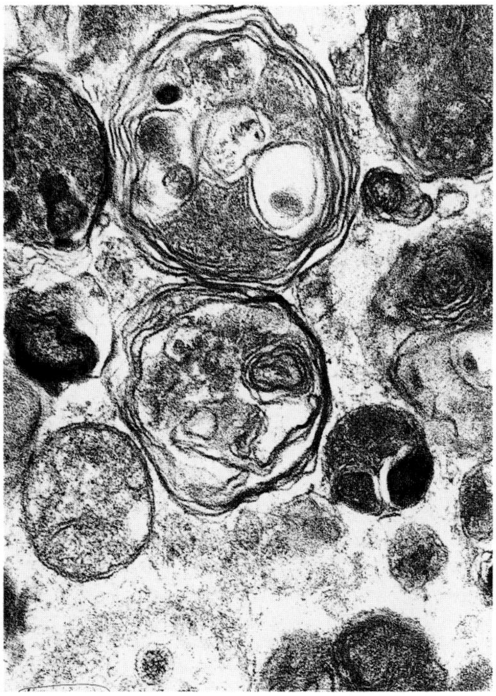

116

116 GM1 gangliosidosis. Membranous cytoplasmic bodies in ganglion cells. Same case as **115**, × 15,000.

117

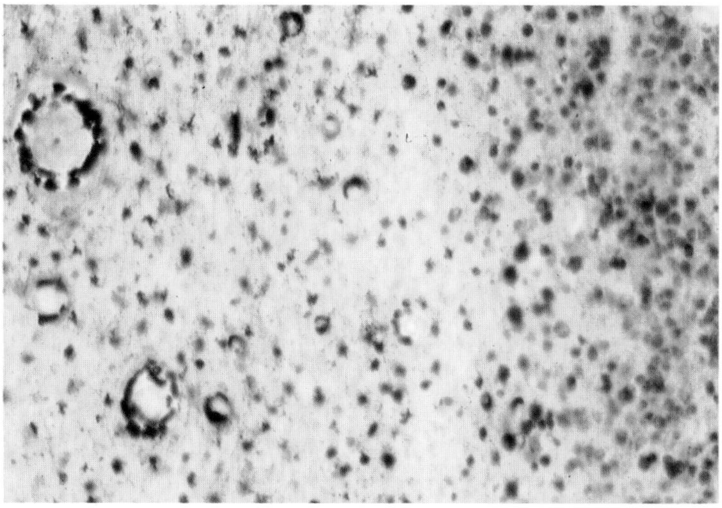

17 GM2 gangliosidosis (Tay-ach's disease). Massive lipid torage within cerebral macrophages/ nicroglia. Sudan black, × 60.

118

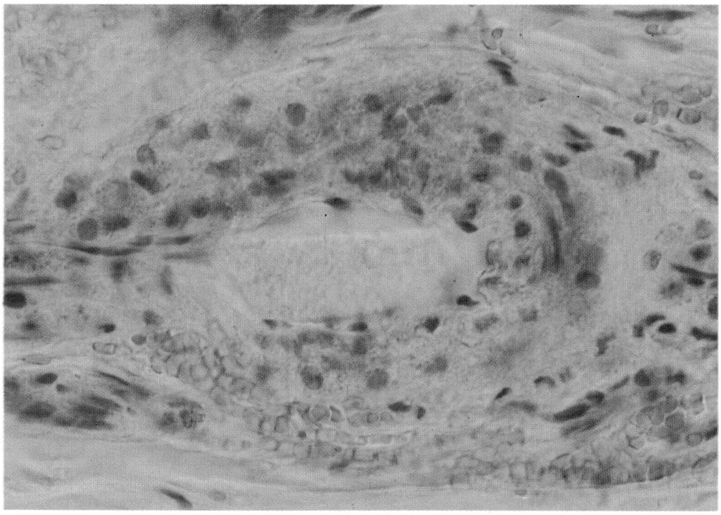

18 Fabry's disease. (Angiokeratoma orporis diffusum.) Sudanophilic lipid vithin wall of small artery. Biopsy pecimen. Oil red O. × 100.

119

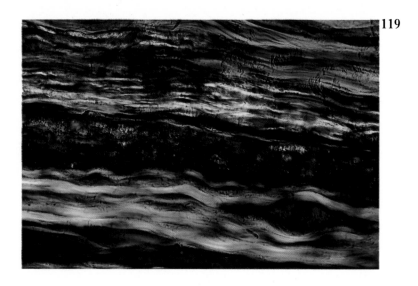

19 Fabry's disease. Ceramide exoside deposits (yellow) in eripheral nerve. Polarized light with etardation/acceleration plate, 100. (*Courtesy of Professor .O. Weller*)

120

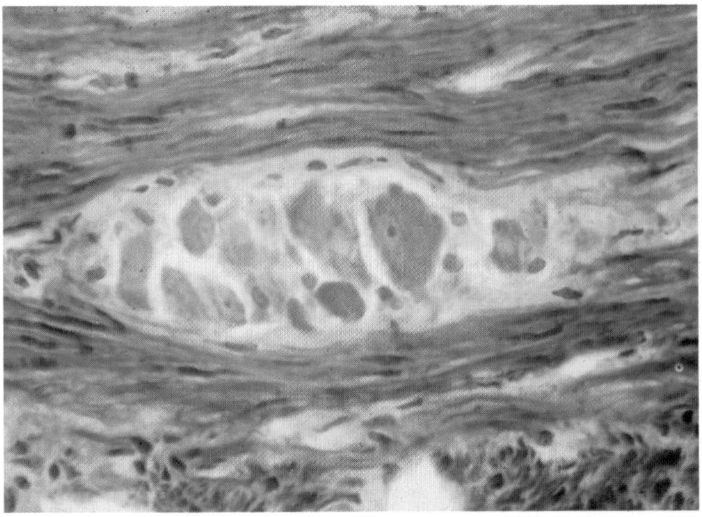

120 Batten's disease (lipofuscinosis, juvenile form). Staining of ceroid in myenteric ganglion cells. Appendix biopsy, Luxol fast blue, × 300.

121

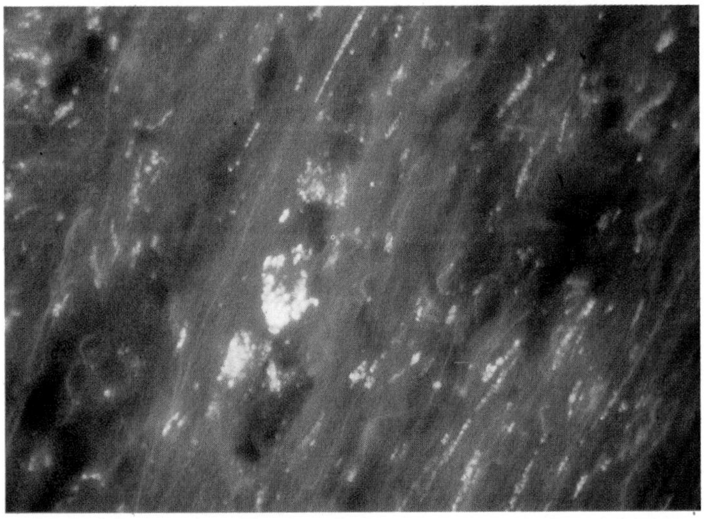

121 Batten's disease, same case as in **120.** Autofluorescence of accumulated ceroid, × 200.

122

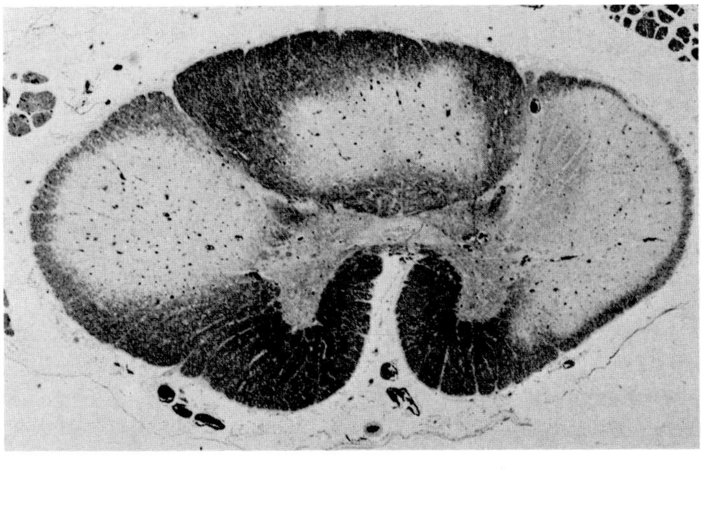

122 Subacute combined degeneration (vitamin B_{12} deficiency). Demyelination of lateral columns and central areas of posterior columns. Sudan black, × 6.

123

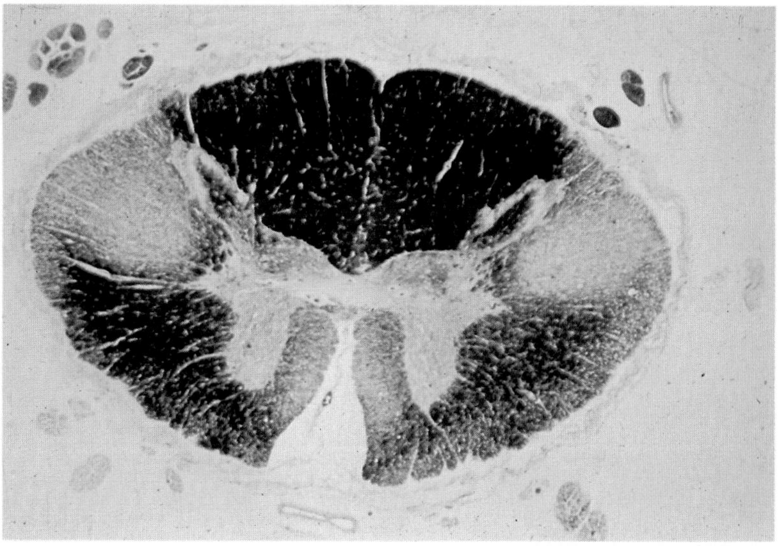

23 Motor neurone disease. Vallerian degeneration of lateral .nd ventral motor tracts. Loyez, × 5.

124

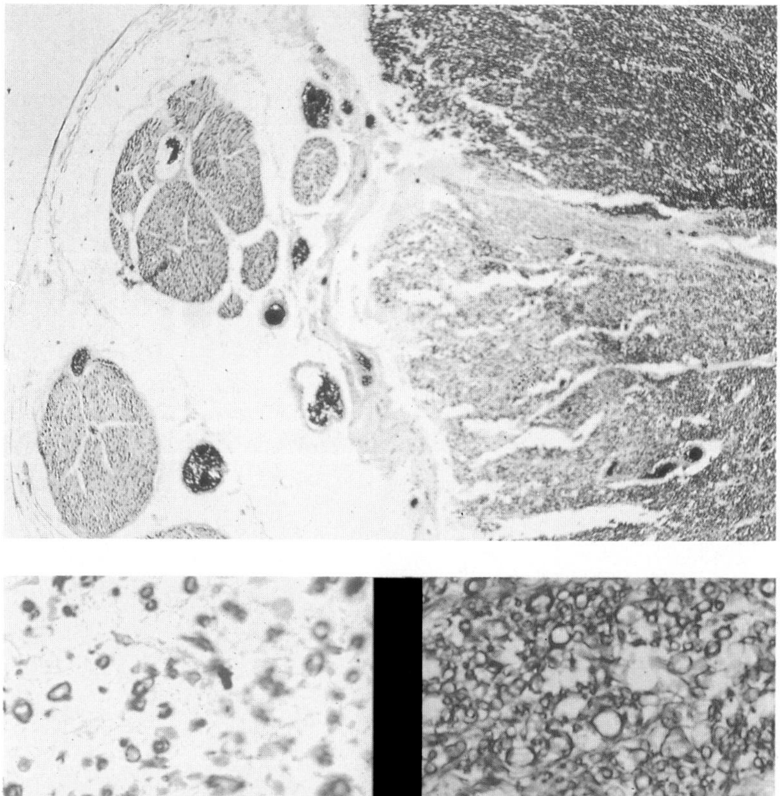

24 Motor neurone disease. Vallerian degeneration of motor oots (at left) of spinal cord. Luxol ast blue, × 10.

125

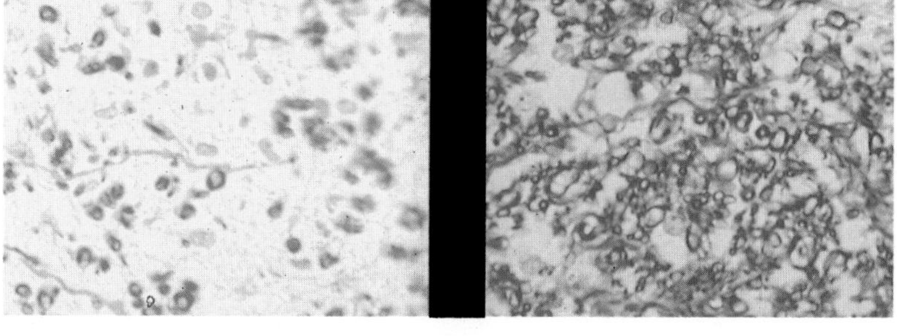

25 Spinal cord in tabes orsalis. Left: Wallerian egeneration and loss of axons ı posterior columns. Right: ıtact anterior columns. Loyez, × 80.

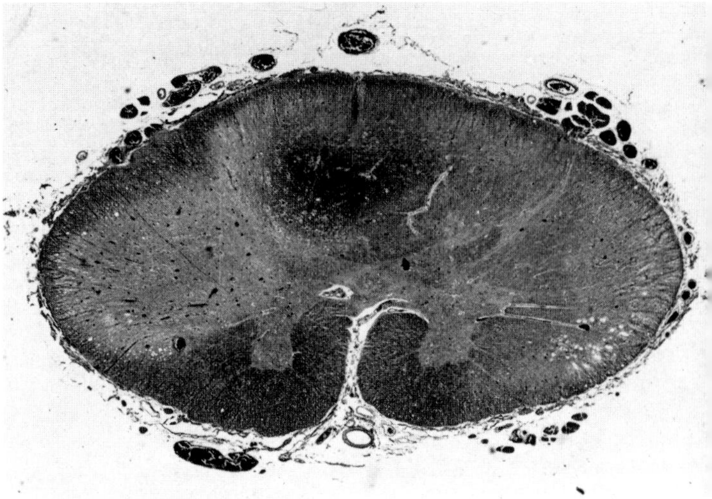

126 Friedreich's ataxia. Wallerian degeneration of lateral columns and patchy involvement of posterior columns. Loyez, × 5.

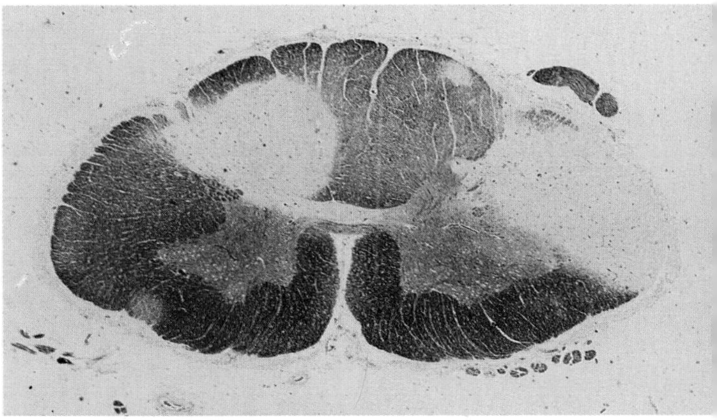

127 Spinal cord in multiple sclerosis. Plaques in posterior, lateral and anterior columns. Note that the lesions are not confined to particular tracts and there is an absence of symmetry. Loyez, × 5.

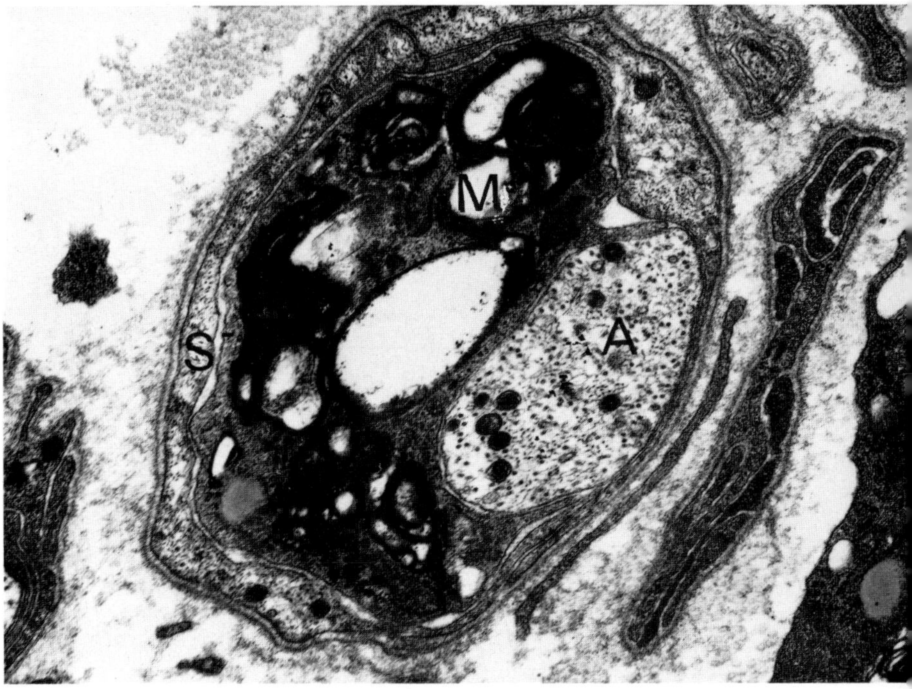

128 Guillain-Barré syndrome. Demyelinated axon (A) separated from a sleeve of Schwann cell cytoplasm(S) by an invading macrophage containing myelin debris (M), × 11,000. *(Courtesy of Dr Susan Hall)*

129

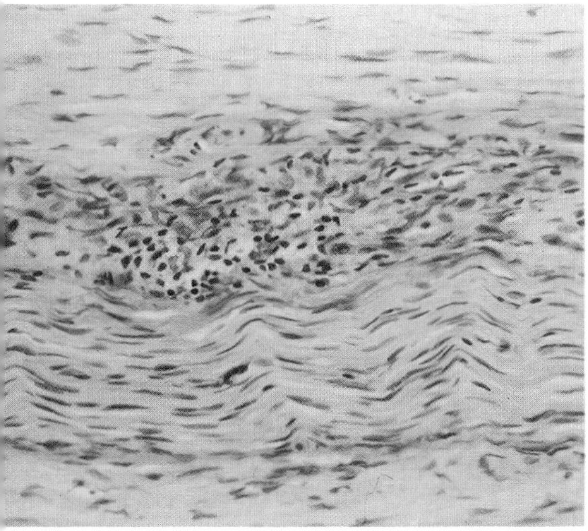

129 Tuberculoid leprosy. Chronic inflammatory focus with demyelination and marked epineurial fibrosis in a hyperimmune subject. Sural nerve, haematoxylin-eosin, × 100.

130

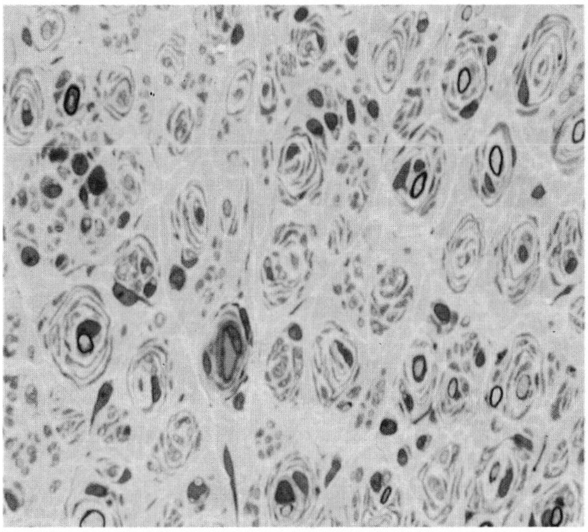

130 A condition resembling the demyelinating form of Charcot-Marie-Tooth disease. Multiple onion bulb formation, with frequent incomplete myelination. Sural nerve, toluidine blue, plastic embedded section, × 300.

131

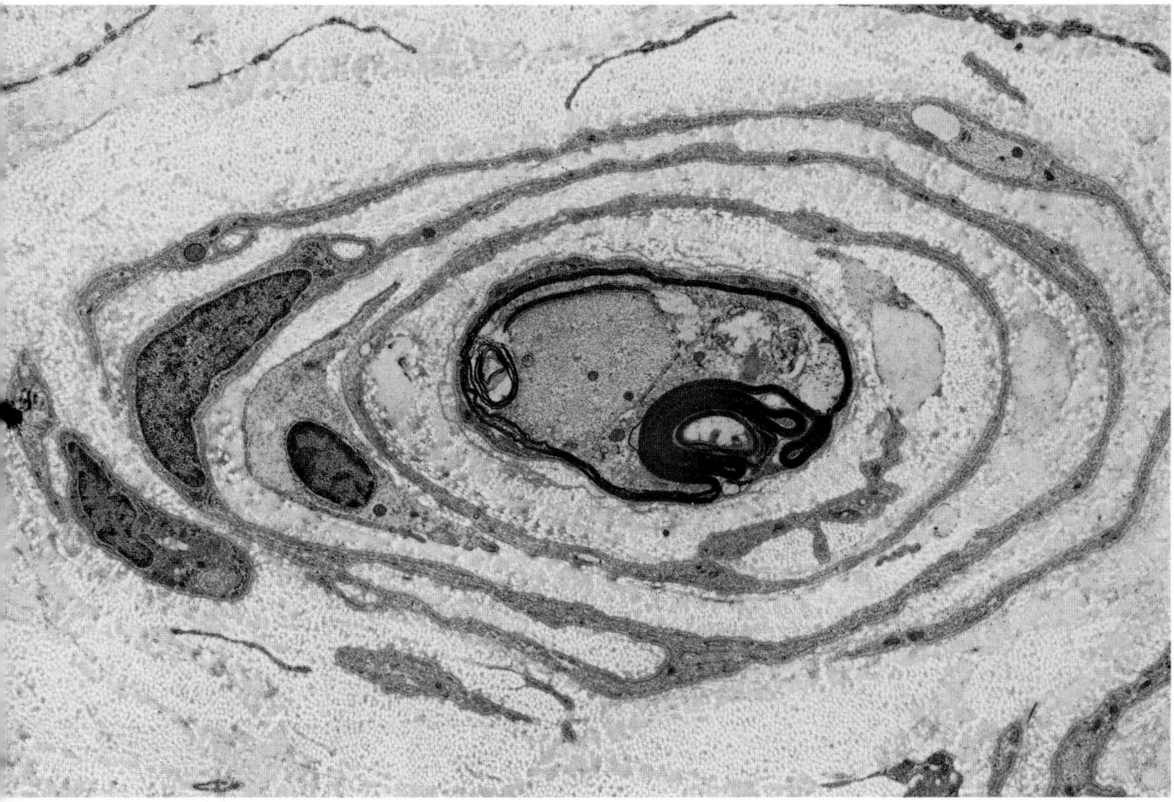

131 Charcot-Marie-Tooth disease, demyelinating form. Onion bulb with scanty thin partly remyelinated sheath, sural nerve × 9,000. *(Courtesy of Professor R.A.C. Hughes)*

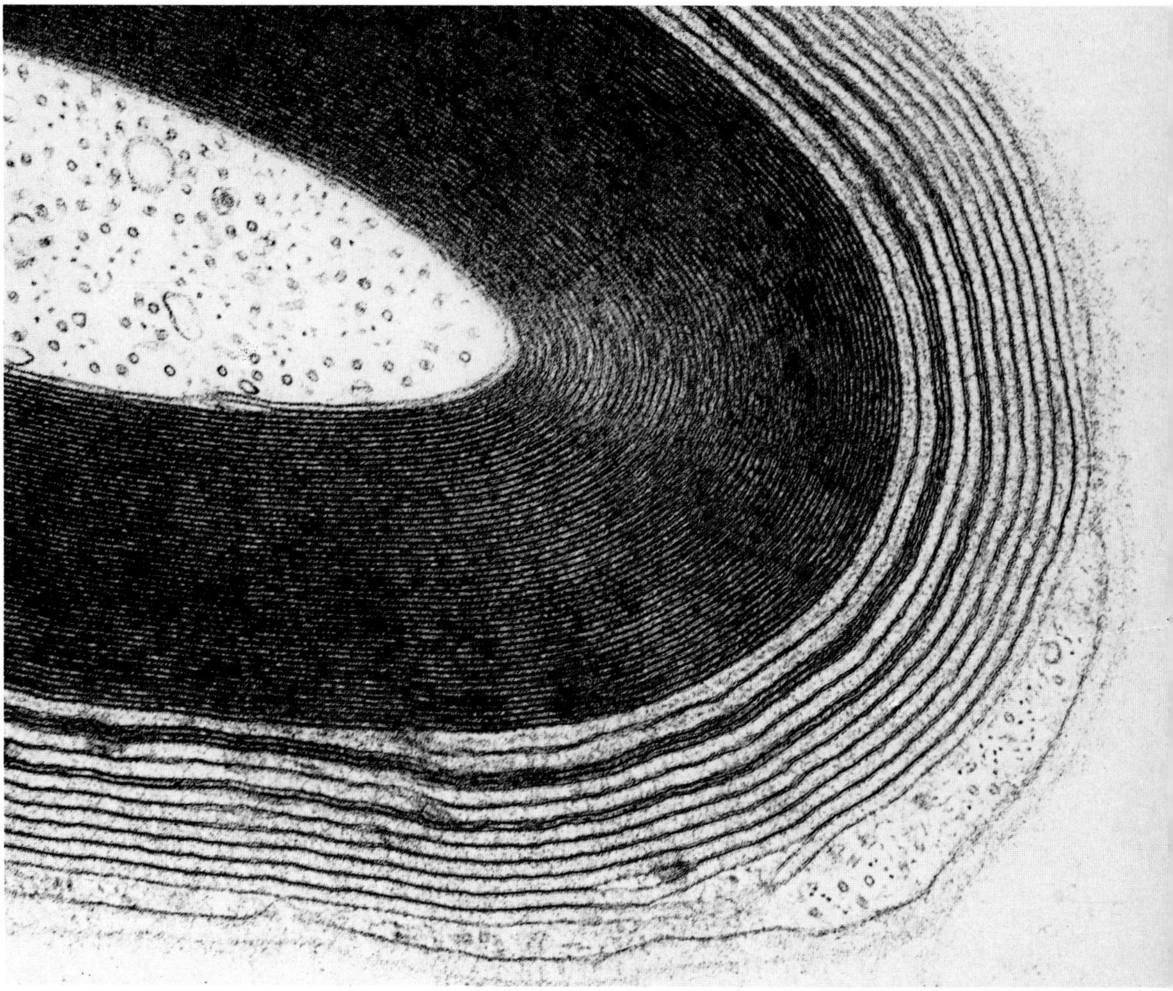

132 Paraproteinaemia, IgM type, in peripheral nerve with antibodies against myelin-associated glycoprotein (MAG). Note prominent non-compaction of outermost myelin lamellae, × 70,000. *(Courtesy of Professor R.A.C. Hughes and Dr S. M. Hall)*

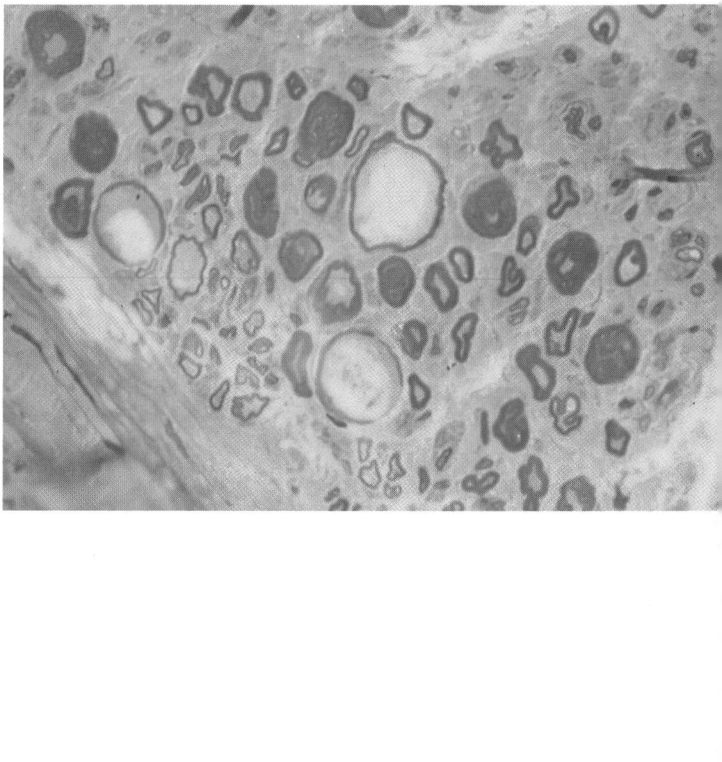

133 Giant axonal neuropathy, familial type. Note thin sheaths over four axonal expansions, caused by accumulation of intermediate filaments. Toluidine blue, plastic-embedded section, × 300.

134

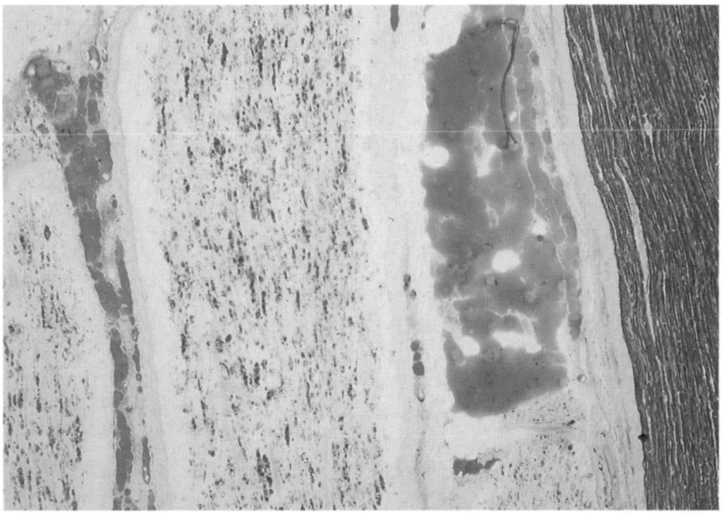

134 Wallerian degeneration in two fascicles of sciatic nerve (left), with normal fascicle at right. Droplets of ester cholesterol are stained red in the degenerating fascicles. Epineurial depot fat is bright red. Solochrome cyanin – oil red O, × 30.

135

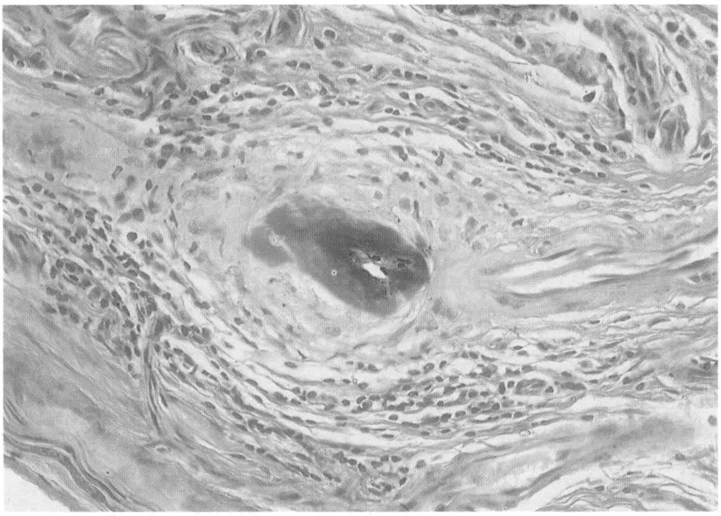

135 Peripheral neuropathy, systemic lupus erythematosus. Fibrin (red) in lumen and wall of small epineurial artery, with surrounding marked mononuclear inflammatory infiltrate. Sural nerve biopsy, Mallory trichrome-MSB, × 60.

136

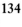

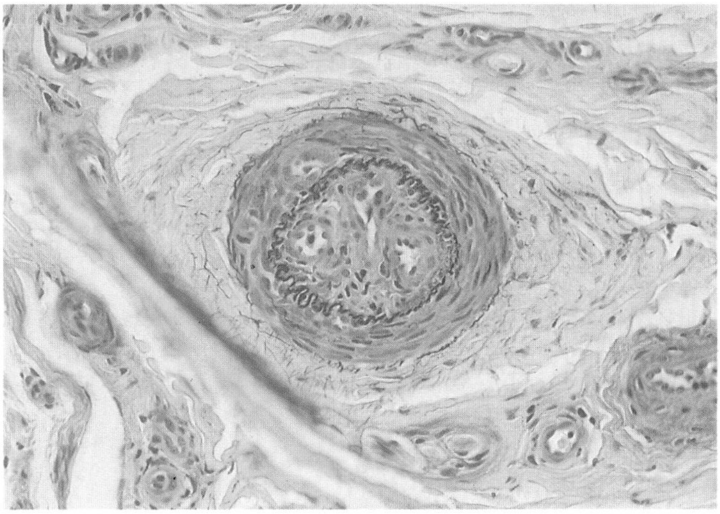

136 Peripheral neuropathy, Wegener's granulomatosis. Organising thrombus in epineurial artery. Other arteries showed surrounding focal inflammatory infiltrate. Sural nerve biopsy. Mallory trichrome-MSB, × 60.

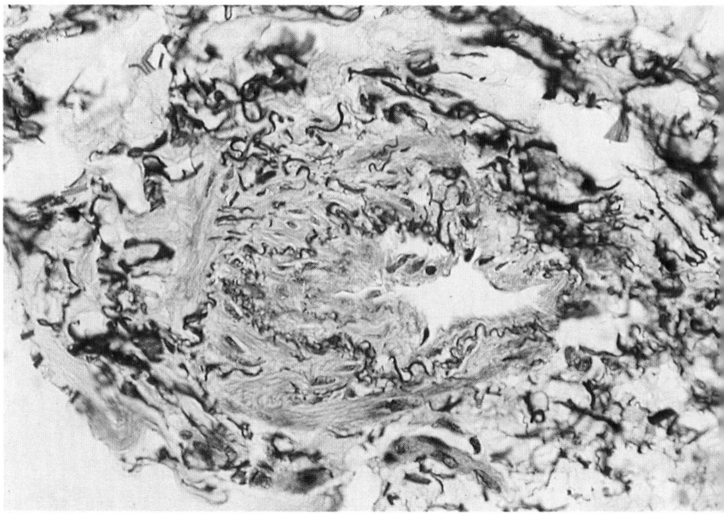

137 Chronic peripheral neuropathy, old healed vasculitis. The arterial wall is ragged and shows elastic reduplication and medial thinning. The tunica media on the right is excessively thinned, suggesting healed arteritis. Sural nerve biopsy, Mallory-trichrome-MSB, × 60.

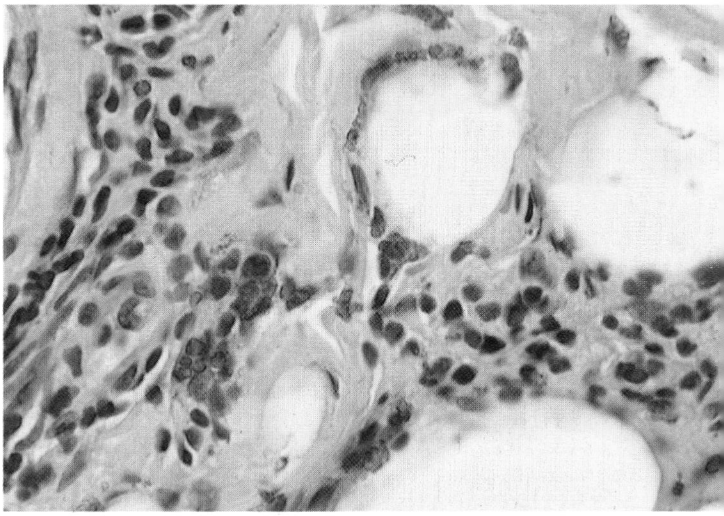

138 Wegener's granulomatosis. Same case as **136** to show haemosiderin deposition indicative of past haemorrhage into the nerve. Haematoxylin-eosin, × 150.

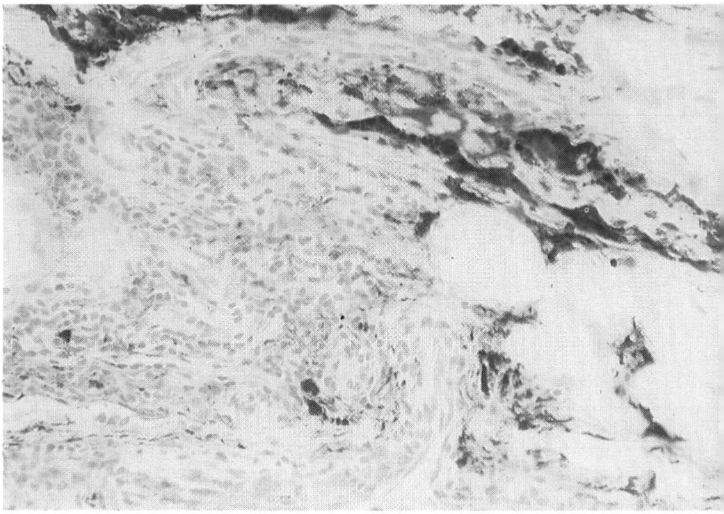

139 Wegener's granulomatosis. Same case as **136** and **138**. Iron deposition among inflammatory infiltrate, shown as Prussian blue reaction (ferric ferrocyanide). Severe vasculitis in the peripheral nerve often leaves evidence of past haemorrhage on testing for iron (haemosiderin). Sural nerve biopsy. Perl's ferrocyanide, × 60.

140 Peripheral neuropathy, old healed vasculitis. Wallerian degeneration with moderate axon loss. Palmgren's silver stain, × 300.

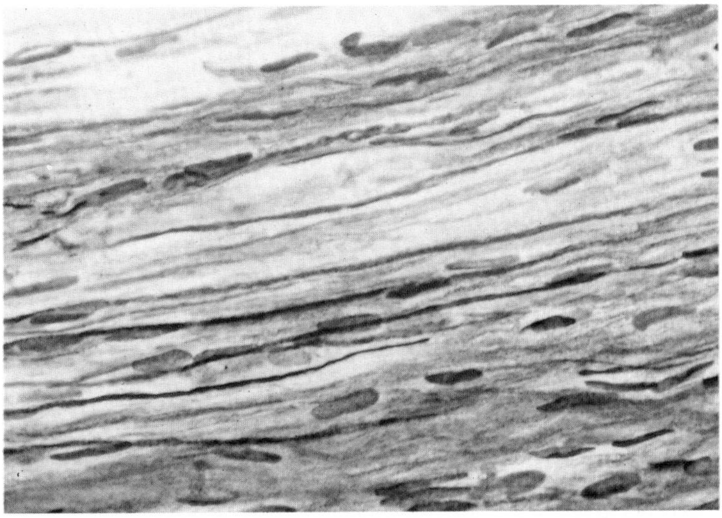

140

141 Hypomyelinogenesis or dysmyelinogenesis in peripheral nerve. Hypomyelination neuropathy in a 3½-year-old girl. The axons are too few and two small to stimulate the Schwann cells to myelinate, × 7,500.

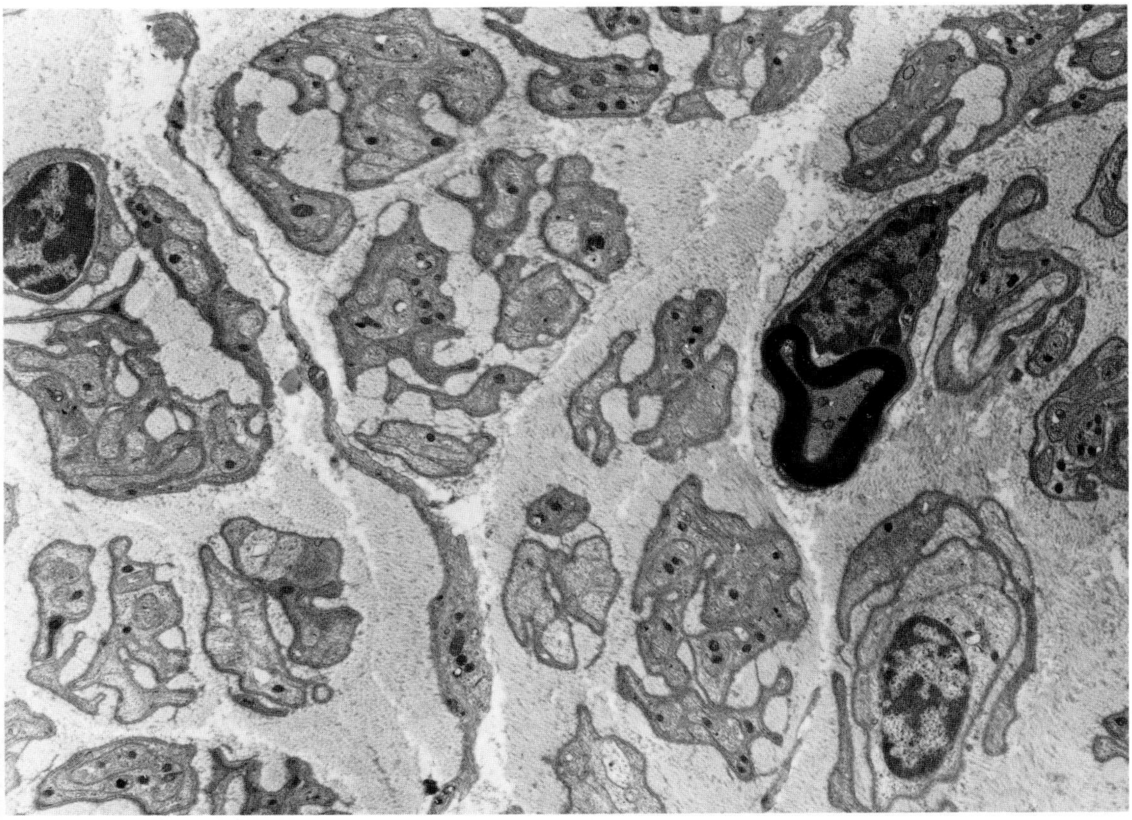

141

3 Spontaneous demyelinating and other myelin diseases in animals

Viral diseases

A number of spontaneous demyelinating diseases are encountered in domestic or wild animals. These diseases are associated with viral infections, often involving the oligodendroglia. These include JCM disease in mice, Theiler's murine encephalomyelitis, canine distemper, visna in sheep and Semliki Forest virus disease (Table 3).

JCM virus (mouse hepatitis virus type IV) infects the oligodendroglia in mouse brain and cord to cause focal demyelinating lesions (**142** and **143**; Knobler and Oldstone, 1983; Knobler *et al.*, 1983; Johnson, 1983). The disease is usually self-limiting and recovery of the oligodendroglia is usually accompanied by nearly complete remyelination (Herndon *et al.*, 1977; Harrison, 1983). In rats, the JCM virus causes an acute encephalomyelitis, but 6 months or so later persistent virus may cause further demyelinating lesions (Knobler and Oldstone, 1983). Immunosuppressive drugs have no effect, which suggests that the disease is caused by intracellular (oligodendroglial) virus replication (**143**), and is not an autoimmune disorder. JCM virus is a coronavirus of RNA type (the term corona refers to surface projections on the virus).

JCM virus DNA has been introduced into the fertilised egg to produce transgenic mice. The viral genome is expressed in oligodendroglia and this results in dysmyelination in the young mouse (Small *et al.*, 1986; *see* hypomyelinogenesis congenita below). The syndrome of tremor and dysmyelination is very similar to that seen in the 'jimpy' and 'quaking' mouse (see below).

Theiler's murine encephalomyelitis is a relapsing demyelinating disease caused by a picovirus (Dal Canto and Lipton, 1975, 1977). Although this virus infects oligodendrocytes, the established disease appears to be of an autoimmune nature as immunosuppressive agents inhibit development of the disease (Rodriguez *et al.*, 1986). Oligodendrocytes do not degenerate, while the damaged myelin is removed by macrophages (**144**). Its relapsing course has similarities to that of multiple sclerosis, and its ultrastructural appearances are similar to those of experimental allergic encephalomyelitis. Remyelination occurs during remission: the peripheral parts of the cord are remyelinated by invading Schwann cells while the central parts are variably remyelinated by oligodendrocytes (Dal Canto and Lipton, 1980; Dal Canto and Barbano, 1984). An antiserum to spinal cord stimulates oligodendroglial remyelinating activity in Theiler's disease (**145**; Rodriguez *et al.*, 1987), but the mechanism remains to be explained.

In canine distemper, an acute encephalomyelitis is characteristic of the early stages but, at a later stage focal demyelinating lesions are encountered (Wisnewski *et al.*, 1972; **146** to **148**). The very earliest events are accompanied by little inflammation around the neurones (Raine, 1976), which is also a feature of the early stages of anterior poliomyelitis (*see* Chapter 1; **46** and **47**). However, a degree of perivenular lymphocytic infiltration is noted in this early phase (Summers *et al.*, 1979), and the demyelinating stage ensues about 3-4 weeks after onset of the illness. The virus concerned in distemper is a paramyxovirus, closely related to measles (morbilli) virus.

There has been some suspicion that canine distemper may be associated with multiple sclerosis (Cook *et al.*, 1978a); the most persuasive evidence being the temporal relationship between the epidemics of MS in man and distemper in dogs in the Faroe Islands from 1940-1960, following the import of pet dogs by the British garrison during World War II (Cook *et al.*, 1978b). However, the initial correlation between the keeping of domestic pets and the prevalence of MS has been difficult to substantiate (Krakowka and Koestner, 1978; Alter *et al.*, 1979; Bunnell *et al.*, 1979; Kurtzke and Priester 1979): the slightly raised canine distemper antibody level in MS patients may represent cross-reactivity with measles virus (Hughes *et al.*, 1980; Madden *e* al., 1981). The suggestion has been made that antibodies to morbilli virus-like structures in the cat brain react with a non-myelin component of the MS plaque (Cook *et al.*, 1986), but this idea requires further investigation.

Visna is a relatively rare neurological complication of the lentivirus infection that causes the pneumonic disease maedi in Icelandic sheep. The disease may also occur in goats and be accompanied by synovitis and mastitis. The primary event is infection of the monocyte precursor, leading to chronic infection of the monocyte and lymphoproliferation (Kennedy *et al.*, 1985). Production of interferon by inflammatory cells leads to increased expression of Ia antigens by macrophages, and down-regulation of viral proliferation. This regulatory mechanism could be the reason for the 'slow' nature of visna-maedi. Inflammatory exudates, macrophages and lymphocytes are seen in the interstitial pneumonia of maedi and in the pre-visna stage of necrotising encephalomyelitis (**149**). Demyelinating lesions subsequently develop and these show characteristic axonal preservation (**150** and **151**; Nathanson *et al.*, 1983; Narayano *et al.*, 1983). Remyelination is effected by Schwann cells or oligodendroglia (Nathanson *et al.*, 1983).

Semliki Forest virus infection produces a chronic demyelinating disease in rats (**152** and **153**), but in the early stages a more necrotic encephalomyelitic lesion may be produced. Again a relapsing demyelinating course may occur, with a similarity to that in MS. The demyelinating stage is thought to result from the action of cytotoxic T-cells formed in an autoimmune reaction to host glycolipid cell-membrane antigens which have become incorporated into the viral envelope as it proliferates and buds from the surface of glial cells (**154**; Webb *et al.*, 1984; Khalili-Shirazi *et al.*, 1986).

Defective myelination (hypomyelinogenesis congenita; congenital tremor) is seen in the progeny of sows infected with the swine cholera virus (toga virus; pestivirus) (**155**). This is a dysmyelinating rather than a demyelinating disease (Done, 1976). Oligodendroglia are defective from an early stage, but the Schwann cells in the PNS are unaffected. Border disease is a similar condition in lambs, causing trembling, defective wool and severe hypomyelination (**156** to **159**), with thin myelin sheaths that contain only a few lamellae and there is marked astrogliosis (Barlow and Dickinson, 1965; Cancilla and Barlow, 1968). Little or no esterified cholesterol is present (**156** and **157**), which suggests that demyelination is a minor or absent feature. Border disease is caused by a pestivirus or mucosal virus infection in the pregnant ewe (Anderson *et al.*, 1987) which is transmitted to the lamb in utero (Dickinson and Barlow, 1967). Infection of thyroid epithelium by pestivirus leads to reduced thyroxine production and it could be that the absence of this hormone results in impaired myelin synthesis by oligodendroglia. Hypomyelinogenesis congenita is also seen in calves, young goats and Samoyed pups (Cummings *et al.*, 1986).

The viral infective nature of these various diseases distinguishes them from MS, where no one clearly causative organism or transmissibility has been established. Indeed it has been said by a well-known virologist that claims to have identified viruses in MS is the graveyard of many virologists' reputations. The poetic hyperbole highlights the frustration and inherent difficulties in this area of work (*see* Chapter 5).

In spite of the above comments, the recurrent or chronically progressive autoimmune nature of Theiler's, Semliki Forest and visna virus diseases suggests that these demyelinating disorders do have some relevance to MS. As will be discussed later, MS may be a syndrome that is the autoimmune end-result of a number of different sorts of injury or viral disease in youth. Theiler's, visna and the Semliki Forest virus diseases may be models for this suggested pathogenesis.

Nutritional defects

Copper deficiency in pastures in certain parts of the United Kingdom, China, South America and Western Australia results in a form of dysmyelination in developing lambs, a disease known as swayback (Innes and Shearer, 1940; Barlow, 1963a; Howell *et al.*, 1964; Howell, 1971; Done, 1976). The disease also occurs in goats (Howell *et al.*, 1981). The disease seems to arise as a result of deficient copper in the grazing fields, so that pregnant ewes have an insufficient supply of this mineral to provide for the developing lamb. The fault may also lie in leaching of soil elements by inclement weather and, possibly, a genetic defect.

The brain in swayback may show a large defect in the central white matter (**160** and **161**), akin to a sudanophilic leucodystrophy, developmental defects in the cerebellum (**163**; Howell *et al.*, 1981), demyelination and chromatolysis in the cord (**163** and **164**) and demyelination/Wallerian degeneration in the peripheral nerve (**165**). Brainstem and cord lesions occur consistently, but the cerebrum is not always involved (Barlow *et al.*, 1960).

Copper levels and cytochrome oxidase activity are reduced in swayback lambs (Howell and Davison, 1959). Copper is an essential component of the enzyme monoamine oxidase and may be concerned with cross-linking of aldehydes in the formation of connective tissues (Partridge, 1969). However, the role of this oxidase or its analogues in CNS development is uncertain, and the serum copper levels are normal in patients with multiple sclerosis (Mandelbrote *et al.*, 1948; Thompson, 1961). Another oxidase, cytochrome oxidase, has been shown by histochemical means to be deficient in the neurones in swayback (Barlow, 1963b), presumably as a result of the lack of copper. The occurrence of probable, transitional or confirmed MS in four members of a research team investigating swayback (Campbell *et al.*, 1947; Dean *et al.*, 1985) can only be regarded as tragic but coincidental.

It is of interest concerning swayback that copper deficiency has been reported in the dysmyelinating mutant Quaking mouse (*see* Guenet, 1980), while induced copper deficiency leads in young rats to hypomyelination or myelin deficit (Dipaolo *et al.*,1974; Zimmerman *et al.*, 1976). Cuprizone, which seems to cause demyelination through a toxic action on oligodendroglia (**41** and **42**; Blakemore, 1973; Ludwin, 1978; *see* Chapters 1 and 4) is also a copper chelator, but it has not been shown that this copper chelation is relevant to the demyelination.

Genetic dysmyelination

In the genetically determined (mutant) dysmyelinating disorders of mice, there is either a defect in synthesis of particular myelin lipids/proteins or a failure in the metabolism of the Schwann cell/ oligodendrocyte or both (see Baumann, 1980). These defects produce a deficiency or absence of myelin (dysmyelination, leucodystrophy). However, this definition of dysmyelination is complicated by the additional occurrence in some instances of myelin breakdown, which is the hallmark of a leucoencephalopathy or demyelinating neuropathy. There are a number of these genetic disorders in mutant mice that lead to the development of characteristic bizarre neurological defects with equally bizarre appellations, namely, quaking, jimpy, shiverer, twitcher and trembler mice (Table 3 see reviews by Guenet, 1980; Lyon and Goffinet, 1980; Hogan and Greenfield, 1984).

Quaking mice are hypomyelinated autosomal recessives and suffer from a failure of myelin compaction and from a deficiency of CNS myelin lipids (particularly cerebroside) and myelin-associated enzymes (Sidman *et al.*, 1964; Hogan, 1977; Hogan and Greenfield, 1984). Jimpy mice show a similar but more severe CNS disorder (Nussbaum *et al.*, 1969; Galli *et al.*, 1969; Kurihara *et al.*, 1970). Oligodendroglia are abnormal and necrotic (Koeppen *et al.*, 1988), and myelin breakdown may occur with the appearance of sudanophilic cholesterol esters. This mutant is sex-linked and the locus is on the X-chromosome (reviews in Baumann, 1980). Both the 'jimpy' and 'quaking' mice resemble the transgenic mouse infected in ovo with JCM virus with regard to dysmyelination, tremor and their pathology (see above; Small *et al.*, 1986).

Recent work indicates that a transcription fault (DM20) for proteolipid synthesis is the basic defect in the Jimpy mouse (Morello *et al.*, 1986), as well as in the myelin-deficient rat (see below) and in Pelizaeus-Merzbacher disease (Chapter 2; Koeppen *et al.*, 1987).

Shiverer (md) mice have an autosomal recessive genetic defect, an inability to synthesise myelin basic protein (MBP), and consequent disordered formation of CNS myelin membranes. Southern blot (cDNA probes) shows that the DNA/mRNA sequences for MBP synthesis are deleted in these shiverer mutants (Roach *et al.*, 1983; brief review by Martin, 1984). Electronmicroscopy of the scanty CNS myelin in shiverers reveals failure of compaction, splitting at, and absence of, the major dense line which results in a triplet appearance (**166**), attributable to the lack of MBP. The peripheral nerve in shiverer mice is also deficient in MBP, but does not show abnormal dense lines or disordered compaction (**166**; Ganser and Kirschner, 1980). Hence, it is concluded that the structural integrity of central myelin depends on different factors to those in peripheral myelin, a feature that might be very relevant to the contrasting aetiologies of human demyelinating diseases in the CNS and PNS. The myelin-deficient mouse (MLD) has a very similar disorder, but with a more limited penetration (Ginalski *et al.*, 1980).

Twitcher mice have an autosomal recessive disorder of galactocerebroside metabolism, resulting in defective myelination (**167** and **168**) and a globoid-cell dystrophy (**169**; Duchen *et al.*, 1980), similar to that seen in Krabbe's leucodystrophy (**108** and **109**, Chapter 2). As with human Krabbe's disease and the canine form, the twitcher mouse shows a defect in galactosylceramidase activity (galactosylceramide-B-galactosidase; Suzuki and Suzuki, 1970; Scaravilli and Suzuki, 1983), leading to the typical storage of galactosylcerebroside in the distended sometimes binucleate modified macrophages known as globoid cells (**169**; *see* Chapter 2). The storage bodies are angulated tubules and crystalline structures, similar to those seen in the human disease. Peripheral nerves from young twitcher mice grafted in young trembler mice (with defective Schwann cells) myelinate and develop normally because they are able to take up galactosylceramidase from the host and, thus, overcome the metabolic block (Scaravilli and Jacobs, 1982; Scaravilli and Suzuki, 1983). Globoid-cell leucodystrophies are also seen in the cat and dog (**170** and **171**; Suzuki *et al.*, 1970; Howell and Palmer, 1971).

Myelination in the myelin-deficient (MD) rat is defective or absent in the optic nerve and elsewhere in the CNS. The oligodendroglia are dystrophic, showing accumulation of lipid droplets, and are focally necrotic (**172** and **173**; Barron *et al.*, 1980). Synthesis of CNS myelin components is depressed, notably that of proteolipid protein (the major CNS myelin protein), myelin basic protein, myelin-associated glycoprotein and 2′, 3′-cyclic nucleotide-3′-phosphoesterase (Yanagisawa *et al.*, 1986; Duncan *et al.*, 1987). Compact myelin is abnormal in MD rat; a defect in the period line is attributed to proteolipid protein.

Other storage disorders in animals resulting in leucodystrophy include metachromatic leucodystrophy (mink), gangliosidoses GM_1 and GM_2 (dog, cat and cattle), Niemann-Pick-like disease (cat) and ceroid lipofuscinosis (dog and cat) (see review by Done, 1976).

Trembler mice are dominant mutants with a defect in the Schwann cell that leads to hypomyelinogenesis (dysmyelination) and hypertrophic neuropathy (onion bulb formation, aborted myelination) in peripheral nerves (Darriett *et al.*, 1978; Hogan and Greenfield, 1984). Schwann cells show reduced activity of UDP-galactose: ceramide-galactosyltransferrase (White *et al.*, 1986).

A genetic neuropathy with focally swollen axons in Boxer dogs seems to promote segmental demyelination followed by remyelination, a form of remodelling of the myelin sheath in response to the increased size of the axon (Griffiths *et al.*, 1987). This evidence indicates that myelin has a greater capacity for remodelling and growth than is customarily considered to be the case. Similar attenuation is seen in the myelin covering the axonal swellings of giant axonal neuropathy (**133**; *see* Chapter 2).

Some further genetic models of myelin disorders are summarised in Table 3 in Chapter 2.

Conclusions

The various viral and mutant animal conditions described in this section clearly show that diseases involving the oligodendroglia (or Schwann cell) will cause demyelination. However, the added factor of an autoimmune response in Theiler's disease and Semliki Forest virus disease, and possibly in chronic visna, results in relapsing episodic diseases with some resemblance to multiple sclerosis.

142

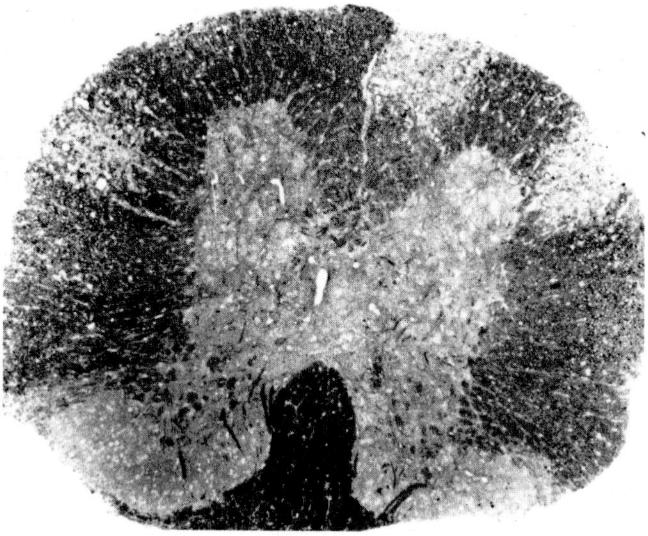

142 JCM virus leucoencephalitis. Scattered demyelinating lesions in mouse spinal cord. Luxol fast blue, × 40. *(Courtesy of Dr R.L. Knobler)*

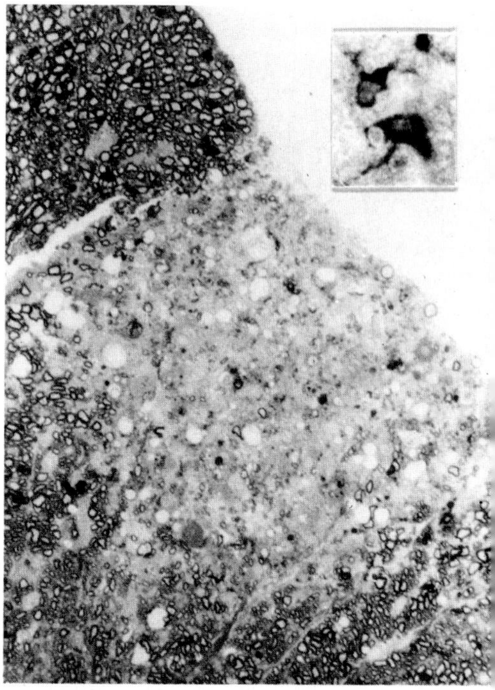

143 JCM virus. Detail of demyelinating lesion in mouse spinal cord. Toluidine blue, × 120. Inset: oligodendroglia stained by anti-JCM virus peroxidase. *(Courtesy of Dr R.L. Knobler)*

144 Demyelination in a mouse persistently infected with Theiler's virus. Four axons (a) are shown in the picture which have no surrounding myelin. The axons in the centre are actively undergoing demyelination. Two axons (b) still have their normal myelin sheaths (arrows). A macrophage (m) is seen in intimate contact with the demyelinated axons (a), × circa 6,000. *(Courtesy of Dr M. Rodriguez)*

144

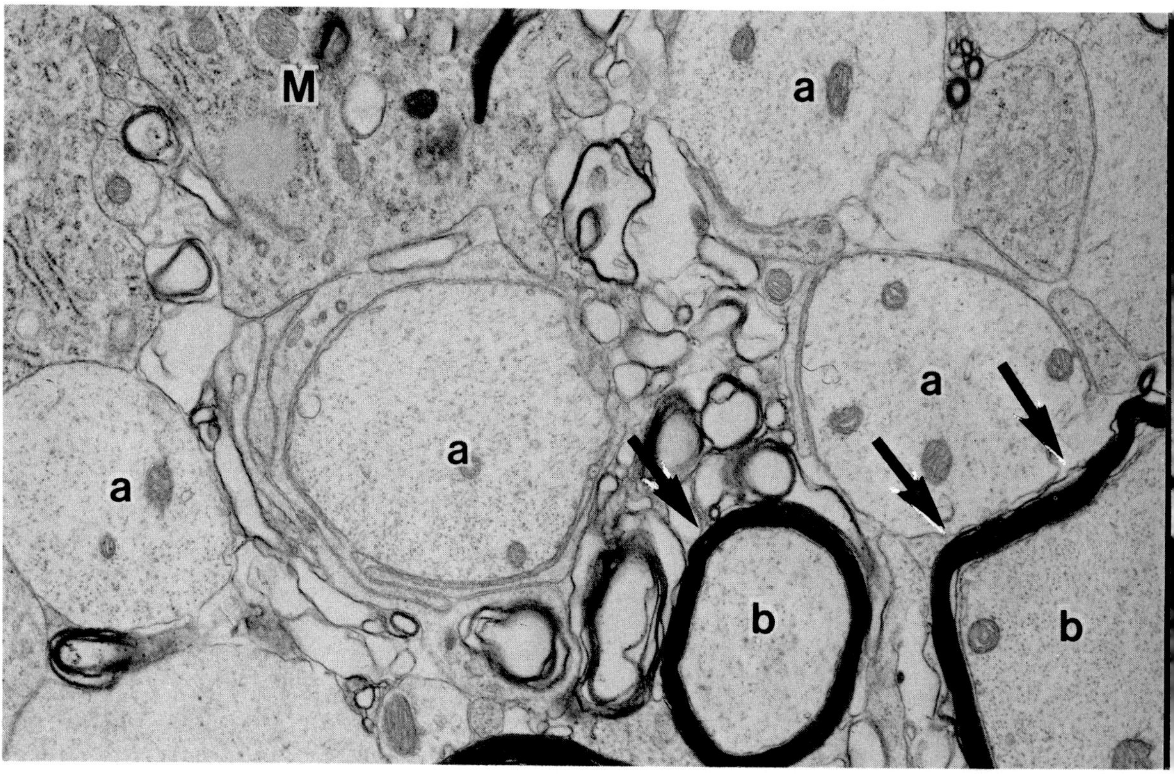

145

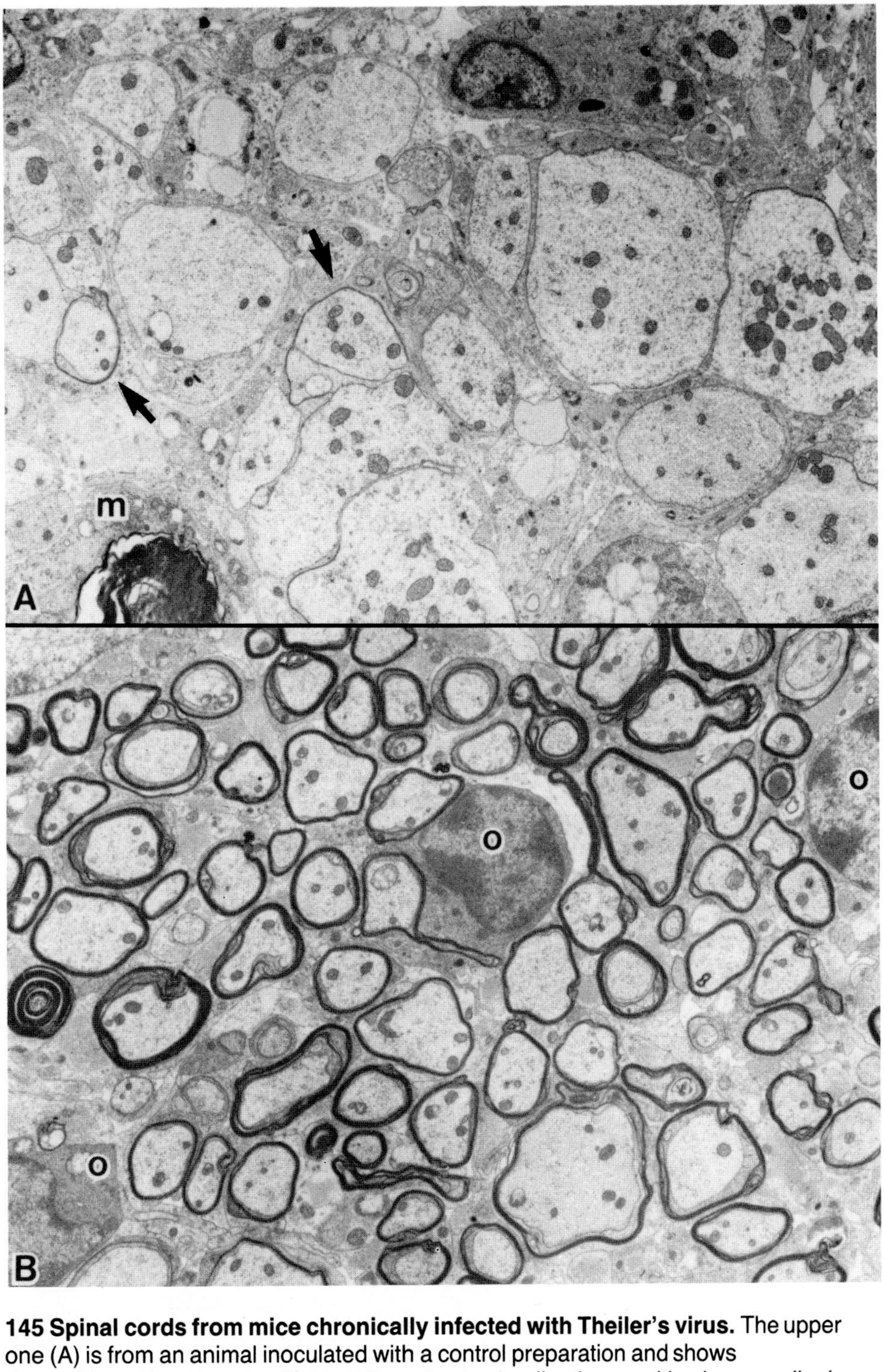

145 Spinal cords from mice chronically infected with Theiler's virus. The upper one (A) is from an animal inoculated with a control preparation and shows demyelinated bare axons with two attempts at remyelinating resulting in exceedingly thin myelin (arrows). A macrophage is seen containing lipid debris (M). The lower one (B) is from an animal inoculated with an antiserum to spinal cord. Nearly all axons show newly formed thin myelin. The three dark cells (O) are oligodendrocytes and have probably remyelinated the many axons seen. Both circa × 6,000.
(Courtesy of Dr M. Rodriguez)

146

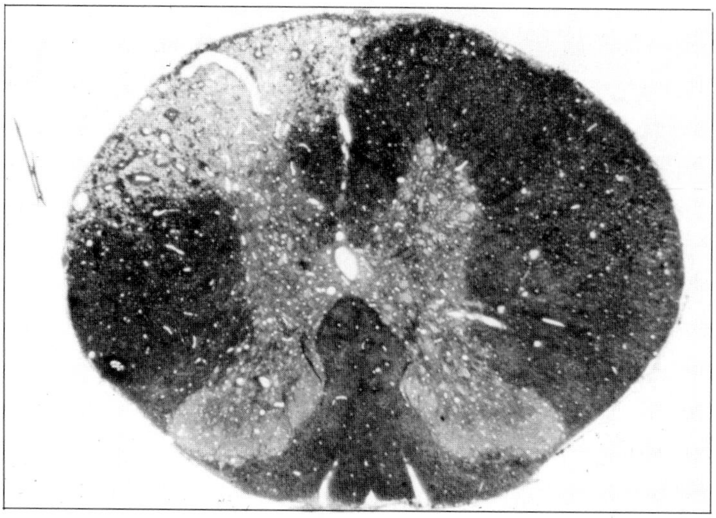

146 Canine distemper. Large demyelinated plaque in posterolateral column of spinal cord, × 6. *(Courtesy of Professor Cedric Raine)*

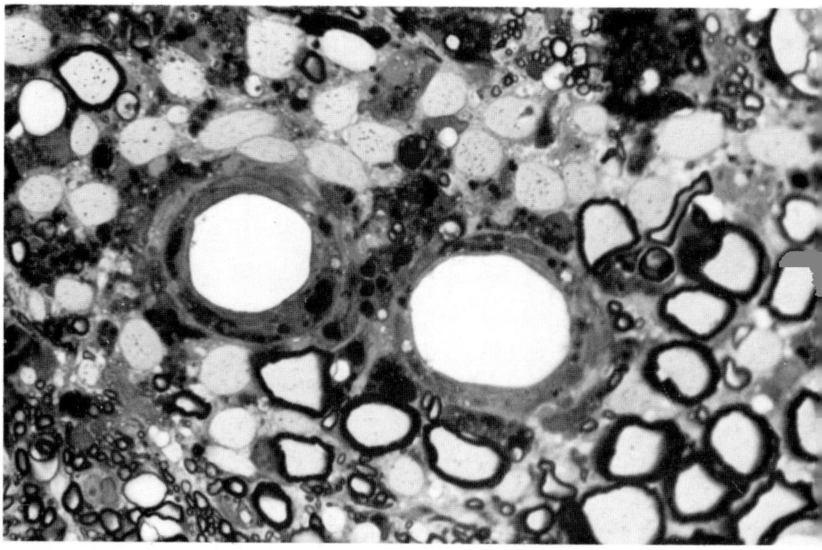

147 Canine distemper, 2 weeks after onset. Demyelinated axons, and modest perivascular infiltration. Toluidine blue, plastic section, × 560. *(Courtesy of Professor Cedric Raine)*

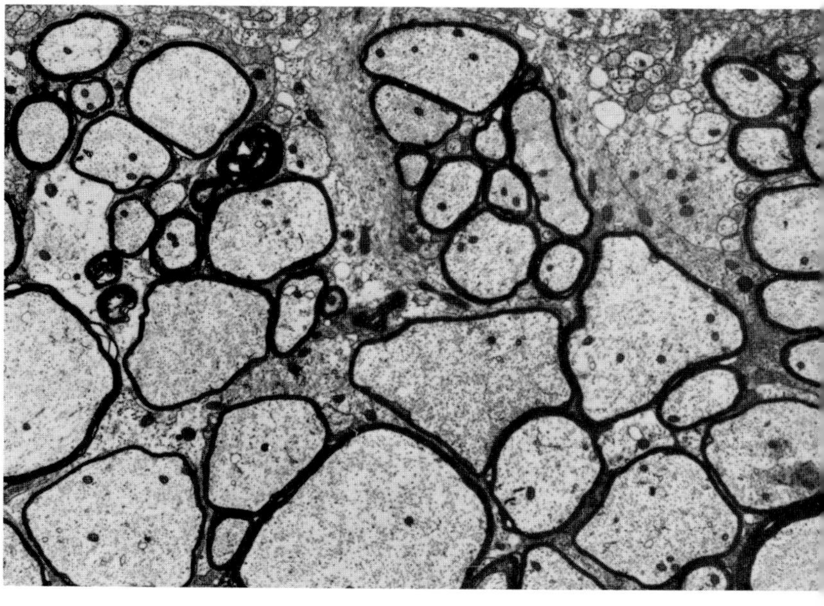

148 Canine distemper. Apparent remyelination of axons (inappropriately thin myelin sheaths), with oligodendrocyte cytoplasm surrounding groups of fibres, × 10,000. *(Courtesy of Professor Cedric Raine)*

149

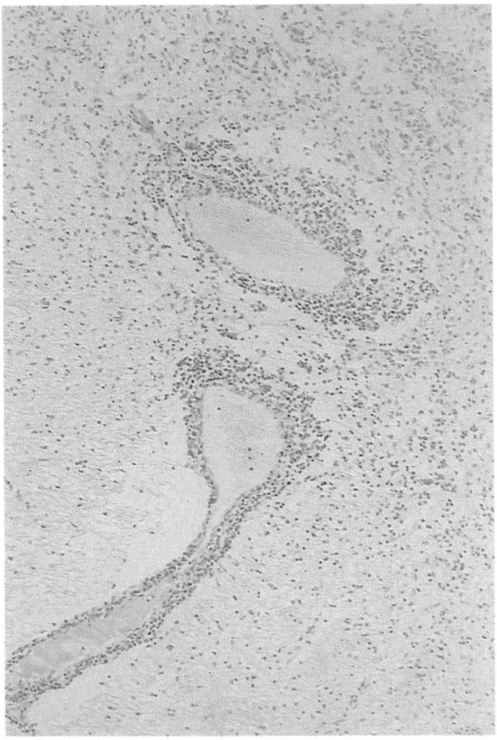

150

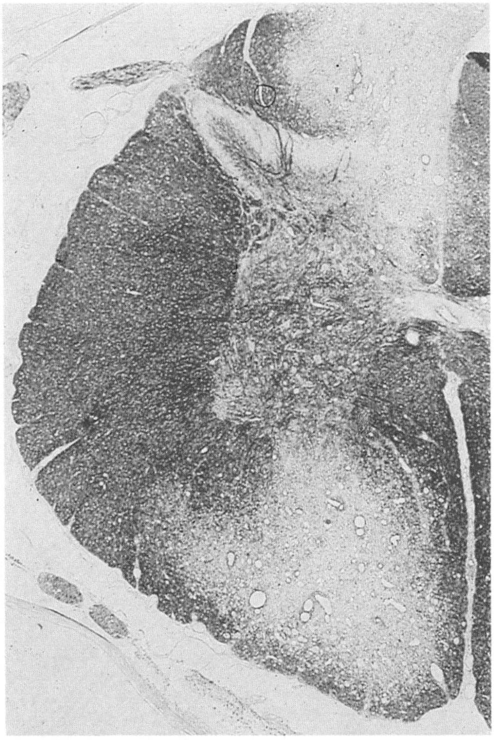

149 Visna. Early stage of necrotising encephalomyelitis. Note loss of structure, necrosis and marked perivascular lymphocytic infiltrate. Haematoxylin-eosin, × 50. *(Courtesy of Professor J. Mc. Howell)*

150 Visna in sheep. Demyelinating lesions in posterior and anterior columns of right side of spinal cord. Luxol fast blue, × 5. *(Courtesy of Dr G. Petierson)*

151 Visna. Small focus of demyelination in anterior column of cord. Luxol fast blue, × 70. *(Courtesy of Dr G. Petierson)*

151

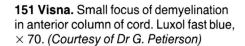

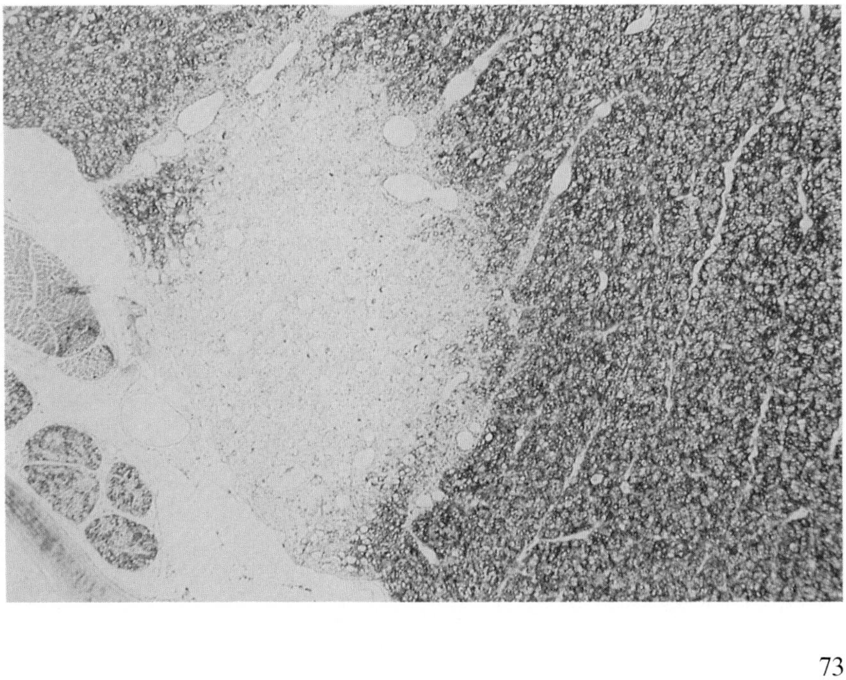

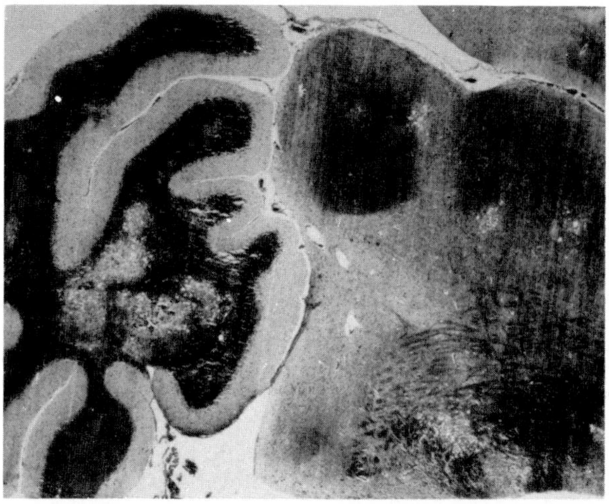

152

152 Semliki Forest virus disease. Rat cerebellum showing a cluster of demyelinating lesions in white matter. Further scattered lesions in the midbrain. Luxol fast blue, × 20. *(Courtesy of Professor H.E. Webb)*

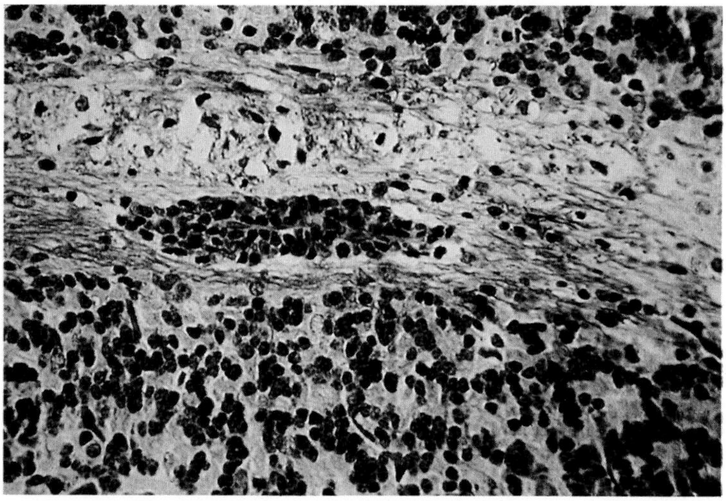

153

153 Higher power view of 152 to show perivascular inflammation and vacuolar myelin degeneration. Luxol fast blue, × 200. *(Courtesy of Professor H.E. Webb)*

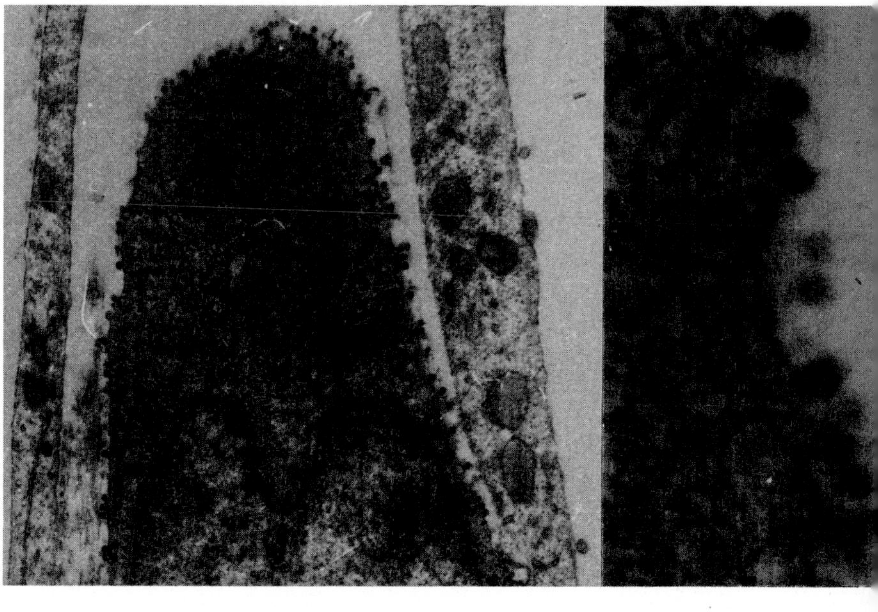

154 Semliki Forest virus. Astrocyte in culture infected with the virus. Note budding of virus from cell membrane. Left, × 20,000. Right, enlargement of budding virus, × 50,000. *(Courtesy of Professor H.E. Webb)*

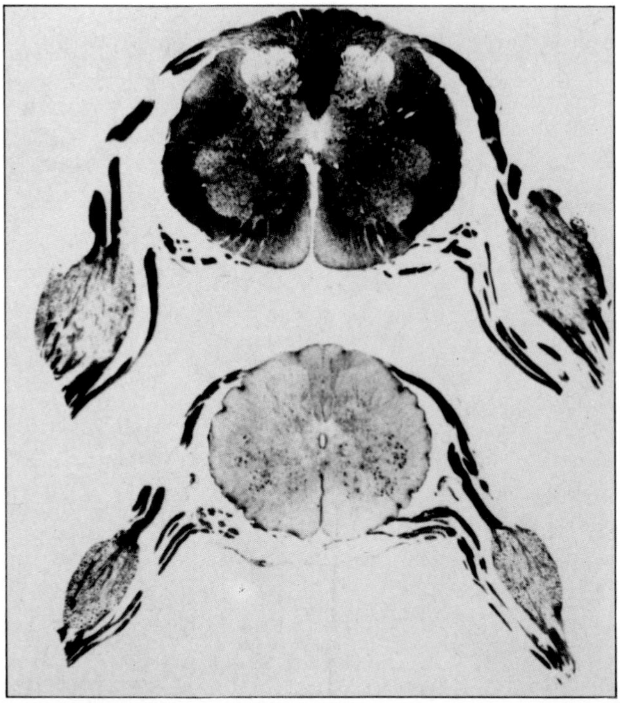

155

55 Hypomyelinogenesis congenita n pig spinal cord. The top specimen s normal, while the affected cord at the ottom shows nearly complete lack of nyelin. The spinal roots, including the osterior root ganglia are normal, × 4. Courtesy of Dr J.T. Done)

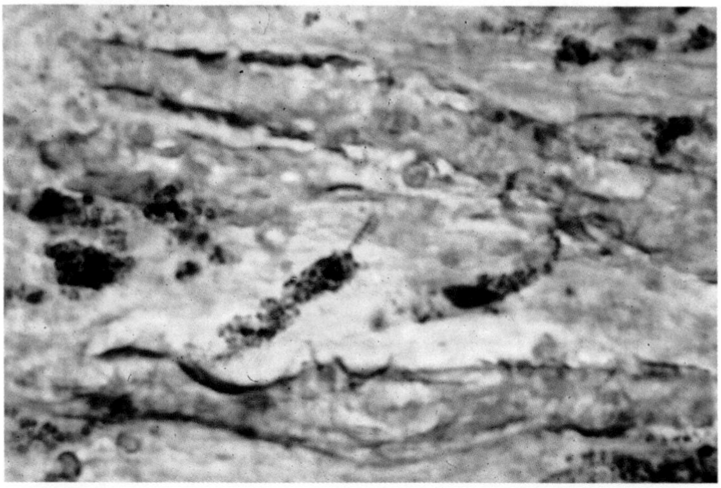

156

56 Border disease in foetal lamb. Scanty myelinated tracts n spinal cord as a result of ypomyelination. There are only traces f Marchi-positive lipid (black; sterified cholesterol). Osmium extroxide-α naphthylamine (OTAN), × 300. *(Courtesy of Professor R.M. Barlow)*

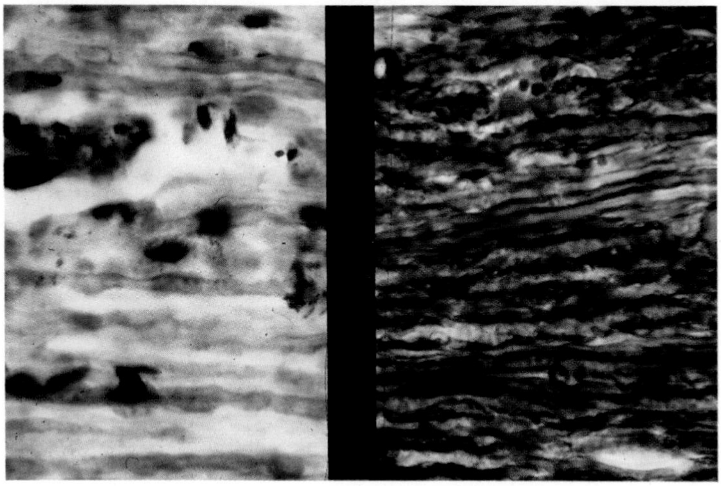

157

57 Spinal cord in Border disease. Left: spinal cord in lamb to show small amounts of esterified cholesterol (black) in scanty hypomyelinated nerve ibres. Right: numerous myelinated ibres in control lamb to show normal dark red reaction. OTAN, × 150. *(Courtesy of Professor R.M. Barlow)*

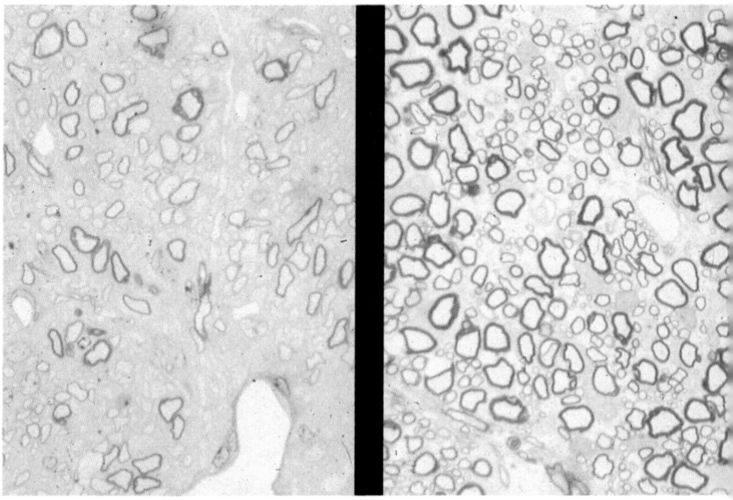

158 Spinal cord in Border disease. Left: variable but reduced myelination in scanty fibres in 135-day foetal lamb. Right: normally myelinated fibres in control animal. Toluidine blue, plastic section, × 150. *(Courtesy of Professor R.M. Barlow)*

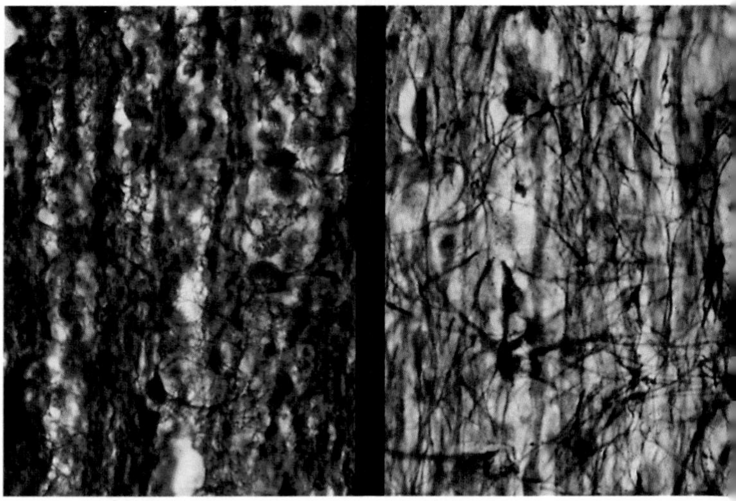

159 Spinal cord in Border disease. Left: astroglial proliferation in diseased animal. Right: control animal. Cajal's gold sublimate, × 150. *(Courtesy of Professor R. M. Barlow)*

160

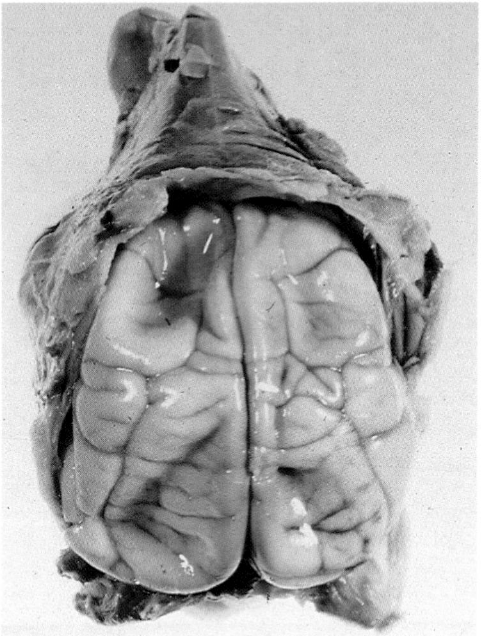

160 Swayback in the goat causing cerebral cavitation with collapsed surface of brain. *(Courtesy of Professor J.McC. Howell)*

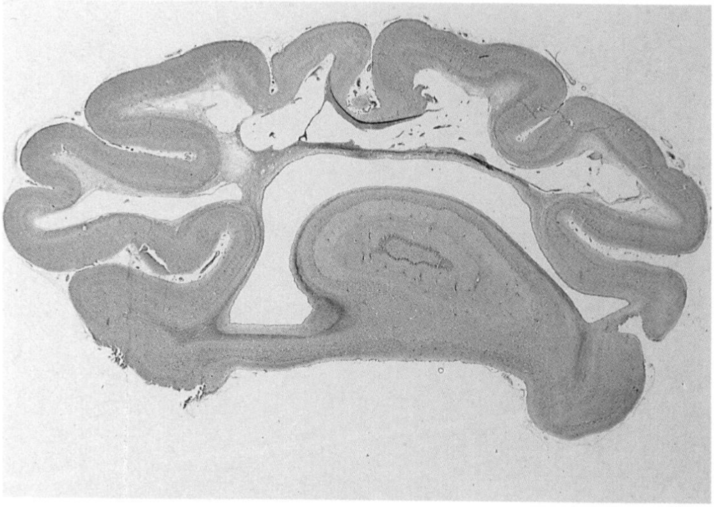

161

161 Swayback in the lamb. Note cavitation in the brain with gross myelin deficiency. Luxol fast blue, × 1. *(Courtesy of Professor J.McC. Howell)*

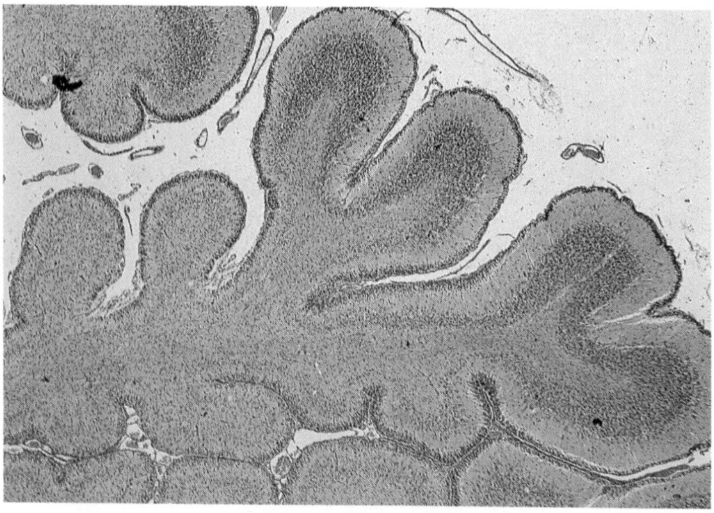

162

162 Swayback in the lamb. Cerebellum to show defective formation of cerebellar folia. Haematoxylin-eosin, × 6. *(Courtesy of Professor J.McC. Howell)*

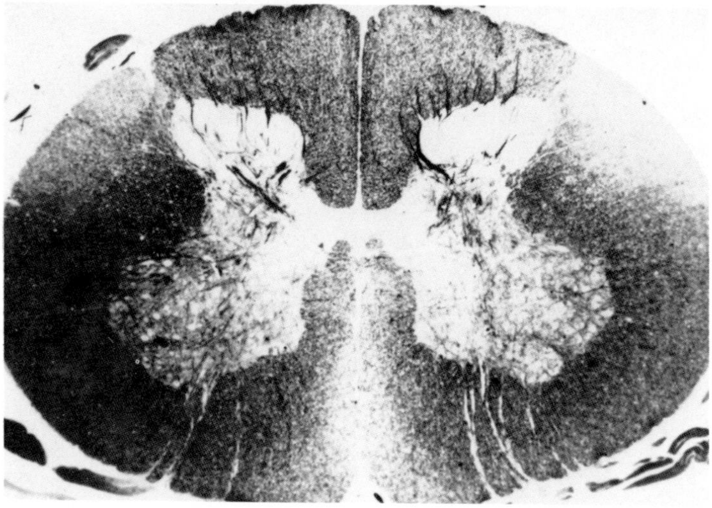

163

163 Swayback in the lamb, with dysmyelinating lesions in dorsolateral and anterior columns. Loyez method, × 6. *(Courtesy of Professor J.McC. Howell)*

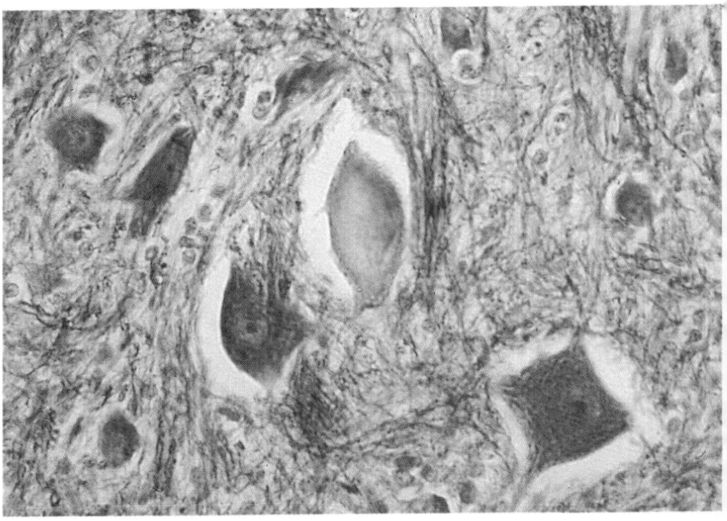

164 Swayback in the lamb. Anterior horn cells, one of which shows chromatolysis. Cresyl violet-Luxol fast blue, × 225. *(Courtesy of Professor J. McC. Howell)*

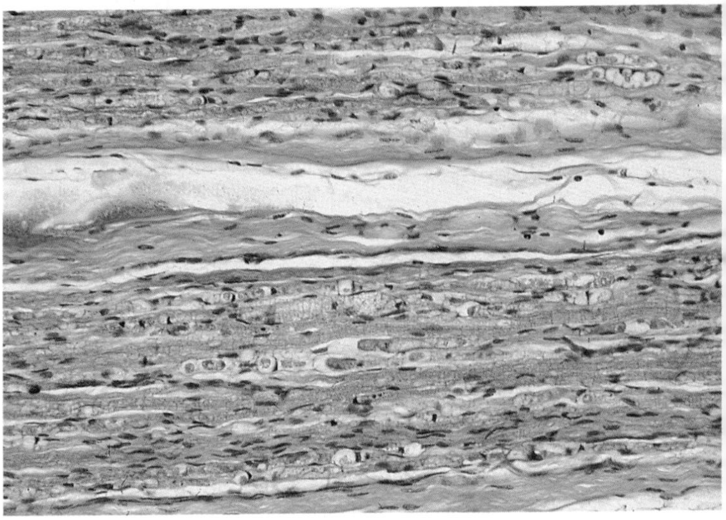

165 Swayback in the goat. Wallerian degeneration in sciatic nerve. Haematoxylin-eosin, × 100. *(Courtesy of Professor J.McC. Howell)*

166 *(facing page)* **CNS and PNS myelin in Shiverer and normal mice:** Shiverer mice fail to code for basic protein (MBP). a, b = normal mouse CNS; c, d = Shiverer mouse CNS; e, f = Shiverer mouse PNS. Note defective CNS myelin (c) and double major period lines (d) in Shiverer mouse. This reflects loss of MBP with absent interperiod line from CNS myelin. By contrast, PNS myelin in the Shiverer shows normal structure (e) and normal major and interperiod dense lines (f). *(Reproduced from 'Neurological Mutations Affecting Myelination' (1980), by courtesy of Drs.A.L. Ganser and D.A. Kirschner and of Elsevier/North Holland)*

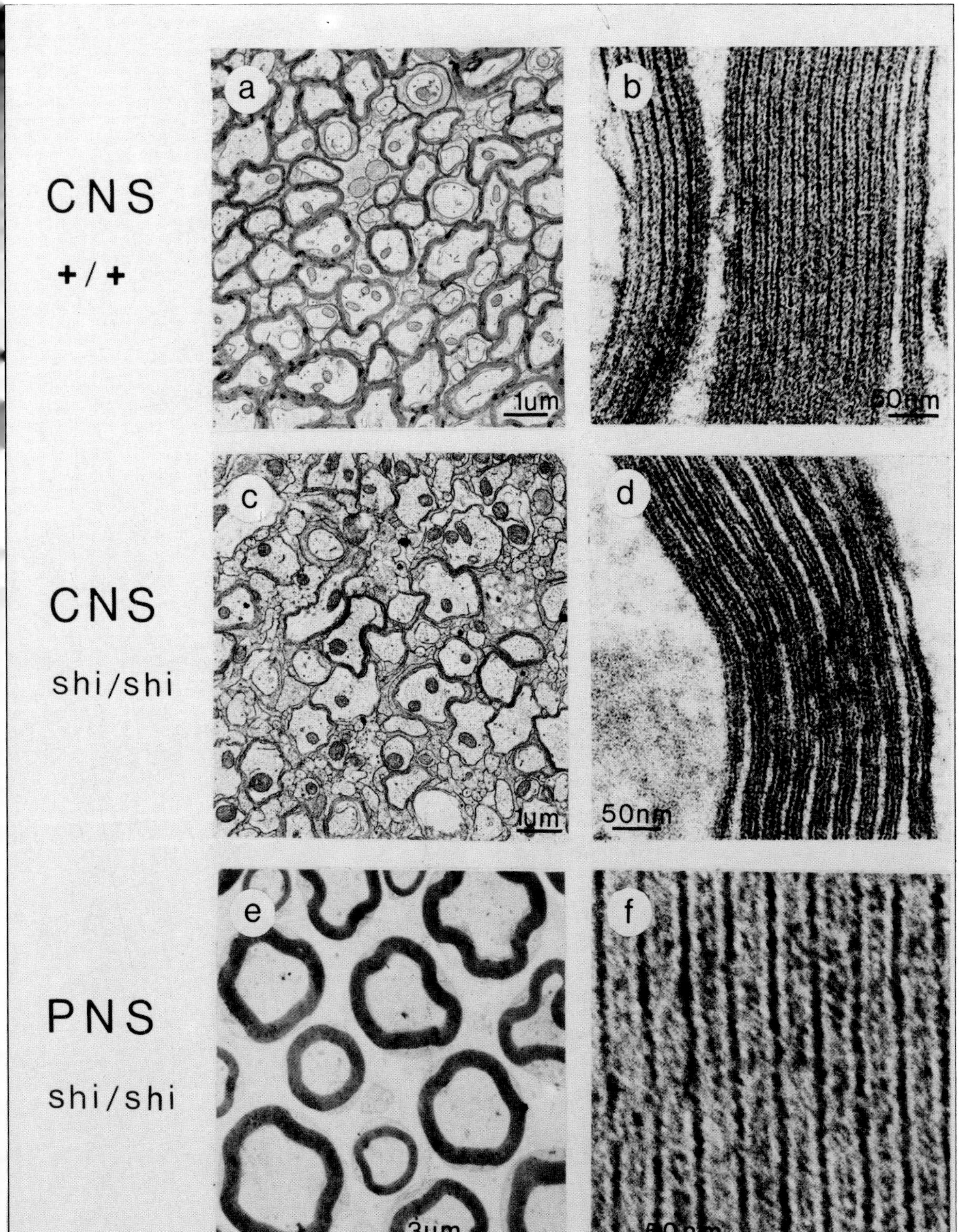
CNS
+/+
CNS
shi/shi
PNS
shi/shi
a
b
c
d
e
f
1um
50nm
1um
50nm
3um
50nm

167 Twitcher mouse. Thoracic spinal cord showing focal myelin loss in lateral and posterior columns. Luxol fast blue and cresyl violet, × 30. *(By courtesy of Professor L. Duchen)*

168 Twitcher mouse. Spinal cord showing two large axons and smaller axons with no myelin sheaths. Some smaller axons are imperfectly myelinated with prominent tongues of oligodendroglial cytoplasm, × circa 10,000. (*Courtesy of Professor L. Duchen)*

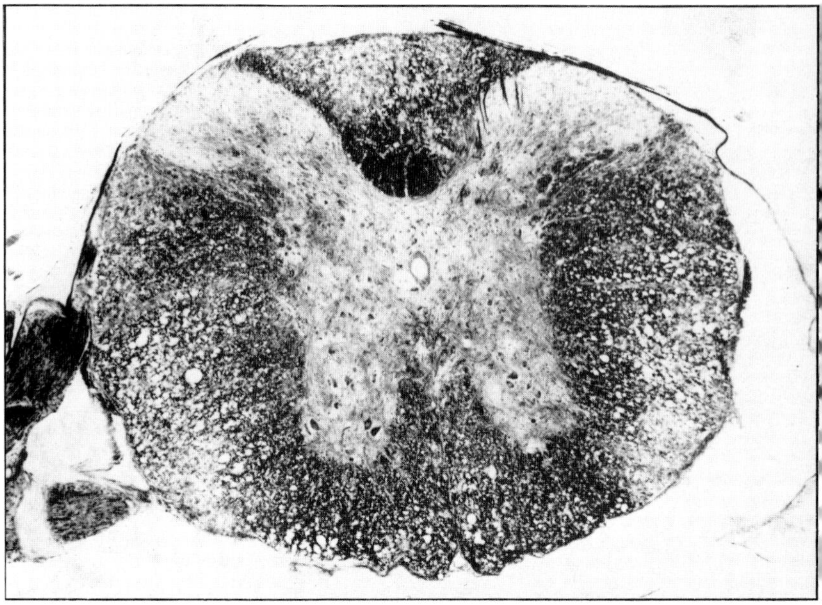

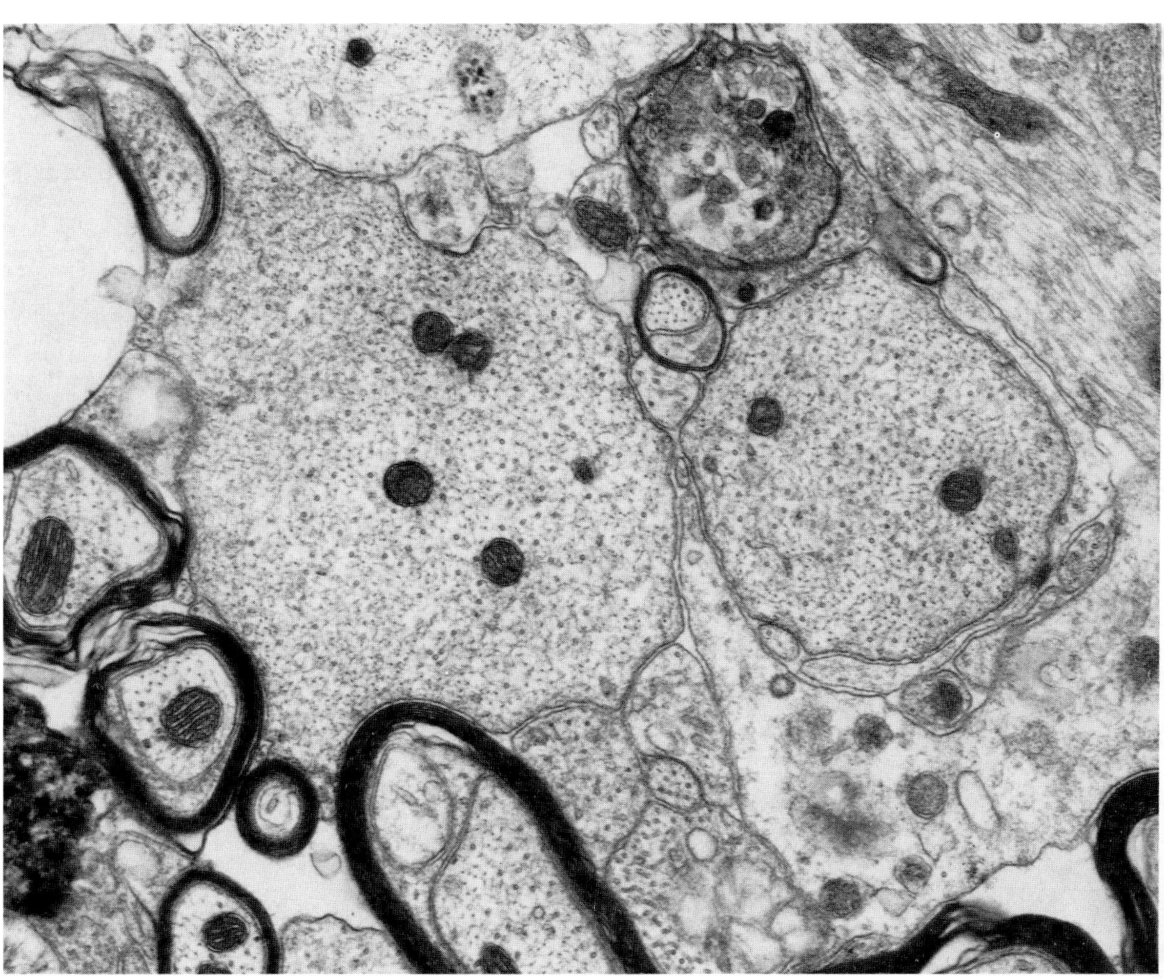

169

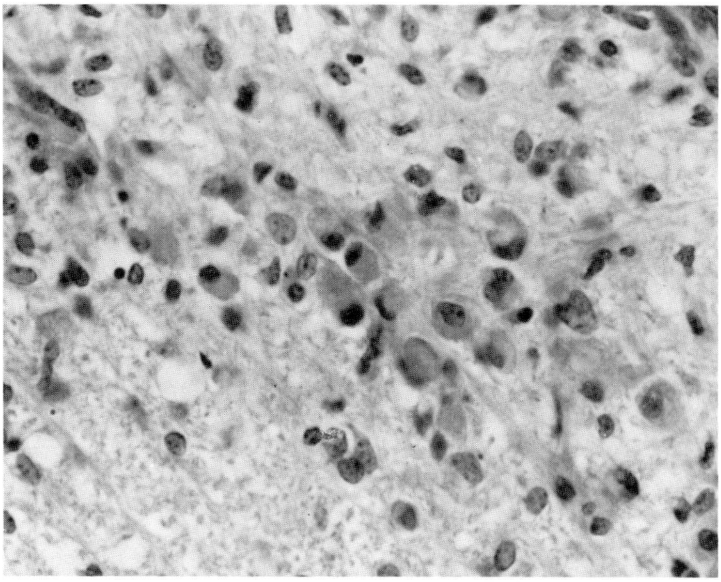

169 Twitcher mouse. Focal accumulation of globoid cells in cerebrum. Compare with **108** and **109**. PAS-haematoxylin, × 200. *(Courtesy of Professor L. Duchen)*

170

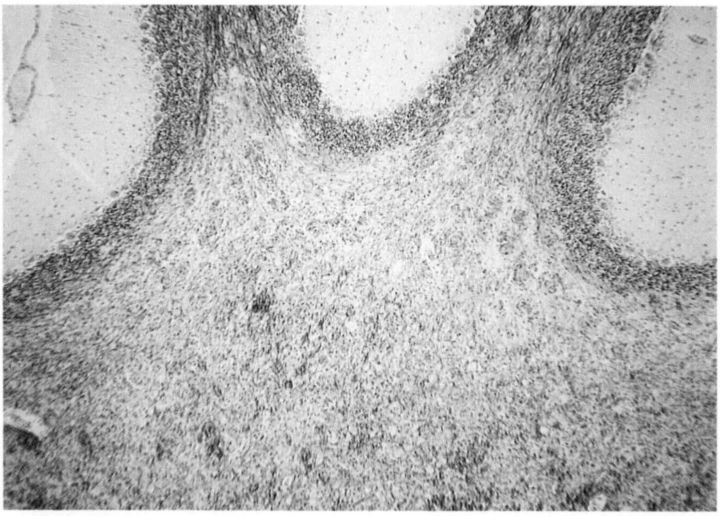

170 Globoid cell leucodystrophy in the dog. Note demyelination in cerebellar white matter. Luxol fast blue and crystal violet, × 20. *(Courtesy of Professor J.McC. Howell)*

171

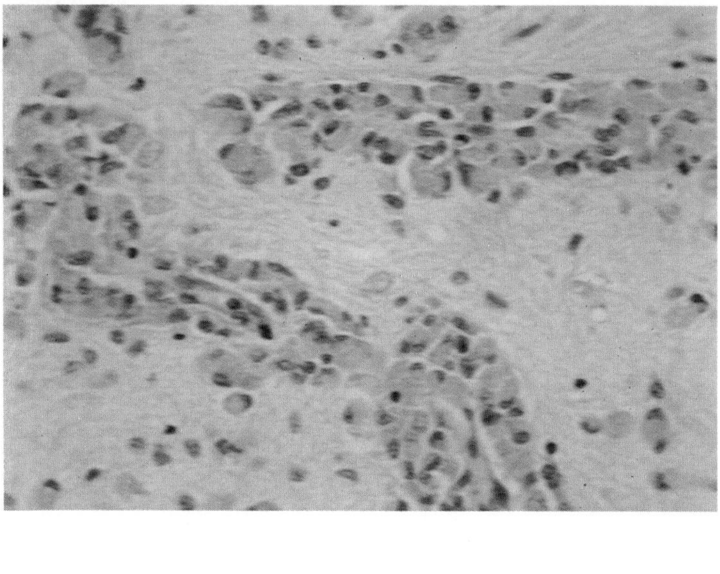

171 Globoid cells in leucodystrophy in the dog. Compare with **108**, **109** and **169**. Haematoxylin-eosin, × 200. *(Courtesy of Professor J.McC. Howell)*

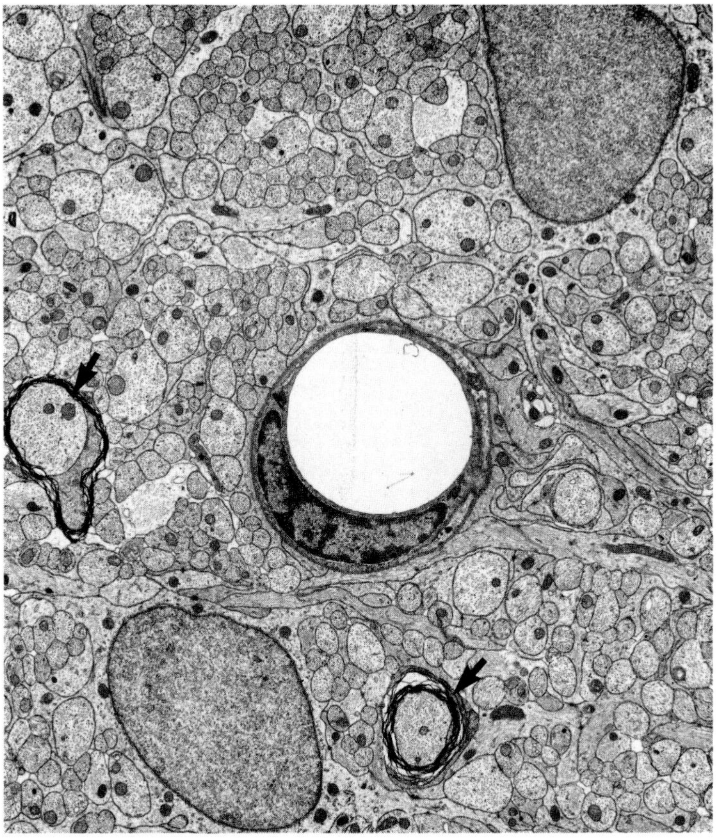

172

172 Myelin deficient (MD) rat. Most axons are nearly unmyelinated, but two dysmyelinated axons are seen (arrows). Three abnormal oligodendroglia (dark cells) are seen, one containing a large lipid vacuole, optic nerve, × 8,600. *(By courtesy of Dr K.D. Barron)*

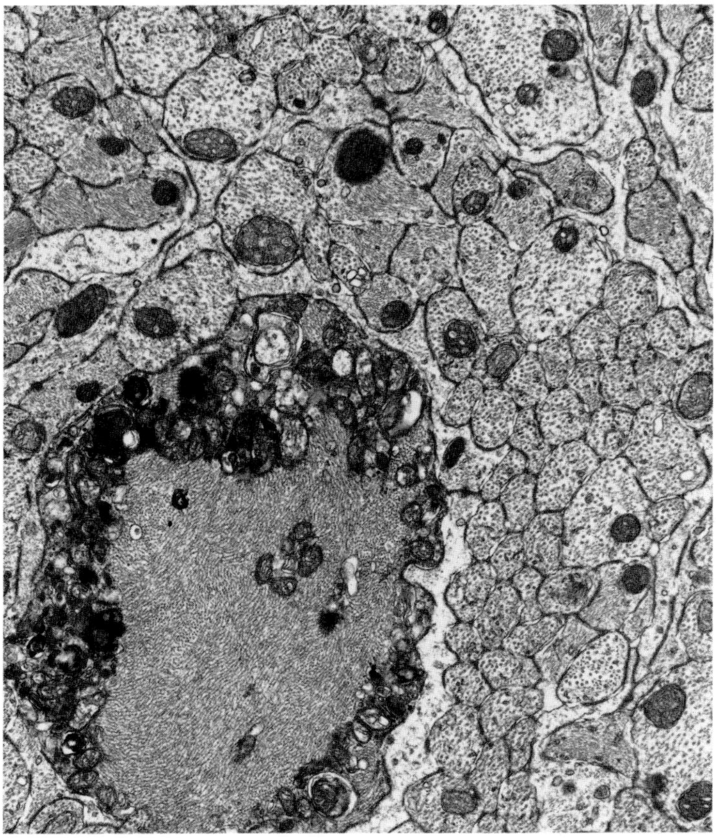

173

173 Myelin deficient (MD) rat. Most axons are thinly myelinated, while a few are unmyelinated. The lone oligodendrocyte contains a rim of myelin bodies, representing abortive attempts at myelination, optic nerve, × 21,900. *(By courtesy of Dr. K.D. Barron)*

4 Experimental and laboratory studies on myelin diseases

The pathogenesis of demyelination can be considered from two aspects: (a) the local mechanisms of myelin disruption and breakdown (b) the conditions which initiate the demyelinating process.

Myelin disruption and breakdown

The mechanism of myelin breakdown appears to depend on physical destruction or structural disintegration of the sheath, followed by a slower process of chemical degradation of the myelin lipids.

An important feature of myelin breakdown is that the lipids are degraded slowly (Table 4). In the peripheral nerve, it takes 1½ to 2 weeks before any substantial lipid changes are seen (**174** to **176**) and about 3-4 weeks to remove all the lipid debris by endocytosis and lysosomal degradation. In the CNS, lipid removal takes much longer (McCaman and Robins, 1959; Bignami and Rolston, 1969; Bignami and Eng, 1973; Perry *et al.*, 1987), and may be incomplete after a year. The initial structural breakdown is most likely to be due to alteration or destruction of the protein layers of the sheath (Adams, 1962a, b; **177**). Basic myelin proteins seem to be particularly vulnerable to lysosomal proteolytic enzymes (Einstein *et al.*, 1968; Roytta *et al.*, 1974; Marks *et al.*, 1976; Berlet *et al.*, 1984), and disappear early in the course of Wallerian degeneration (Adams *et al.*, 1972; **178**) and multiple sclerosis (Einstein *et al.*, 1972; **193**). Basic myelin protein also seems to be particularly vulnerable to autolytic digestion and exposure to oedema (Smith and Sedgewick, 1975; Smith, 1977: Ansari *et al.*, 1975, 1976). Another possibility is that lysophosphatides, formed by the action of lysosomal phospholipase A, cause disintegration of the sheath by their surface-active cytolytic membrane-destructive action (Gregson and Hall, 1973, see below). Lysophosphatides also cause the release of lysomal enzymes, including proteases, from brain tissue (Marples *et al.*, 1959). Thus, the possible roles of lysolecithin and proteases can be unified.

Enzyme extracts from degenerating peripheral nerves cause in vitro demyelination when applied to sections of both PNS and CNS myelin (**179** and **180**): inhibitor studies suggested that the enzyme concerned is cathepsin D (Hallpike *et al.*, 1970a). This accords with the finding that trypsin releases lipid from myelin in brain sections (Tuqan and Adams, 1961). Recent work in our laboratory has shown that application of purified proteolytic enzymes to cerebral white matter causes lipid loss, but no loss of axonal staining (**181** and **182**; Adams, C.W.M. and High, O.B. 1984, unpublished.) Application of lysolecithin to brain sections also causes focal loss of lipid, presumably as a result of its cytolytic action on myelin membranes (Adams, C.W.M. and Webster, G.R. 1961, unpublished). The demyelinating action of lysolecithin (Gregson and Hall, 1973) is discussed later in this section; lysolecithin can also be formed in vivo by the action of another lysosomal enzyme, phospholipase A.

To add credence to the idea that lysosomal proteolytic and other enzymes in the inflammatory infiltrate may promote myelin breakdown, acid and neutral proteolytic enzyme activity has been shown to increase in the early stages of Wallerian degeneration (Porcellati and Curti, 1960; Adams and Bayliss,

Table 4 Lipid changes after peripheral nerve section (see Adams, 1965)

Days after section	free cholesterol	ester cholesterol*	phospholipid	cerebroside
0	100	0	100	100
4	99	1	101	103
8	92	5.3	99	96
14-14	62	31.4	46.5	52.5
32-45	36	25	20.5	25
64	17	15	12	20
96-100	9	14.7	13.5	1.5

*% of free cholesterol as at day 0.

1961; Adams and Tuqan, 1961; Hallpike *et al.*, 1970a; **183** and **184**) and at the edge of active plaques of multiple sclerosis (**185** and **186**; Table 5; Adams, 1968, 1969; Hallpike and Adams, 1969; Einstein *et al.*, 1970; Riekkinen *et al.*, 1970, 1971; Hirsch *et al.*, 1976). Opinions differ about the extent of increased proteolytic activity in the surrounding 'normal' white matter around MS plaques: levels vary between different studies (Riekkinen *et al.*, 1970; Einstein *et al.*, 1972; Cuzner and Davison, 1973). A problem with working on 'normal' white matter outside MS plaques is that small foci of Wallerian degeneration may be present, or very small lesions may have escaped detection. The esterified cholesterol level is increased in such 'normal' white matter, and this is an indication of active demyelination therein (Wender *et al.*, 1973).

With regard to Wallerian degeneration, there is also a marked increase in acid phosphatase activity in the first week of degeneration (Hallpike and Adams, 1969; Hallpike *et al.*, 1970b): this enzyme and acid lipase/esterase can be regarded as markers for lysosomal enzyme activity (**187** and **188**). Presumably, the source of these lysosomal enzymes are the activated macrophages (**189**) which play a prominent role in the digestion of the myelin sheath during Wallerian degeneration. In multiple sclerosis, the source of these lysosomal proteolytic enzymes is not so clear-cut, but the probability is that they are again derived from lysosomes in macrophages (see Chapter 7; Norton *et al.*, 1978) and, possibly, astrocytes (Arstila *et al.*, 1973; Allen *et al.*, 1979a; McKeown and Allen, 1979). Although lysosomal acid proteinase and acid phosphatase is increased in and around MS plaques, acid-lipase or esterase is reduced in the plaque (Hirsch *et al.*, 1976).

It has been suggested that plasmin (plasma fibrinolysin) may gain entry to the brain through leaking blood vessels and cause myelin breakdown (Adams, 1972). Blood fibrinolytic activity is increased in patients with active MS (Menon *et al.*, 1969). Cammer *et al.* (1978) found that plasmin activated by a macrophage fibrinolysin-activator would digest MBP in vitro: P_o, P_1 and P_r proteins in the PNS were digested but not P_2 (Cammer *et al.*, 1981). Using Todd's fibrin film method, Hirsch *et al.*, (1981) found that plasmin activity in plaques was mainly located around vessels, as to be expected from its plasmatic origin. In this connection serum tryptic activity is increased in MS patients (Huszak, 1972).

Table 5 Acid proteinase activity in multiple sclerosis lesions (after Einstein *et al.*, 1972) (Number of cases in parentheses)

Control white matter	100 (5)
Multiple sclerosis white matter	139 (10)
Plaque edge	192 (8)
Plaque	198 (4)
Active plaque	283 (3)

The role of basic myelin protein (P_1) as a major target for lysosomal proteolytic digestion in both Wallerian degeneration and multiple sclerosis (**190** and **191**) is supported by histochemical evidence of an early loss of basic protein staining in the earliest stages of Wallerian degeneration (Adams *et al.*, 1972; **178** and **192**) and around active early plaques of multiple sclerosis (Hallpike *et al.*, 1970c; **193**). These histochemical observations are supported by a number of biochemical studies on MS showing loss of basic myelin protein from the centre and edges of plaques and, in several instances, from apparently normal white matter (Table 5, Einstein *et al.*, 1970, 1972; Reikinnen *et al.*, 1970, 1971). Active plaques show more loss of MBP extending out from their edges than do inactive or burnt out lesions; this probably reflects ongoing damage to myelin in a zone of active demyelination.

Proteolytic enzyme and other lysosomal enzyme activities increase in the acute stage of experimental allergic encephalomyelitis (Benetato *et al.*, 1965; Govindarajan *et al.*, 1974; Smith *et al.*, 1974; Hirsch and Parks, 1975; Gabrielscu, 1978; Smith, 1979; Einstein, 1982) and some but not all proteinase inhibitors suppress or ameliorate the disease (Boehme *et al.*, 1978; Brosnan *et al.*, 1980; Smith, 1980; Smith and Amaducci, 1982). However, the applicability of proteinase inhibition to preserve myelin in the treatment of multiple sclerosis is uncertain. It is of interest that MBP increases proteolysis by inhibiting proteolytic enzyme inhibitors (Van der Veen *et al.*, 1985).

Acid and neutral proteases leak into the CSF in acute MS (Cuzner *et al.*, 1978; Hulberg and Olsson, 1979; Inozuka *et al.*, 1987) but CSF proteinase inhibitors are reduced (Price and Cuzner, 1979). The presence of myelin basic protein in CSF relates to active demyelination only. It occurs in patients with new symptoms and signs, but not in those with a relapse or with a recurrence of previous symptoms and signs (Mastin-Mordiere *et al.*, 1987).

The field of proteolytic enzymes in demyelination has been reviewed from various aspects and at greater or shorter length by Hallpike and Adams (1969); Adams (1972); Hallpike (1972); Norton *et al.*, (1978); Adams (1983); Smith and Benjamins (1984) and others. Myelin proteins have been recently reviewed by Einstein (1982).

Experimental demyelination

There are a number of experimental techniques for inducing demyelination (Table 2). The mechanism depends either on damaging the myelin maintenance cells or on causing direct damage to the myelin sheath.

i) Cytotoxic agents

Local injection of diphtheria toxin induces segmental demyelination of the peripheral nerve by a toxic effect on Schwann cells (Jacobs *et al.*, 1966). The toxin has a similar effect on oligodendroglia in the CNS when applied locally as a demyelinating agent to the cord or optic nerve; Wisniewski and Raine, 1971; Harrison *et al.*, 1972; McDonald, 1974; **194** and **195**). Vesicular demyelination is prominent and macrophages resorb debris, but perivascular cuffing is not seen. Diphtheritic neuropathy was a common condition when diphtheria was an endemic disease but, because of active immunisation, it is now rare in the Western world. Diphtheria toxin is thought to damage Schwann cells and neuroglia by suppression of protein anabolism, engendered by defective RNA template production (Collier, 1967).

Cuprizone has been used by a number of workers to induce CNS demyelination through its cytotoxic action on oligodendroglia (Blakemore, 1973, 1983: Ludwin, 1978, 1981, 1987; **41** and **42**). Cuprizone inhibits carbonic anhydrase (Komaly *el al.*, 1987); its effect on oligodendroglia might be mediated through such inhibition as the enzyme is concentrated in oligodendroglia (*see* Chapter 7). However, there is an unexplained anomaly in the delay between inhibition of the enzyme and the onset of demyelination. Recovery occurs rapidly when cuprizone administration is stopped, and remyelination commences within a week (Ludwin, 1978, 1987; Blakemore, 1978; Hall, 1988).

Lysolecithin has a local disruptive action on cell membranes and, as mentioned above, is a very effective demyelinating agent (Gregson and Hall, 1973). Its specific mode of action seems to be to split the intermediate period line of myelin, which represents the point of fusion between successive layers of membrane secreted around the axon. Subsequently, the myelin undergoes vesicular changes leading to marked intramyelin oedema (**196**). The process first starts at the paranodal region and spreads into the internodal part. In the central nervous system, lysolecithin seems to have the additional action of being cytotoxic for oligodendroglia. Macrophages take up the damaged myelin, but this secondary response can be inhibited by reticuloendothelial blockade with silica quartz (Triarhou and Herndon, 1985). The experimental technique used is the direct local injection or application of lysolecithin into the peripheral nerve or cord (Hall, 1988). In addition to lysolecithin, phospholipase A may be used, as this lysosomal enzyme hydrolyses myelin phosphoglycerides to the relevant lyso-derivative (Gallai-Hatchard *et al.*, 1962), which has a 'clearing action' on brain suspensions (Webster, 1957) and on sections of brain tissue (see above).

Experimental sublethal chronic cyanide intoxication results in demyelinating lesions (**197** and **198**), but overdosage readily causes necrotic lesions and the technique is not easy (Ibrahim *et al.*, 1963).

ii) Viruses

Certain viruses directly infect oligodendroglia, as for example the polyoma virus in progressive multifocal leucoencephalopathy (Chapter 2), the slow incomplete measles infection of oligodendroglia in chronic sclerosing panencephalitis (Chapter 2) and a paramyxovirus in canine distemper (Chapter 3).

As experimental tools, JCM virus, canine distemper virus, Theiler's murine encephalomyelitis virus and the visna virus have been used to produce demyelination in various species (Table 3). It is not difficult to understand the pathogenesis of the demyelination produced by these viruses, which inter alia directly infect oligodendroglia and cause a characteristic viral inflammatory response. Theiler's virus, the Semliki forest virus and visna seem in addition to produce relapsing autoallergic diseases, comparable in some ways to multiple sclerosis. These conditions have been more fully discussed and illustrated in Chapter 3.

The provirus or prion causing scrapie in sheep has now been discredited as the cause of multiple sclerosis. Initial experimental studies on injecting MS brain into Icelandic sheep apparently led to the development of scrapie. However, repeat investigations showed that the development of scrapie after injection of MS material was purely fortuitous (Dick *et al.*, 1965; Chapter 2). Furthermore, scrapie is a disease of grey matter, a spongiform encephalopathy like Creutzfeldt-Jakob disease, and does not cause demyelination.

iii) Trauma

Local intermittent modest pressure on the spinal

cord by CSF barbitage (repeated removal and replacement of CSF) is another experimental technique that has been used to induce demyelinating lesions in the spinal cord (Bunge *et al.*, 1962). Cord compression has a similar effect (Harrison and McDonald, 1977). The effect is presumably due to direct damage to myelin or oligodendroglia by pressure insufficient to affect the axon directly. Remyelination occurs after recovery of the oligodendroglia. Comparable segmental demyelination in the peripheral nerve can be experimentally produced by application of a sphygmomanometer arm band inflated to 500-1000 mm Hg (Gilliatt, 1975) or by incising the perineurium (perineurial 'window') so that the nerve fascicle herniates and, thus, locally damages the myelin (Spencer *et al.*, 1975). Extreme trauma results in axonal death or Wallerian degeneration. Here, the myelin vesiculates and dies; it is then rapidly attacked by macrophages that unpeel and digest the lamellae (Lampert, 1983).

iv) Alterations in permeability

Since local oedema has been linked with MS plaques, attention has centred on the permeability of vascular endothelium which is known to be increased in both experimental allergic encephalomyelitis (EAE) and in MS plaques (EAE: Leibowitz and Kennedy, 1972; MS: see Chapter 9). It is of interest that Snyder *et al.*, (1975) found vascular fenestrations in the cord of guinea pigs with chronic EAE, and this may relate to the above permeability changes. However, destruction of cerebral vascular endothelium by the intracarotid injection of Forsmann antibody results not in demyelination, but in a local necrotic lesion (Leibowitz *et al.*, 1961: **199** and **200**). Complete destruction of endothelium would seem to be a too massive event to cause the restricted and subtle lesion of demyelination. Administration of small amounts of antibody does not produce damage restricted to myelin (Aleu *et al.*, 1963).

Induction of myelin oedema by administration of triethyltin or hexachlorophene (see Smith and Benjamins, 1984) or calcium ionophores (Schlaepfer, 1977; Smith *et al.*, 1985) leads to gross vacuolation and vesiculation of myelin, accompanied by very limited breakdown of the sheath. (Trimethyltin is different in that it is neurotoxic.) The mechanism of triethyltin oedema appears to be damage to the control of water uptake, but astrocytes and oligodendroglia could be involved. The typical appearance of this myelin oedema is shown in **201**. Electron microscopy shows a similar picture and confirms that the oedema is located in vesicles within the myelin sheath (**202**). No Marchi-positive lipid breakdown products (cholesterol esters) are seen within macrophages (Ibrahim *et al.*, 1965; **201**), so it is unlikely that the myelin is severely damaged. Repair (remyelination) occurs when the triethyltin is withdrawn. Relatively low doses of triethyltin first leads to reduction of protein metabolism in the peripheral nerve but, after a month, such metabolism is markedly increased as the nerve is being repaired (Smith and Benjamins, 1984).

v) Autoimmunity

Experimental allergic encephalomyelitis (EAE) has attracted research workers in the MS field for many years. Originally, this allergic perivenular inflammatory condition was induced by multiple injections of homologous brain (Rivers and Schwentker, 1935), but the response was then found to be accelerated and increased by the simultaneous administration of a single injection of brain and of Freund's complete adjuvant (Kabat *et al.*, 1947). The lesion is essentially a mononuclear allergic infiltration (lymphocytes and macrophages) around small veins, with a limited degree of perivenular demyelination (**203** and **204**), including vesicular demyelination (Dal Canto *et al.*, 1975; Lampert, 1983). As with Wallerian degeneration and MS, EAE shows increased proteolytic activity in the perivascular infiltrate (**205**) and more diffusely in the parenchymal lesion (**206**; Gabrielescu, 1978).

In most respects EAE is similar to acute disseminated encephalomyelitis (post-viral allergic encephalomyelitis or post-vaccinial encephalomyelitis), as sometimes occurred after the older style of rabies inoculation or as an occasional complication of vaccinia vaccination; *see* Chapter 2.

It was later shown that the major encephalomyelitic activity of brain was located in the myelin basic protein (MBP) fraction of myelin. The antigenic sequence and determinants of MBP have been extensively investigated, yet no unequivocal common ground has been shown between EAE and MS as regards any specific pathogenic role of this protein. CSF anti MBP-antibody levels are raised in both MS and other neurological patients (*see* Chapter 9).

Classical EAE in smaller animals (namely, the guineapig) has only limited resemblances to MS, mainly in the scanty demyelination and nature of the acute inflammatory reaction in acute cases. Large demyelinating plaques in the guineapig spinal cord can be produced by preimmunisation with ovoalbumin prepared in water-soluble adjuvant (Colover,

1980). A chronic relapsing form of EAE (CREAE) has been induced in Hartley or strain 13 guinea pigs (**207** and **208**) and this has rather more resemblance to MS, in that some lesions have similarities to the MS plaque and that the disease has a relapsing remittent course (Lassmann and Wiskniewski, 1978, 1979; Raine, 1983). However, in other ways CREAE differs from MS, the most noticeable being that, in CREAE, plaques are relatively small, inflammatory foci are more severe and the anatomical distribution is different. MBP administered to mice together with Freund's adjuvant results in a necrotising encephalomyelitis. The presence of a myelin lipid hapten in the inoculate seems to be required to produce a demyelinating lesion (Wayne Moore *et al.*, 1987).

Antigalactocerebroside antibody induces EAE-like demyelination in the peripheral nerve (Saida *et al.*, 1979a, b). Antiglucocerebroside antibody has a lesser effect, as the lipid is the glucosyl analogue and not a myelin lipid. The antibody to galactocerebroside seems mainly to damage the Schwann cell, which is the site for synthesis of this lipid. Injection of antigalactocerebroside into the optic nerve causes CNS demyelination with damage to oligodendroglia and vesiculation of myelin (Carroll *et al.*, 1985). Likewise, injection of a monoclonol antibody to myelin-associated glycoprotein (MAG) into the optic nerve of the guineapig produces optic nerve demyelination (Sergott *et al.*, 1988).

Conclusions

Although many of the experimental conditions discussed above are of much academic interest, only a few have direct relevance to MS. Those where the oligodendrocyte is infected could model for certain aspects of progressive multifocal leucoencephalopathy, while EAE is very relevant to acute disseminated encephalomyelitis. However, if MS starts as an acute encephalomyelitis, as some acute cases seem to suggest, then EAE does have some relevance to the initial pathogenesis of MS. It follows that chronic relapsing EAE (CREAE) has a more extended relationship to MS. Nevertheless, it seems unlikely that hypersensitivity to brain antigens, particularly MBP, is going to be the agent that initiates MS. The autoimmune demyelinating diseases, produced by Theiler's virus, Semliki Forest virus and visna virus, are of somewhat variable incidence and intensity and are produced after primary viral damage to the CNS. It can be argued that these are more akin to the unpredictable relapsing course of MS than the other models considered.

To summarize: The mechanism of myelin breakdown in the various *experimental diseases* discussed above ranges at one extreme from (1) the reversible intramyelin oedema seen with triethyltin intoxication; through (2) the vesiculation and intra-lamellar splitting produced by lysolecithin and calcium ionophores with subsequent removal of myelin by macrophages and remyelination; through (3) the autoimmune inflammatory infiltrates occuring in EAE, CREAE and EAN and with antigalactocerebroside serum to (4) the primary oligodendroglial (or Schwann cell) disease seen in mouse hepatitis virus (JCM) disease and distemper. Some diseases (5) start as primary viral diseases infecting the oligodendroglia and may end up as chronic relapsing demyelinating diseases: Theiler's disease, Semliki Forest virus disease and visna fall into this category.

Human counterparts of these experimental categories could be designated as follows (the numbers refer to the respective categories above):

1 Canavan's disease and hexachlorophene intoxication (Chapter 2).
2 Segmental demyelination in the PNS (Chapter 2).
3 Post-viral allergic encephalomyelitis (for example, post-rabies vaccine, post-vaccinial vaccine, etc.) (Chapter 2).
4 Progressive multifocal leucoencephalopathy; chronic sclerosing panencephalitis (Chapter 2).
5 Possibly multiple sclerosis in most instances, as well as the variants of MS (*see* Chapters 2 and 6-9). However, involvement of the oligodendroglia in MS is late (Chapter 7) and the primary viral attack (of possibly modest nature) must be directed elsewhere than against the oligodendroglia, for example, possibly against vascular endothelium or the perivascular region (Chapter 8).

17

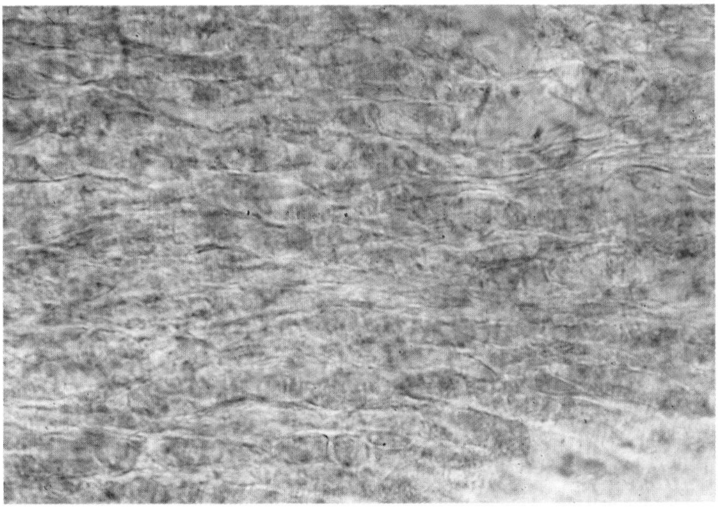

174 Early formation of esterified cholesterol (pink oxazone) in rat sciatic nerve 6 days after nerve section. Myelin phospholipids are stained blue by the oxazine. Nile blue sulphate, × 60.

17

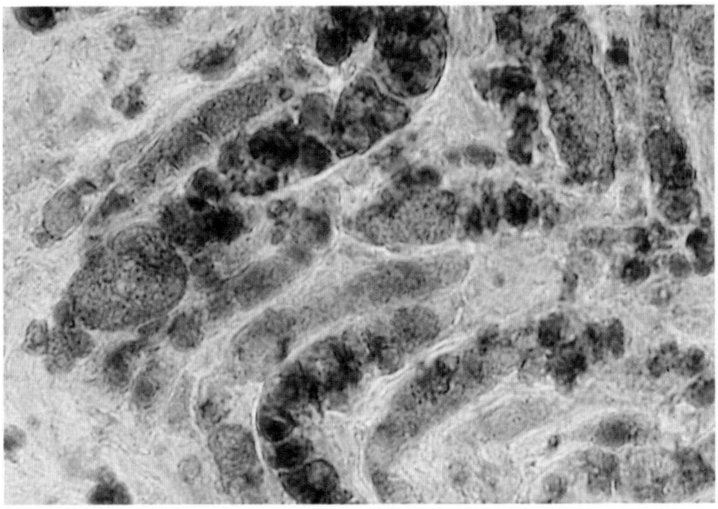

175 Partial degradation of myelin lipids 12 days after section of a rat sciatic nerve. Residual blue phospholipids stained by Baker's acid haematein; cholesterol esters stained by Oil red O, × 150.

176 Degradation of myelin lipids (normally orange-red) and progressive accumulation of esterified cholesterol (black) during Wallerian-degeneration at 0, 6, 12 and 16 days. Rat sciatic nerve, osmium tetroxide-∝-naphthylamine (OTAN), × 150.

17

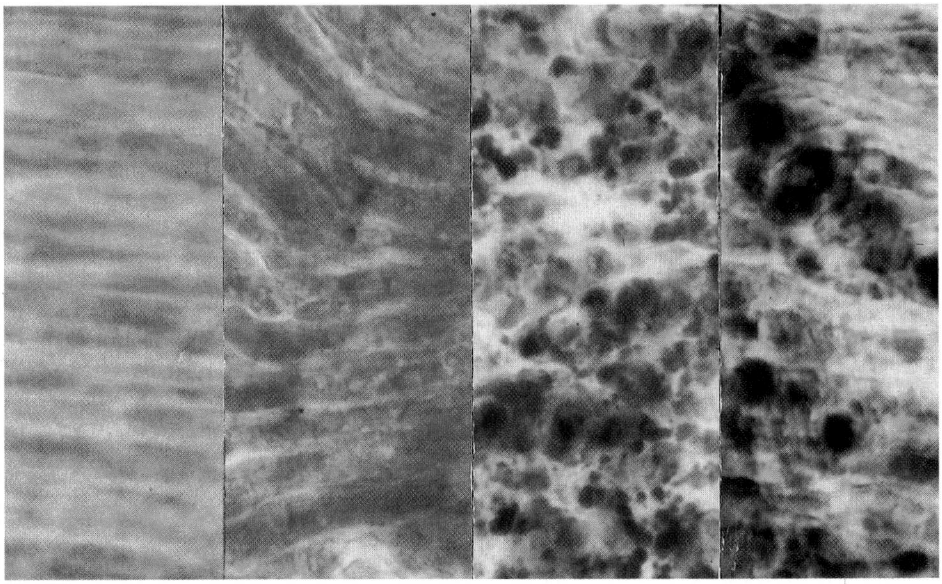

177

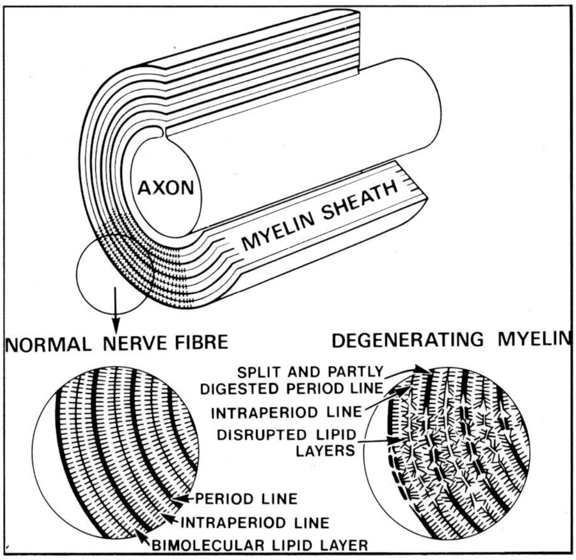

77 Dissociation of lipid from isrupted protein layers in the ıyelin sheath as the mechanism f myelin breakdown (*after dams, 1962b*).

178

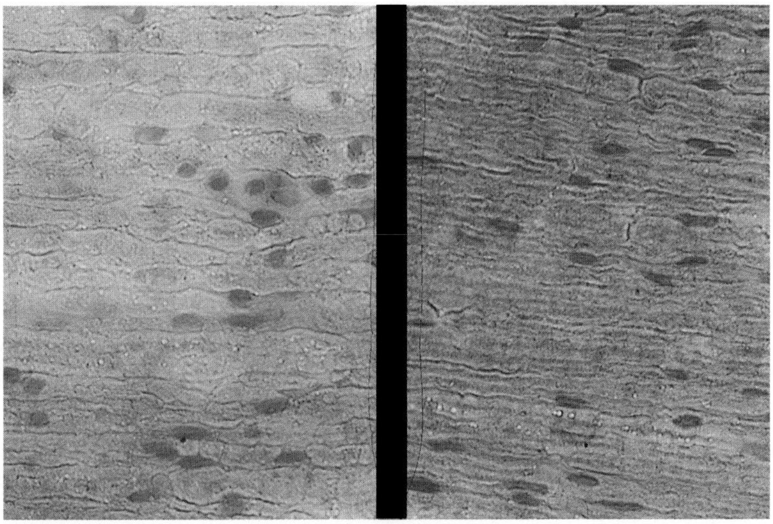

78 Wallerian degeneration. eft: loss of basic protein from a ıt sciatic nerve 2 days after erve section. Right: normal rat ciatic nerve. Trypan blue, × 00. *(Hallpike et al., 1970a)*

179

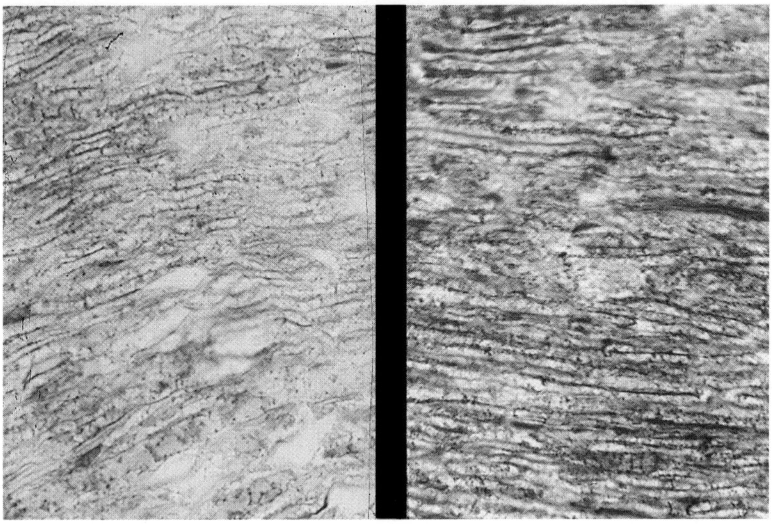

79 Myelin basic protein. Left: ıss of basic protein from a rat ciatic nerve after treatment with xtract of degenerating nerve. ight: control nerve treated with uffer alone. Trypan blue, × 100. *(Hallpike et al., 1970a)*

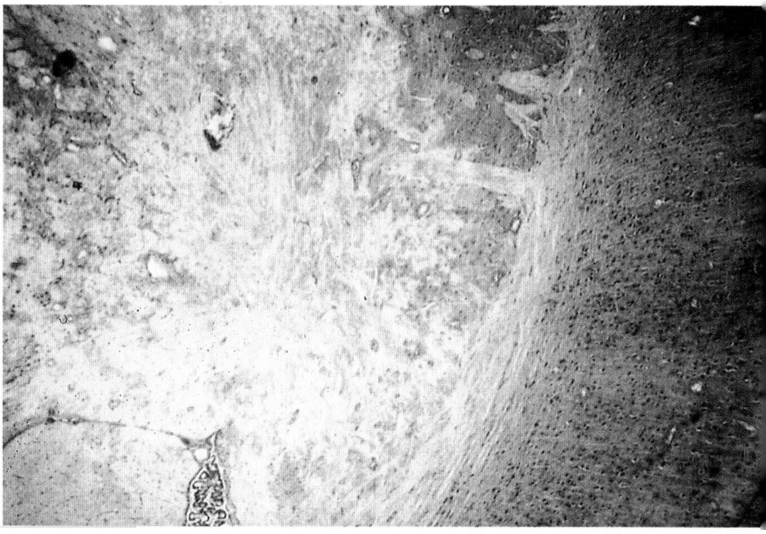

180 Myelin basic protein. Loss of basic protein from myelin in focal area of a rat brain treated with extract of degenerating nerve, as in **179**, × 60.

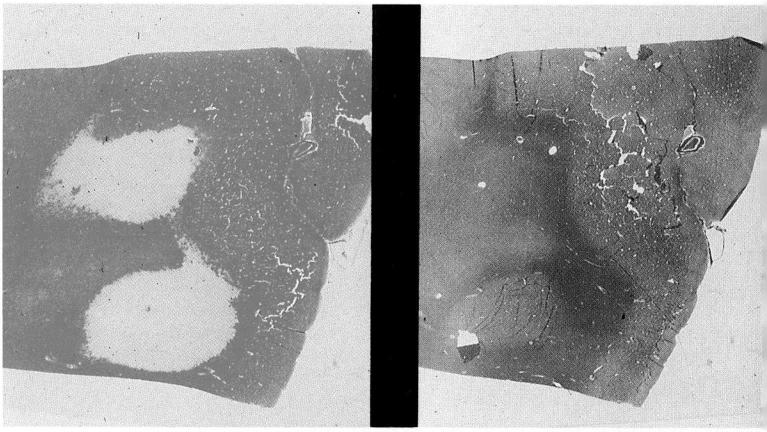

181 Focal effect of 0.01 per cent trypsin on the human brain, incubated for 30 minutes. Left: complete loss of myelin lipids, Luxol fast blue. Right: no loss of axons, Palmgren silver, × 2.

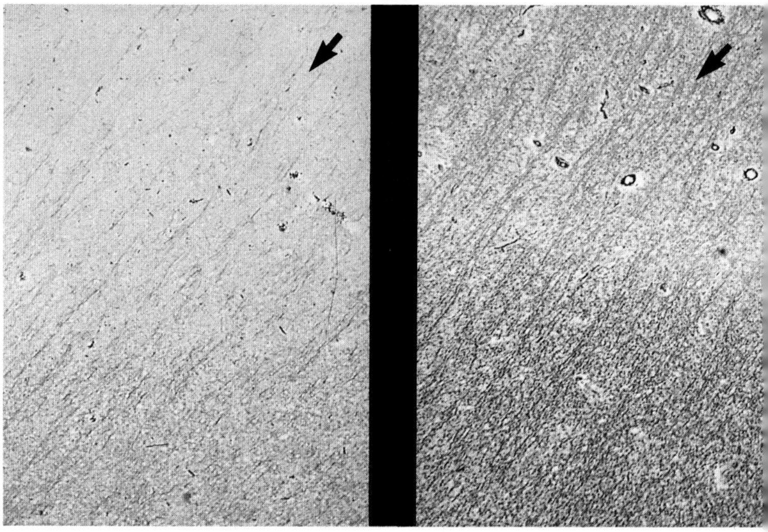

182 Effect of trypsin on the human brain, as for **181**. Left: loss of myelin (arrow), Luxol fast blue. Right: minimal effect on axonal staining (arrow), Palmgren, × 60.

83 Increased acid proteinase ctivity in degenerating rat sciatic erve, 5 days after nerve section. ranslucent areas = digestion of elatin in the gelatin-silver film)lackened photographic plate), : 100.

183

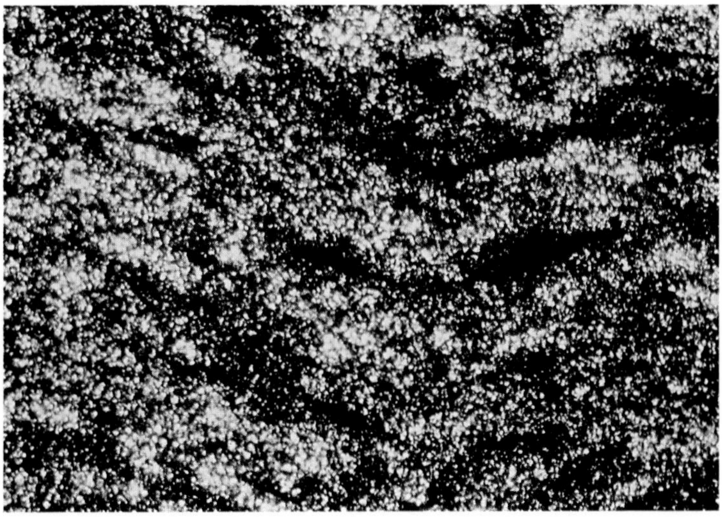

84 Wallerian degeneration a rat sciatic nerve. Changes acid phosphatase, neutral and cid proteinases, and leucine minopeptidase (*after Hallpike t al., 1970b*).

184

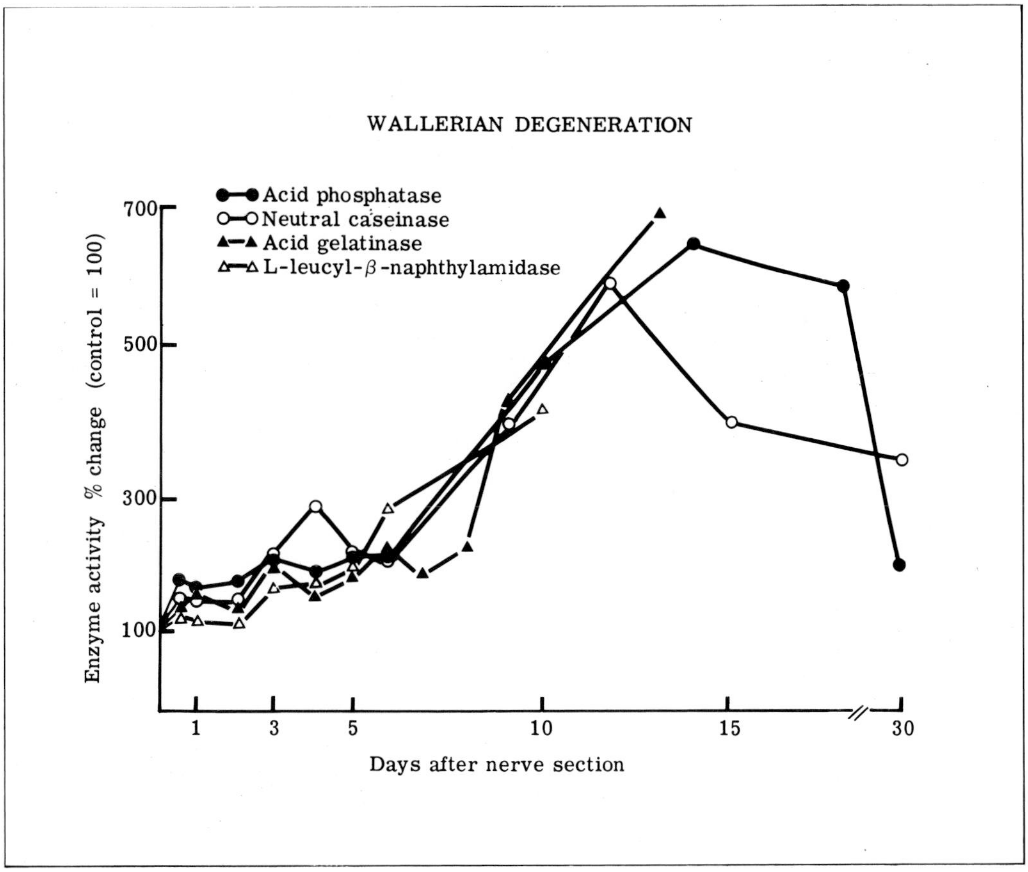

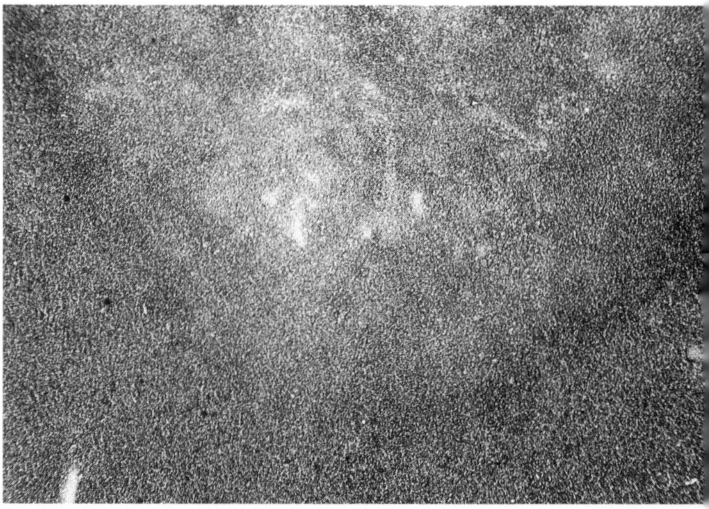

185 Increased acid proteinase activity in active plaque of multiple sclerosis. Gelatin-silver film (as in **183**), × 10.

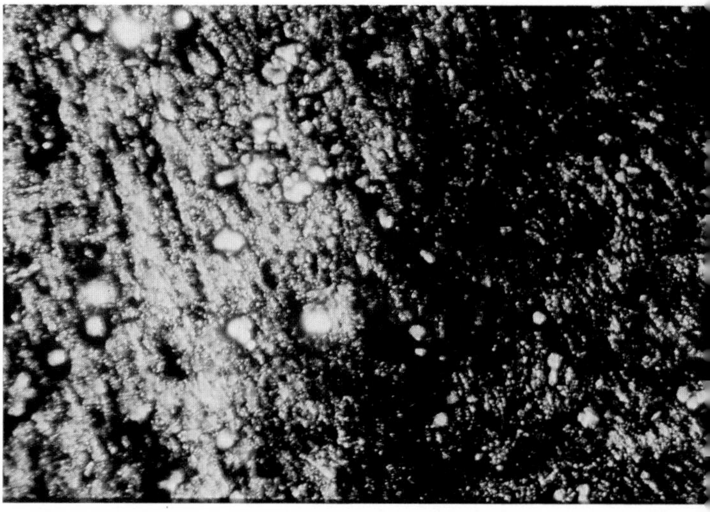

186 Increased acid proteinase activity in active plaque of multiple sclerosis. Note focal activity over glial cells. Gelatin-silver film, × 80.

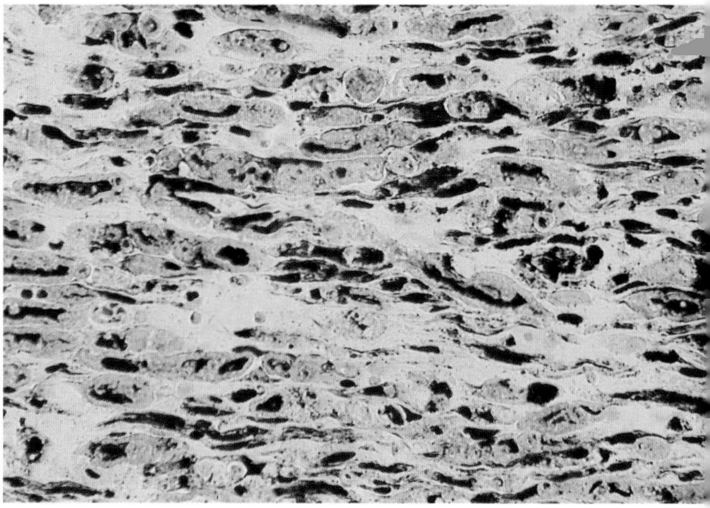

187 Wallerian degeneration. Acid phosphatase in rat sciatic nerve 10 days after section, × 100.

188

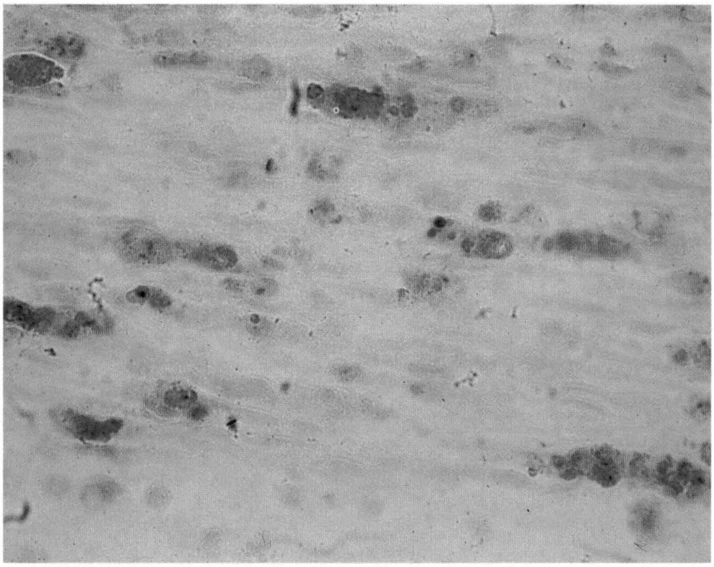

'88 Wallerian degeneration. Acid sterase/lipase in rat sciatic nerve 12 lays after section. Acid naphthyl cetate esterase, × 100.

189

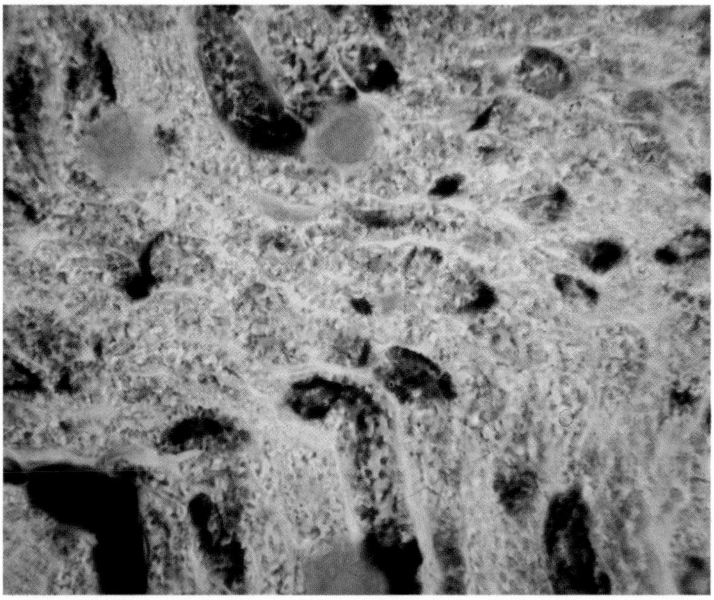

'89 Early Wallerian degeneration. ctivated Schwann cells/ nacrophages. ATPase (Padykula-lermann), × 100.

190

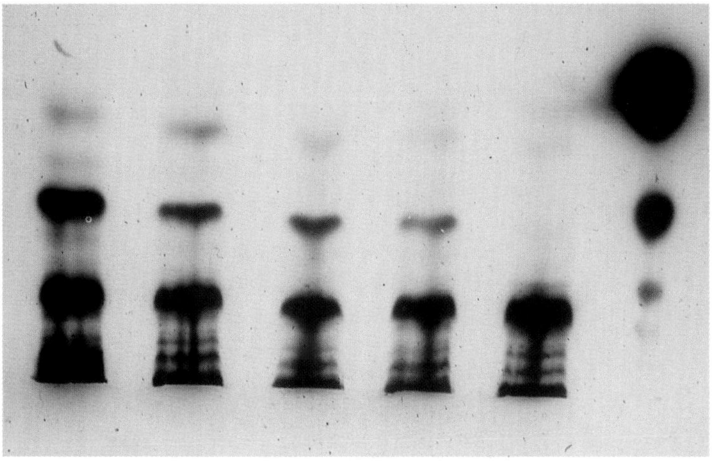

'90 Polyacrylamide gel of myelin roteins in Wallerian degeneration 1 a rat sciatic nerve (left to right) 0, 2, ·, 8 and 12 days after section. Note rogressive early loss of myelin basic roteins P_1 and P_2 (first and second pots from top).

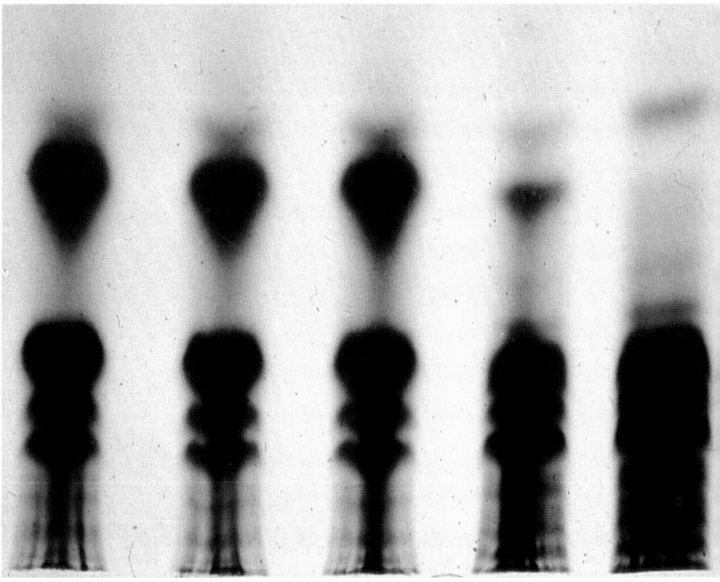

191 Polyacrylamide gel of myelin proteins in multiple sclerosis. From left to right: control white matter, distant MS white matter, close MS white matter, edge of plaque, plaque. Note loss of myelin basic protein (P_1) at edge and in plaque.

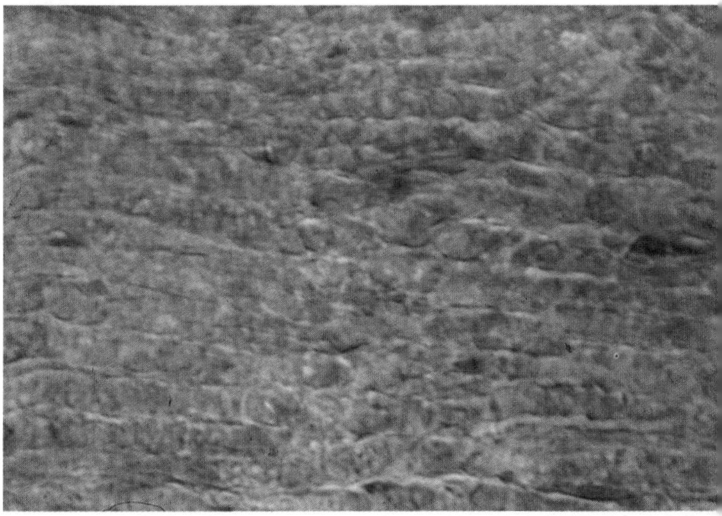

192 Dissociation of lipid (red) from myelin basic protein (blue) in Wallerian degeneration of 6th day. Rat sciatic nerve. Trypan blue, oil red O, × 100.

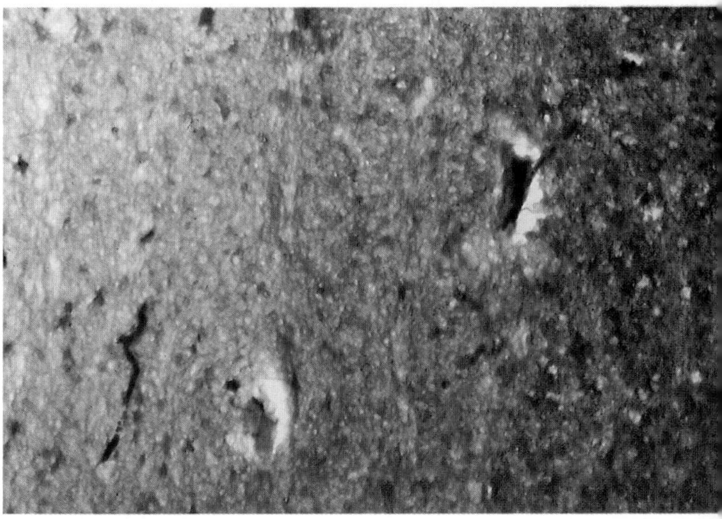

193 Loss of myelin basic protein from edge of multiple sclerosis plaque (left). Trypan blue, × 80.

194

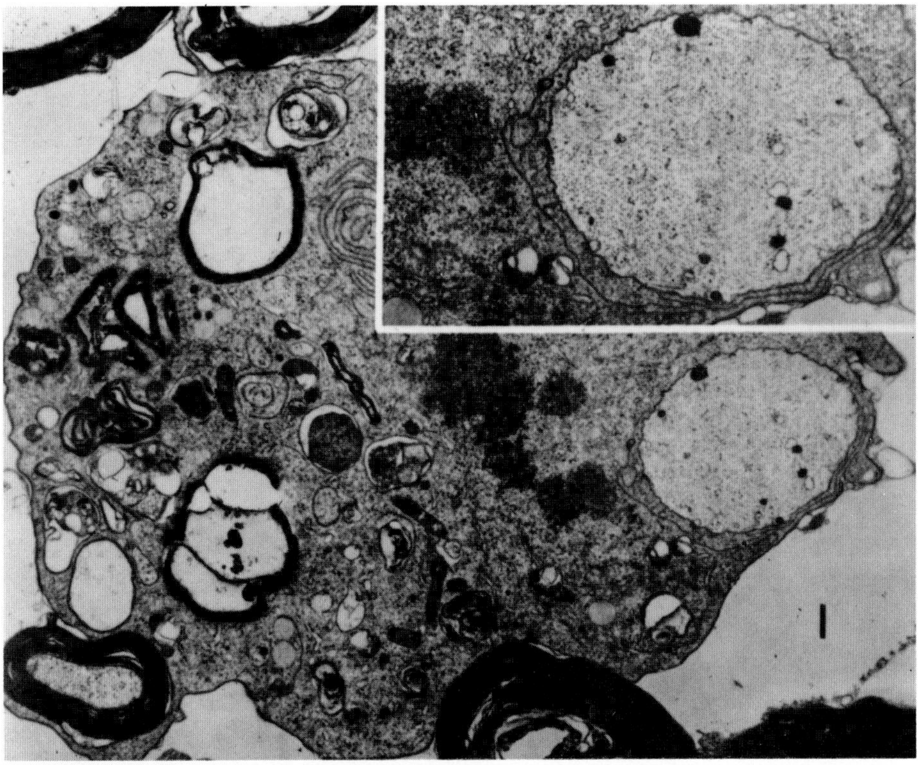

194 Experimental diphtheritic neuropathy in optic nerve. Demyelinated axon surrounded by macrophage with lipid debris, × 2,500. *(Courtesy of Professor Ian McDonald)*

195

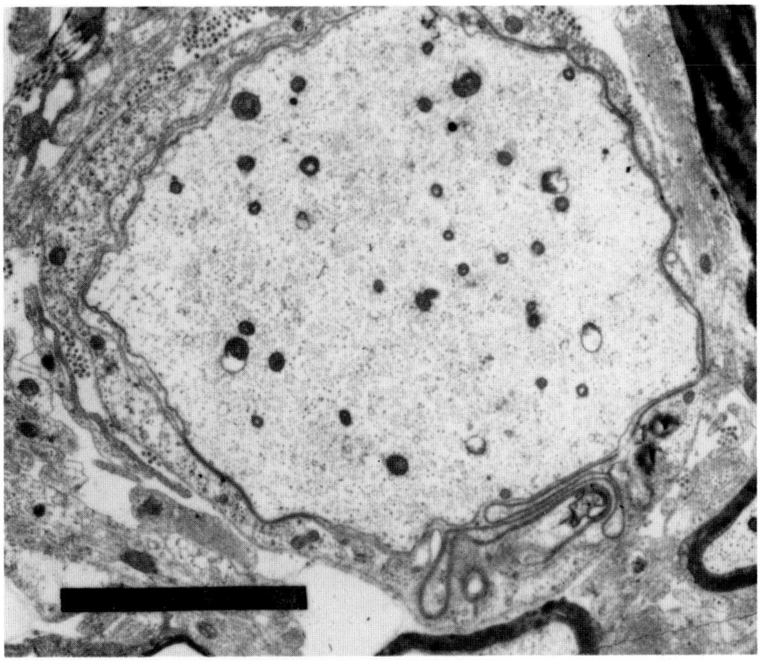

195 Experimental diphtheritic neuropathy in optic nerve. Demyelinated axon, × 6,000. *(Courtesy of Professor Ian McDonald)*

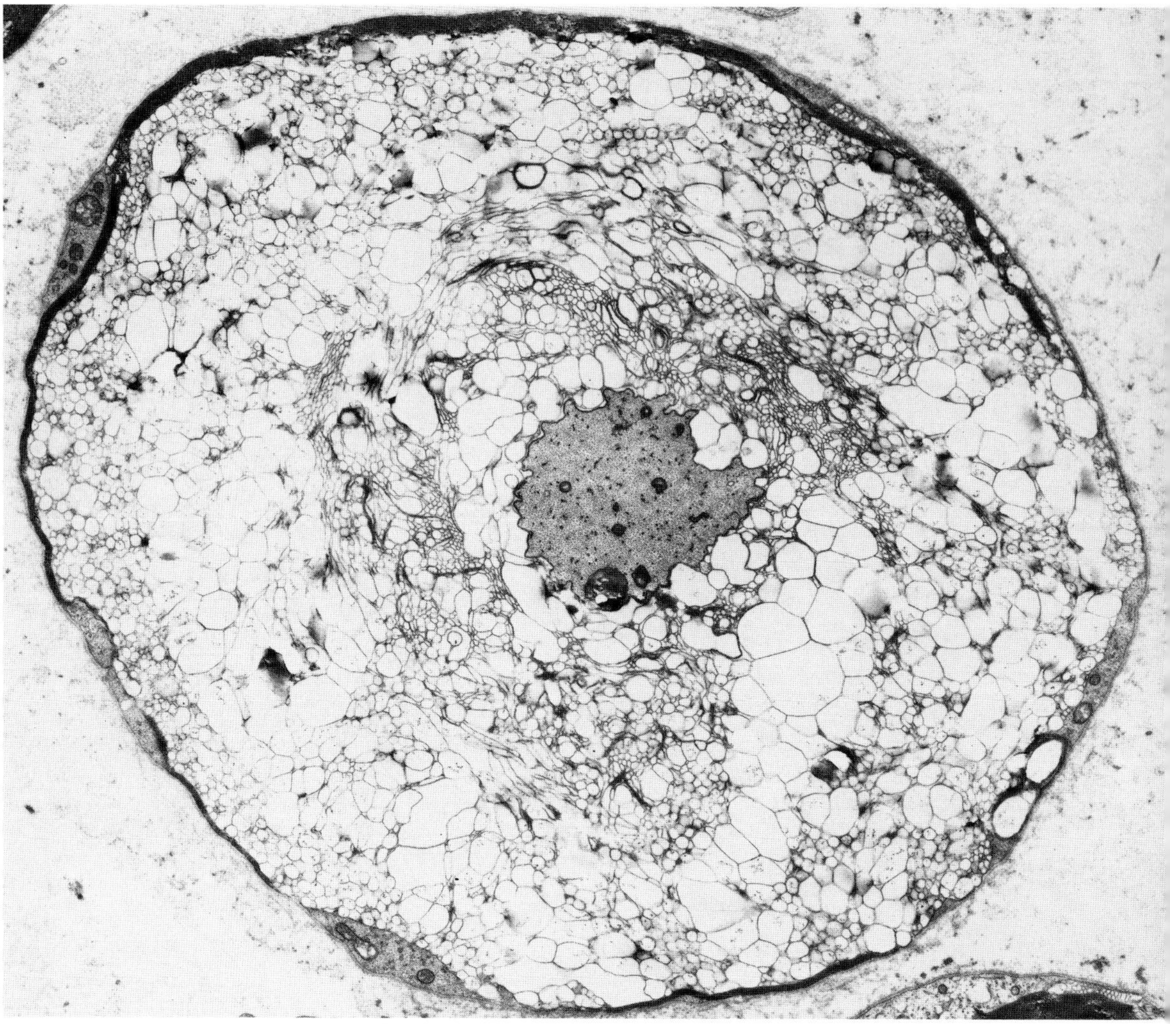

196 Lysolecithin-induced myelin vesiculation in the rat, × 12,000. *(Courtesy of Dr Susan Hall)*

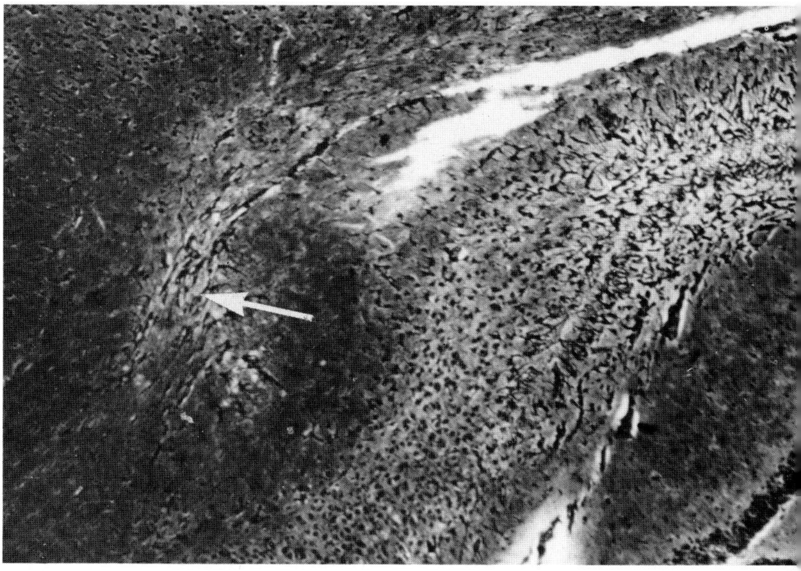

197 Cyanide encephalopathy in rat. Demyelinating lesion in corpus callosum (arrow). Cajal gold sublimate, × 50. *(Ibrahim et al., 1965)*

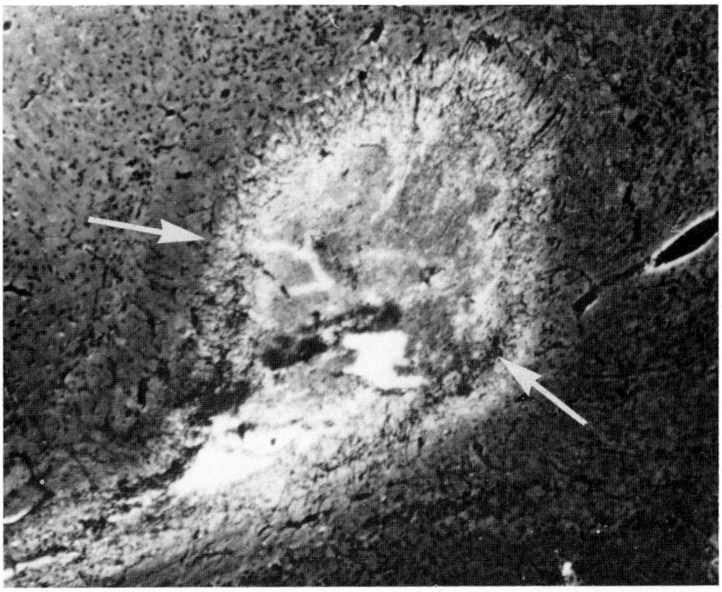

198

198 Cyanide encephalopathy. Larger demyelinating lesion in corpus callosum (arrow). Cajal gold sublimate, × 50. *(Ibrahim et al., 1965)*

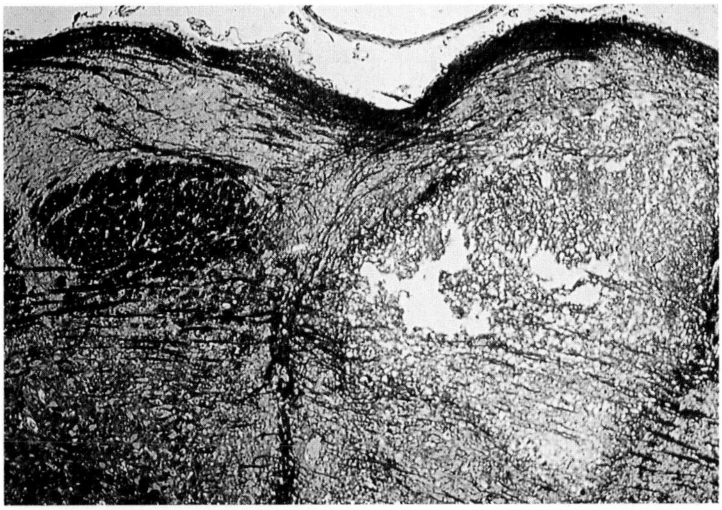

199

199 Focal necrotic encephalopathy in rat medulla/pons after injection of Forsmann antibody. Loyez myelin stain, × 30.

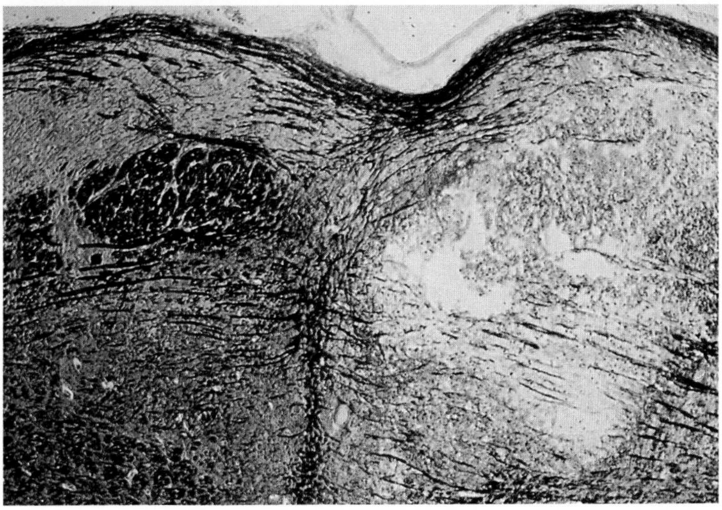

200

200 Same as 199, but Glees and Marsland silver stain to show severe loss of axons, × 30.

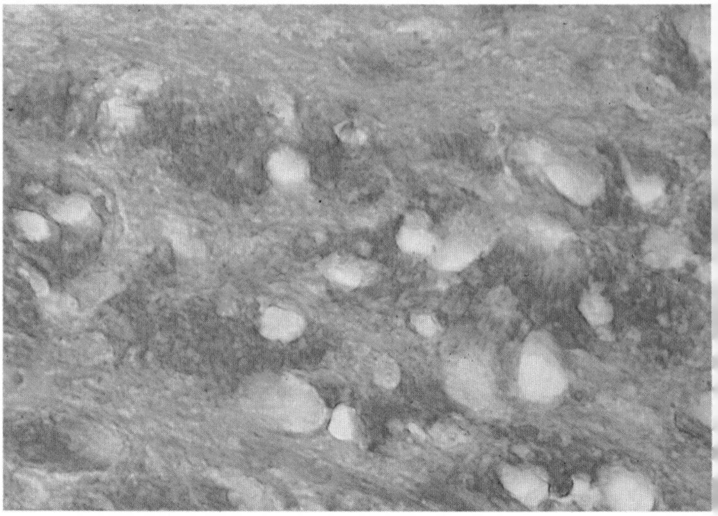

201 Triethyl tin oedema in a rat brain. Note absence of black esterfield cholesterol which is formed in demyelination. Osmium tetroxide-α naphthylamine (OTAN), $\times$ 150.

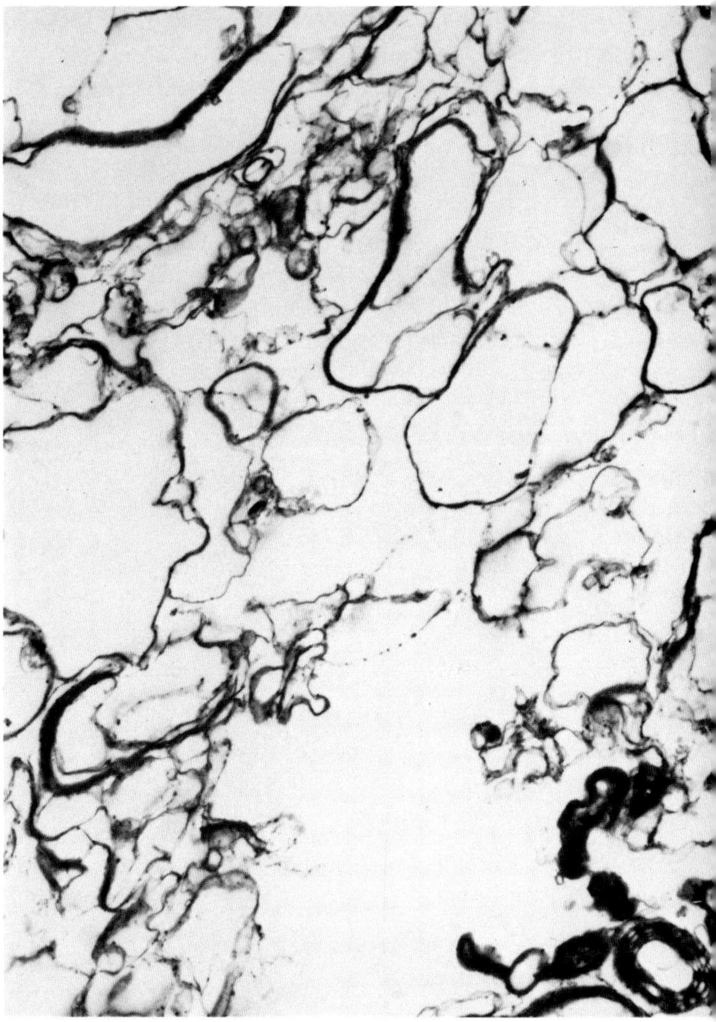

202 Triethyl tin oedema in rat brain. Intense intramyelin oedema, $\times$ 10,000.

203

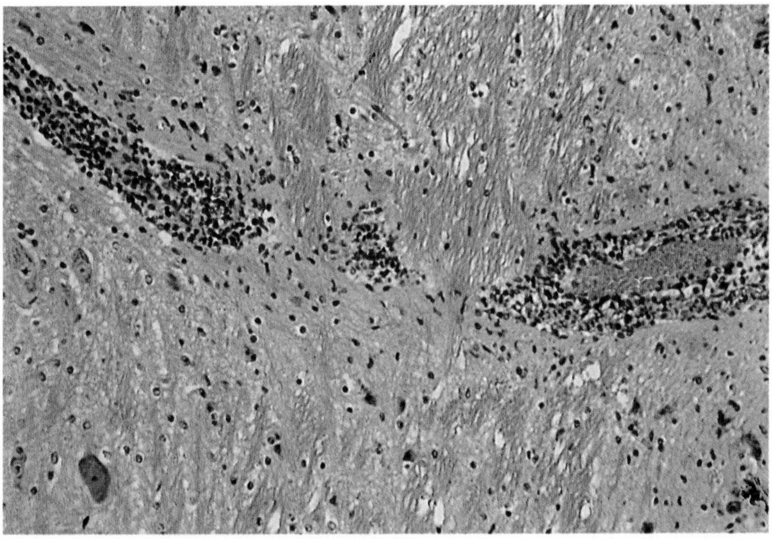

203 Experimental allergic encephalomyelitis (EAE) in guinea pig. Note marked perivascular inflammatory infiltrate. Haematoxylin-eosin, × 50. *(Courtesy of Professor S. Leibowitz)*

204

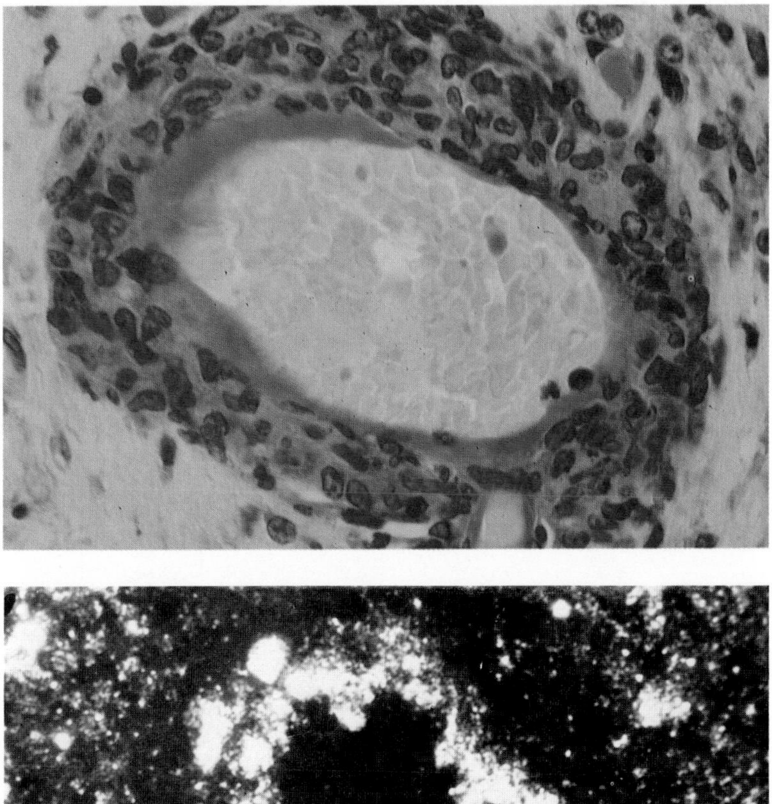

204 Experimental allergic encephalomyelitis (EAE) in guinea pig. Note perivascular mononuclear infiltrate and minimal demyelination. Luxol fast blue-crystal violet, × 250. *(Courtesy of Professor S. Leibowitz)*

205

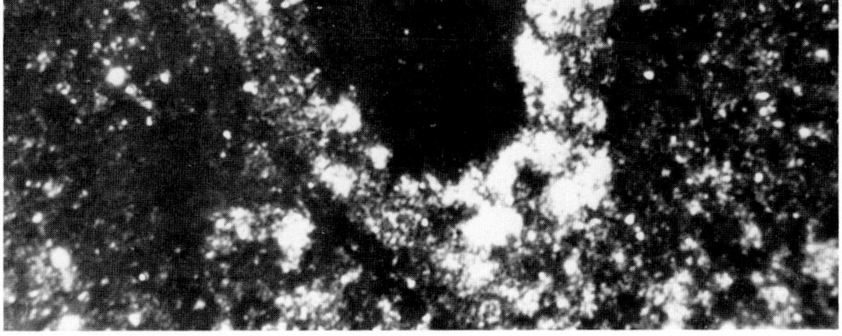

205 EAE. Acid protease (catheptic) activity mainly in the perivascular infiltrate. Proteolytic activity is revealed by opacities caused by digestion of the gelatin film. Nuclear silver emulsion and gelatin, × 100. *(Courtesy of Dr Elena Gabrielescu)*

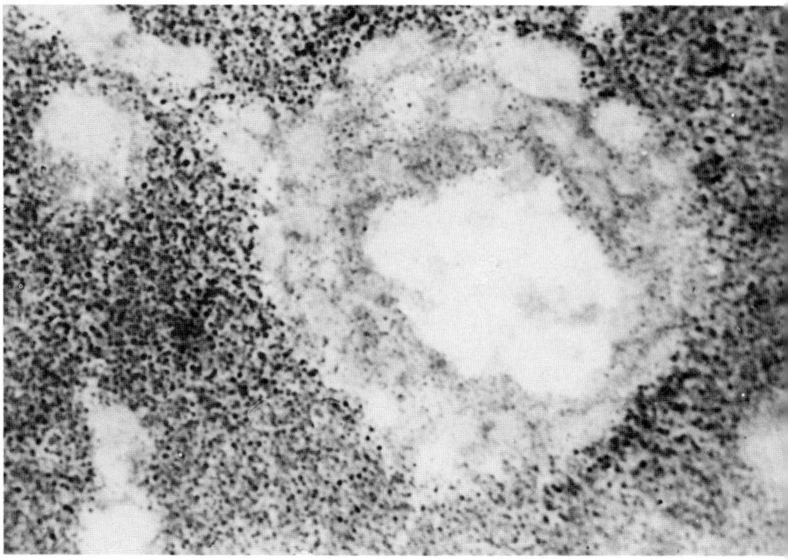

206 EAE. Neutral proteolytic (endopeptidase) activity in perivascular region and surrounding white matter. BANA (naphthylamidase) method, × 100. *(Courtesy of Dr Elena Gabrielescu)*

207

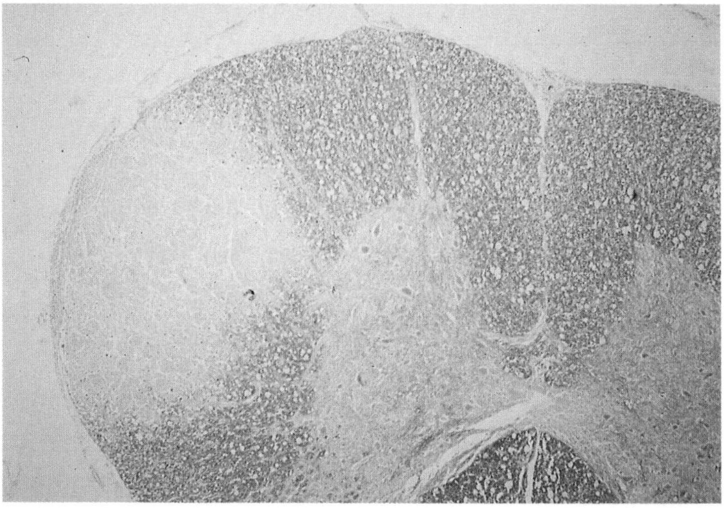

207 Chronic relapsing experimental allergic encephalomyelitis (CREAE). Demyelinating lesion in postero-lateral column of spinal cord. Luxol fast blue, × 10.

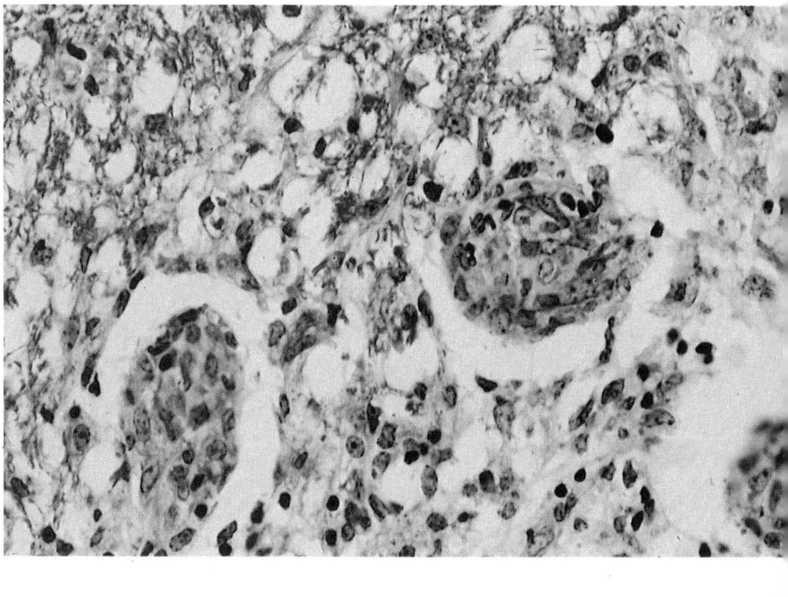

208 CREAE. Perivascular inflammatory infiltrate and demyelination. Haematoxylin-eosin, × 100.

5 Aetiology and epidemiology of multiple sclerosis

Genetic factors

The genetic aspect of multiple sclerosis has been investigated over many years. Older studies were concerned with intra-family and twin studies. These investigations on families led to the conclusion that there is a small but definite familial incidence, which cannot be explained in terms of a common environment during childhood. Subsequent work on tissue histocompatibility antigens has confirmed this genetic factor in MS, and the main associated HLA haplotypes include HLA-A3, B7, DR2, DW2 and DQw1 (Batchelor *et al.*, 1978; Stewart and Kirk, 1983; Francis *et al.*, 1987). It has been suggested that the main haplotype is associated more with raised antibody levels to measles than directly with multiple sclerosis (Visscher *et al.*, 1981), which might indicate that this haplotype determines a raised immune-responsiveness (see below). The DR2 (BT101) histocompatibility antigen confers a four-fold likelihood of developing multiple sclerosis after an attack of optic neuritis (Francis *et al.*, 1987).

Multiple sclerosis is a disease of colder and temperate climates, and is rare in tropical and subtropical countries (**209**). It seems now that the haplotype (or haplotypes) associated with MS are

209 World distribution of multiple sclerosis. Red = high prevalence, yellow = medium, blue = low. *(Courtesy of Dr J.R. Kurtzke)*

209

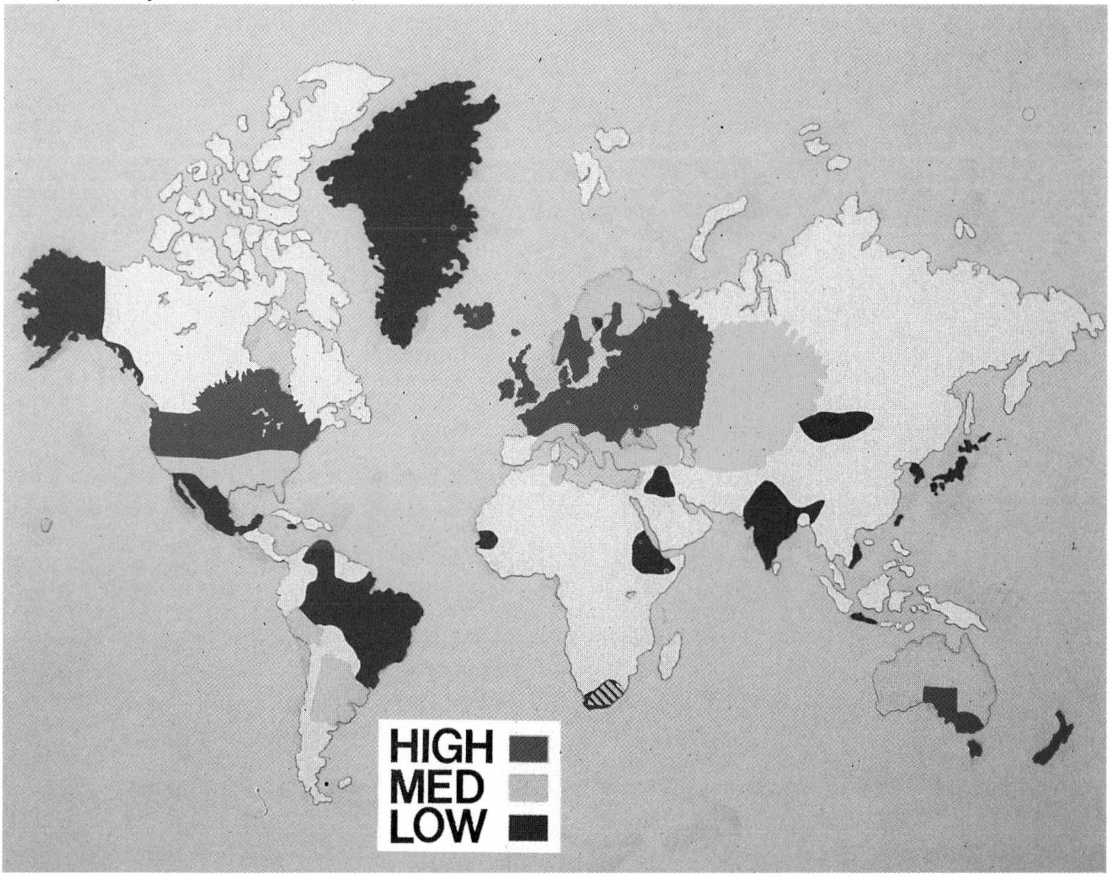

characteristically Scandinavian and, hence, the disease may have originated in this general geographic area (Kurtzke, 1983). Scandinavians have a long history of emigration, mainly to countries with rather less hostile climates but, nevertheless, before the era of air-conditioning, they emigrated to countries with a cooler rather than a hotter climate. In medieval times, the Vikings (Norsemen) emigrated to Scotland, England, Iceland and other Northern islands, to the mainland of Northern Europe (hence the name Normandy) and to Kievan Russia, all of which are areas where MS is prevalent. Some Norsemen penetrated the Mediterranean as far as Sicily and Malta, which latter they colonised (Bowle, 1982). However, Scandinavian genes must by now have become much diluted in these Mediterranean islands, and the prevalence of MS in Malta is actually remarkably low, at 4 cases per 100,000 population (Vassallo *et al.*, 1979), in comparison with the present relatively high prevalence in Sardinia (59 cases per 100,000; Rosati *et al.*, 1987).

Geographic factors

As mentioned above, MS is a disease of temperate climates and is rare in the tropics and subtropics.

The dividing line between areas of high and low prevalence are the longitudes 40°N and 40°S. Japan lies almost entirely below 40°N, and classic MS is rare here. MS is likewise rare in India (Delhi 27°N) and, when the disease occurs, it is often of the fulminating monophasic type, akin to Schilder's disease (see Dastur and Singhal, 1973). Australia is divided from Tasmania by the 40°S parallel and this is reflected in the greater prevalence of the disease in Tasmania than in the rest of Australia. There is also a South-North gradient with an increasing prevalence from Northern Territories, Western Australia, Queensland (Cairns 17°S), South Australia, Tasmania and New Zealand (Acheson, 1972). However, the boundaries at 40°N and 40°S could soon become blurred. If MS is associated with a Scandinavian HLA haplotype, modern comforts such as improved air-conditioning, might encourage emigration of those preferring a cool environment into tropical areas. This could be one explanation for the recently increased prevalence of MS in Queensland (Hammond *et al.*, 1987).

Further instances of this North-South differential can be seen between southern and northern states in the USA (Kurtzke, 1983) and in the prevalence rates in the UK. England and Wales have a lower prevalence rate than Scotland and Northern Ireland; Eire lower than Northern Ireland; and the highest rate in the UK is in the Orkneys and Shetland (Poskanser *et al.*, 1980; Swingler and Compston, 1986). Some doubt has recently been raised about the North-South differential within the United Kingdom, as a prevalence rate of 115 cases per 100,000 population has been recorded in Sutton (S. London) compared with $127/10^5$ in S-E Scotland (Williams and McKeran, 1986). Moreover, the incidence of MS has been declining recently in the Orkneys (Cook *et al.*, 1985). However, the difference between northern Europe at 50 plus cases/10^5 and Mediterranean and Arab countries at 4-10/10^5 speaks for itself (Al Din, 1986; Sosa *et al.*, 1987).

Apart from immigration preferences, another explanation for the North-South gradient in the incidence of multiple sclerosis is that sunlight (particularly in the winter) protects against the disease (Acheson *et al.*, 1960). Although light has profound effects on metabolism, hormone synthesis and diurnal rhythm, there seems to be no clear connection between these climatic factors and the known features of the disease.

Dietary aspects

It has been suggested for many years that lipids may play a role in the development of MS (Swank, 1961; 1970), and deficiencies in polyunsaturated fatty acids (PUFA), particularly linoleic acid, (18:2), have been reported in MS patients (Baker *et al.*, 1966; Fisher *et al.*, 1987). This evidence led to the suggestion that the disease results from a deficiency of PUFA in myelin membranes, in spite of the low metabolic turnover and replacement of most, but not all, of the molecular components of the sheath (Payling Wright, 1961).

Epidemiological evidence has to some extent supported the view that high PUFA intake protects against MS. Thus, the littoral zone of Norway (209) has less MS than the rest of Scandinavia (Swank *et al.*, 1952). The most compelling epidemiological evidence for the inverse correlation between PUFA and MS is the high incidence of the disease in the Shetland and Orkneys (see above), where sheep-rearing is a major agricultural activity. The neighbouring Faroes, by contrast, have had a low incidence of MS since 1960 and before 1940 (Cook *et al.*, 1978a) and rely on fishing and whaling as major sources of food production. However, even though these two communities might be expected, respectively, to eat diets high in animal saturated fat and high in fish or whale polyunsaturated oil, there is no firm evidence on this score. Whether the efforts of Greenpeace will in future years redress the balance remains to be seen.

No study has been made on the incidence of coronary disease and cholelithiasis in the Faroes, Orkney and Shetland islands, both of which might be expected to be influenced by the amount of PUFA in the diet. In fact, if PUFA have any role in MS, the disease should show a positive correlation with coronary disease and a negative correlation with cholelithiasis and other diseases associated with gallstones (see Oliver *et al.*, 1978; Chapter 10). A high polyunsaturated diet has been explored in MS and seems to have a marginal benefit in reducing the severity of relapses, but does not influence the rate of clinical deterioration (Millar *et al.*, 1973, 1975; Liversedge, 1977; Bates *et al.*, 1978; Tourtellotte and Baumhefner, 1983). The possible action of PUFA, particularly linoleic acid, in reducing the severity of a relapse may be due to its slight immuno-suppressive action (Mertin and Meade, 1977).

The other dietary hypothesis that has been aired is that coeliac disease (gluten enteropathy) is a cause of MS, presumably by interfering with the absorption of some essential nutriment. However, two separate biopsy studies on MS patients (Bateson *et al.*, 1979; Jones *et al.*, 1979) show normal histological, histochemical and ultrastructural features in the brush border of the small intestine (a finding quite inconsistent with coeliac disease), while a gluten-free diet fails to influence the course of MS (Liversedge, 1977; Tourtellotte and Baumhefner, 1983). Hence, gluten sensitivity as a dietary factor in multiple sclerosis can, in practical terms, be excluded.

Infective disease

Emigrants from Northern Europe to Israel (32°N) or to South Africa (Cape Town, 34°S) have a higher incidence of multiple sclerosis than those native-born (Dean, 1970; Alter *et al.*, 1978; Kurtzke, 1983). However, those who emigrated as children show the same low incidence as the native-born. The converse situation is that individuals born in the United Kingdom from immigrant parents from the Caribbean islands suffer the same high incidence of MS as the indigenous white population (Elian and Dean, 1987). The general tenor of this evidence has been interpreted to show that MS is a disease which is contracted in late childhood or early adolescence (puberty) and becomes clinically evident some 10 years later. In the Faroes epidemic (see below), the latent period was apparently 5-6 years.

The low incidence of MS in hotter climates has been explained by supposing that children become exposed early to a variety of infective conditions (particularly enteric viruses) in hot climates, and develop immunity to them at an early age, before the critical age at which MS begins (Poskanzer *et al*, 1963). For example, paralytic poliomyelitis is rare in tropical countries, because the disease occurs in infancy when paralytic complications do not develop. Attractive though this view may be to explain the North/South gradient in MS, it is difficult to find any substantial direct evidence for it.

MS patients exhibit raised antibody levels to a wide range of viruses, including measles, varicella and rubella (see Ter Meulen and Stephenson, 1983). A simple view of this observation would be that MS is an inflammatory syndrome caused by a wide variety of viruses. Nevertheless, it seems more likely that these elevated antibody levels reflect an increased immunoresponsiveness in the MS patient, possibly an example of the anamnestic response (Adams, 1972; Sibley *et al.*, 1985; see Visscher *et al.*, 1981 above; Compston *et al.*, 1986).

Further epidemiological evidence in favour of an infective origin for MS has been provided by Kurtzke (1983) in that epidemics of MS have occurred with sudden influxes of populations from high risk areas. The best example of this was an epidemic of MS in the Faroes, confined to the years between 1943-1960, which was related to the occupation of these islands by British troops during World War II and is an example of a 'point-source' epidemic. This epidemic of MS in the Faroes was discussed in Section 3 in relation to a simultaneous epidemic of canine distemper (Cook *et al.*, 1978a).

Acheson (1977) points out that, in general, MS is common in colder and wetter climates, areas where upper respiratory tract infections are common. This could be linked to the recent observation by Gay and Dick (1986) and Gay *et al.*, (1986) that chronic sinusitis and sinus sepsis are common in MS patients. They consider that MS may result from an organism penetrating from the nasal sinuses into the cavernous sinus through the thin bone lining the inner surface of the nasal sinuses. The relationship of the main drainage veins, venous sinuses and the ventricular system to the optic chiasm, periventricular regions and other common sites for MS plaques is discussed in Chapter 8.

A study of infective disease in monozygotic twins showed that where one twin developed MS, this twin had more childhood infections than the unaffected sibling while, where both twins developed MS, the earlier case suffered such diseases at an earlier age (Currier and Eldridge, 1982).

As mentioned in Chapter 3, there have been repeated claims for identifying spirochaetes, viruses and other micro-organisms as the cause of MS, but these have been shown to be unfounded or artefacts (see Ter Meulen and Stevenson, 1983). The brain, in fact, seems to be a repository for a wide range of 'passenger' viruses. The Borrelia of Lyme Disease is the latest micro organism to be considered, but the evidence linking Borrelia burgdorfi to MS is unconvincing (*Lancet* annotation, 1987). In future years, molecular pathology may be expected to resolve the problem but present results are incomplete. An earlier in-situ hybridisation study using a measles virus DNA probe identified measles virus in 1 of 4 cases of MS (Haase *et al.*, 1981), but it was not clear whether or not it might have been an opportunistic infection in a debilitated patient on steroids. However, this work is supported by a study on further MS cases where plaques were shown to contain measles virus by in-situ hybridisation (Allen, I.V. and others, to be published). Another in-situ hybridisation study has been concerned with a DNA probe for human corona virus in MS tissue, but this proved negative (Sorensen *et al.*, 1986).

Most investigators in the MS field have tacitly assumed that viral infection (not necessarily a specific virus) or injury triggers the initial events in MS. Subsequently, an autoimmune response would amplify the process into a major relapsing disease. The suggestion that certain enveloped viruses can both induce (transactivate) Class II antigens in certain cells and incorporate such Class II antigens and the hosts' antigens into the viral envelope, outlines a possible mechanism for an autoimmune reaction in MS (Dalgleish *et al.*, 1987). The cell with the induced Class II antigen would then be recognised by the T lymphocyte as an antigen-presenting cell, presenting its own antigens for the T lymphocyte to attack (*see* Chapter 9).

6 Gross pathology and distribution of MS lesions

Naked-eye appearances and fixation

The lesions of multiple sclerosis are not always easy to see on naked eye inspection of the cut unfixed brain. Active lesions appear pale pinkish-brown, (210 and 211), whereas chronic lesions appear grey brown and often are of a gelatinous texture (212). Indeed, one of the original terms for multiple sclerosis was 'grey degeneration' (Rindfleisch, 1873). In addition, active cases show either focal lesions that are too small to be seen or a diffuse ill-defined friable area usually located in the central white matters of the hemispheres (213; Jellinger, 1969). These ill-defined lesions are very difficult to distinguish and are a non-specific feature, shared with other demyelinating diseases and leucodystrophies, and perhaps representing a 'transitional type' between classic MS and Schilder's diffuse sclerosis (Jellinger, 1969).

Established plaques of any size are rarely completely circular in profile and take on a geographic outline (214). This geographic or serpiginous outline is mainly due to the irregular outward growth of the plaques at its edges in the form of Dawson's fingers (215 and 216). Dawson's fingers are more fully explained in Chapter 7: it suffices here to say that they are extensions of the plaque alongside veins (Dawson, 1916 a,b,c).

For research purposes, it is often necessary to cut the brain unfixed or to compromise with immediate cutting of one hemisphere and leaving the rest of the brain to be fixed in formalin. Undoubtedly, MS lesions are easier to see in fixed brain tissue and, clearly, this is the method of choice for a careful anatomical analysis of lesions. Brains should be fixed in as large a container as possible in 10 per cent formalin (4 per cent formaldehyde), which should be changed several times over 6 weeks to obtain best fixation. During fixation, many brains seem to suffer from the artefacts of either swelling or shrinkage, particularly around vessels. Hence, it is important to ensure that the formalin solution is made up to be isotonic.

The optic pathway

The optic pathway is involved in most MS patients, estimated by Lumsden (1970) at 93 per cent of cases and by Ulrich and Groebke-Lorenz (1983) at 100 per cent of cases. Surprisingly only 44 per cent of patients in the latter study had had clinical optic neuritis. A cursory examination of the optic chiasm is not enough; the full length of the optic nerves and tracts have to be examined. Optic neuritis is, of course, the most common presenting symptom of MS, optic pallor is evidence of its presence (**217**) and the resulting delayed electrical conduction is used in the sensitive clinical test of the visually evoked potential (VEP; **218**). The involvement of the optic pathway may be mild (**219**) or more severe (**220** to **229**). The comparative series of Figures **220** to **229** shows how staining methods distinguish between plaques with retained axons and those with locally destroyed axons. Surprisingly, even when segments of both optic nerves are totally demyelinated, patients may still have adequate vision (Wisnewski *et al.*, 1976).

Gross distribution of lesions in the hemispheres

Most cases of multiple sclerosis show lesions around the lateral ventricles (**210**, **212**, **230**, **231** and **232**). The frequency of these periventricular lesions varies between 82 per cent in our series to 90 per cent in Lumsden's (1970) report.

In the hemispheres, plaques are characteristically seen in the central white or callosal radiation (**233** to **235**), in the corpus callosum (**230** upper right and lower left), in the subcortical white matter or grey-white margin (**236**) and, contrary to popular belief, small lesions may be located in the grey matter or cortex (**237**). Lumsden (1970) records that a majority of lesions in the hemispheres may be in the cortex, but this is not our experience. Lesions in the hemispheres show no special localisation to a particular lobe (see above figures), but frequently show a connection with a periventricular plaque in the form of a Dawson's finger (see above; **238** to **243**).

the form of a Dawson's finger (see above; **238** to **243**).

MS lesions can be detected by Xray computerised tomography (CT; **238** and **239**). Periventricular plaques and Dawson's fingers are particularly well seen by magnetic resonance imaging (MRI; **240, 241** and **243**; Ormerod *et al.*, 1987; Gonzales-Scarano *et al.*, 1987; Hallpike, 1988). Plaques have also been demonstrated by MRI in the swollen cervical cord, corpus callosum (including the subcallosal ependymal-regions) and in the subcortical white matter (Simon *et al.*, 1986; see **230** to **233**).

The hypothalamus and basal nuclei do not often seem to be primarily involved in MS, except by extensions from periventricular lesions (**212**). In the cerebral hemispheres, the prime focus of attack is usually the periventricular region (see Moxon, 1875; Fog, 1965; Adams *et al.*, 1987) and from there the lesions extend outwards into the central white matter in the form of Dawson's fingers (**244** and **245**). It is perhaps at this juncture appropriate to mention that the optic chiasm is in contact with the IIIrd ventricle, in the form of a forward extension that abuts on to the posterior surface of the chiasm (**246**) and, hence, lesions in the optic pathway have a direct relationship to the ventricular system.

The gross distribution of lesions in the brainstem and cerebellum

Plaques are commonly encountered around the IVth ventricle (**247**; 60 per cent in our series) and somewhat less frequently around the aqueduct (**248** and **249**). Lesions are also encountered commonly in the rest of the midbrain and often extend from the aqueduct into the tectum and tegmentum, and may involve the substantia nigra and basis pedunculi (**248** to **250**). The lesions around the aqueduct and IVth ventricle may extend into the cerebral peduncles or pons along the course of veins (**248** and **249, 251** and **252**) in the form of Dawson's fingers (see above).

Multiple pontine lesions are common and were seen in 54 per cent of our original series (**247, 251** to **256**). Sometimes the extent of demyelination in the pons is so extensive that it is difficult to understand how the patient had survived for so long (**255** and **256**). However, Wisniewski *et al.* (1976) showed that complete loss of myelin does not result in complete conduction loss. Other pontine lesions seem to be remarkably small for the symptoms and signs produced (**257**). No doubt this reflects the extent of axonal damage. This is illustrated in **258** and **259**, where the patient suffered from ataxia, and the small demyelinating lesion in the middle cerebellar peduncle showed some axonal loss.

Medullary lesions are common in hyperacute cases (**260** and **261**; see Chapter 7), possibly because they interrupt vital centres at an early stage and, hence, are associated with sudden and early death. Larger and more chronic lesions often involve the olives (**262**).

Lesions in the cerebellar white matter are not as common as might be supposed (6 per cent in our series). The dentate nucleus can sometimes be confused with a plaque (**263**), but true demyelinating lesions can easily be distinguished (**264** and **265**). A small focus of demyelination at the root of a cerebellar folium is seen in **266**.

The spinal cord in MS

Multiple sclerosis in the spinal cord is a common presentation of the disease. Involvement of the long tracts leads to muscular weakness, sensory loss or paraesthesiae, and bladder disturbances and may eventually lead to reduced respiratory efficiency.

The cervical part is the most common site for MS plaques in the spinal cord (**267** to **270**). They can be demonstrated here by magnetic resonance imaging: active plaques may be swollen on account of oedema, whereas chronic plaques are shrunken due to gliosis (Nilsson *et al.*, 1987). Plaques in the cord are clearly circular in outline and do not pick out individual tracts (*see* Chapter 2, **122** to **126**). However, Wallerian degeneration may sometimes be present in a long tract. It is comparatively easy to distinguish between a plaque and Wallerian degeneration, in that the latter is confined to a particular tract or tracts, does not spread into adjacent grey matter, is usually incomplete, does not show perivascular cuffing and the axons have also disappeared. However, this last characteristic can be confusing, as chronic plaques of MS frequently show axonal loss (*see* Chapters 1 and 2). Wallerian degeneration may be seen in the spinal roots if the lower motor or sensory neurone is involved in a plaque before leaving the cord (**271** to **275**). The occurrence of demyelinating neuropathy in the PNS in MS is discussed in the next sub-section.

Lhermitte's sign results from pressure on the posterior columns in the upper cervical cord, and this causes an 'electric shock' or stabbing pain in the extremities. This pressure may result from osteoarhritic protrusions into the spinal canal, particularly compressing the posterior roots, but it may also be encountered in MS where a plaque in the posterior columns of the cervical cord is particularly vulnerable and hypersensitive to the effects of pressure Hallpike, 1983).

It has been claimed that plaques are frequently ymmetrical (Lumsden, 1970), but our series shows only a few partly symmetrical lesions (**276** to **279**). A kissing' plaque across a fissure is a rare variant of ymmetricality: our series shows just one plaque in his category (**279**, bottom left and mid right). Symmetrical lesions are uncommon in MS, so that their occurrence cannot be abscribed any significance apart from coincidence.

Devic's disease (*see* Chapter 2) is a syndrome of monophasic demyelinating, diffuse inflammatory or necrotic disease in the upper cervical cord, associated with optic neuritis (Cloys and Netsky, 1970). Lumsden (1970) held the view that Devic's disease is only the tip of the iceberg and that other demyelinating lesions will be found in the brain at autopsy. However, other workers subscribe to a much wider pathogenesis for Devic's disease: the cases illustrated in **60**, **61** and **280** were diseases of acute onset where both the upper cord and optic pathway showed a diffuse encephalomyelitis, usually of a necrotic rather than a demyelinating nature. No other foci were found in the CNS at autopsy. The range of disorders associated with Devic's disease includes MS, pulmonary tuberculosis, and acute infective diseases (Hughes and Mair, 1977). It seems, therefore, that Devic's disease cannot be directly equated with MS and that an acute encephalomyelitis from other causes may present in the same manner.

In our series (as in others), the cord was not removed in all cases, so it is not possible to adduce accurately the frequency or cord lesions in MS from these cases. However, Lumsden records a frequency of 75 per cent in his autopsies, which accords with the 80 per cent frequency in our cases where the spinal cord had been removed. Although no real substitute for a complete examination of the cord, the upper cervical cord (the most frequent site of MS cord lesions) can be removed at autopsy through the foramen magnum with the aid of a long curved bistoury. This is a particularly useful compromise when only a limited autopsy can be carried out.

The peripheral nervous system in MS

Hitherto, it has been held that peripheral nerves are not directly involved in MS, but Thomas *et al.*, (1987) have recently published a series of 6 cases that suggest that a demyelinating peripheral neuropathy may occasionally occur in MS. Their conclusion depended on the observation of thin myelin sheaths and short internodal lengths of myelin in the peripheral nerves. These findings are hallmarks of demyelination with subsequent incomplete remyelination, and do not occur in Wallerian degeneration.

Demyelinating neuropathy (radicular polyneuritis) has also been recorded in association with MS by Pollock *et al.* (1977), Forrester and Lascelles (1979), Lassmann *et al.* (1981), Sanders and Lee (1987) and by Rubin *et al.* (1987). Hypertrophic neuropathy in MS has been reported by Schoene *et al.* (1977). Hughes (1985) and Poser (1987) reviewed other cases where a demyelinating neuropathy occurred in association with MS (also *see* Chapter 2). Wallerian degeneration in the PNS distal to a plaque in the cord is discussed above.

2

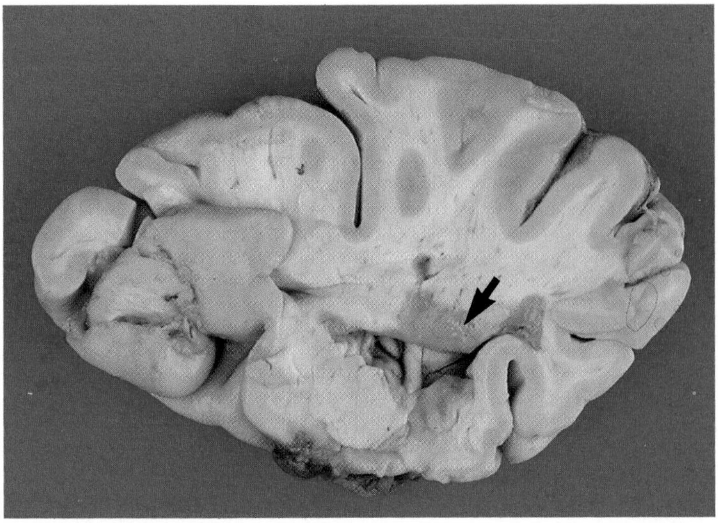

210 Periventricular plaque in lateral ventricle to show typical translucent grey colour of chronic lesion (arrow), × 1.

2

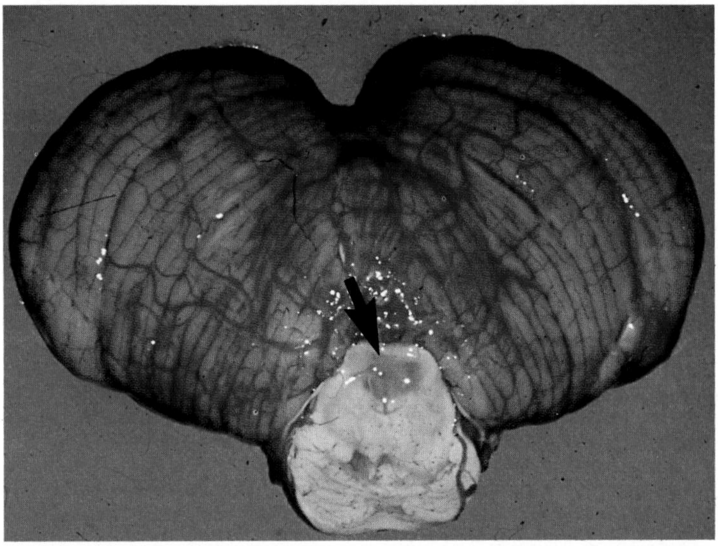

211 Periaqueductal plaque in midbrain (arrow), × 1.

2

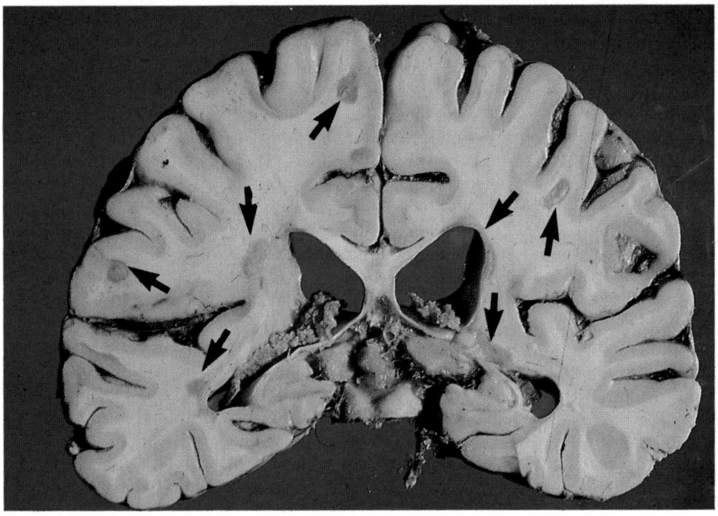

212 A very common pattern of MS. Multiple subcortical, periventricular and central white matter plaques. Note grey translucency of chronic lesions, × ½.

213

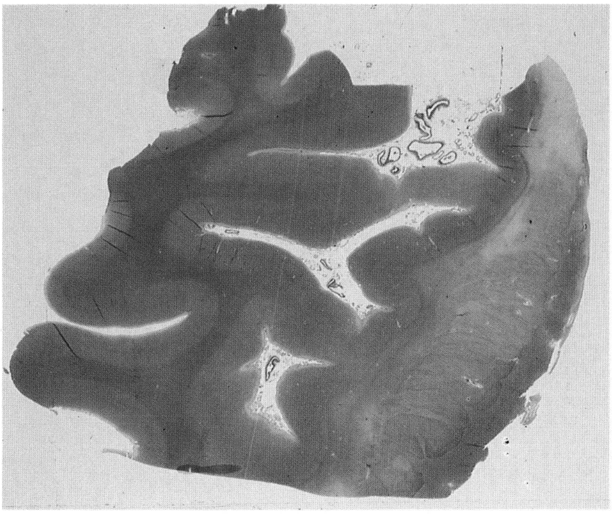

213 Myelin pallor and early ill-defined plaque (top-right). Haematoxylin-eosin, × 2.

214

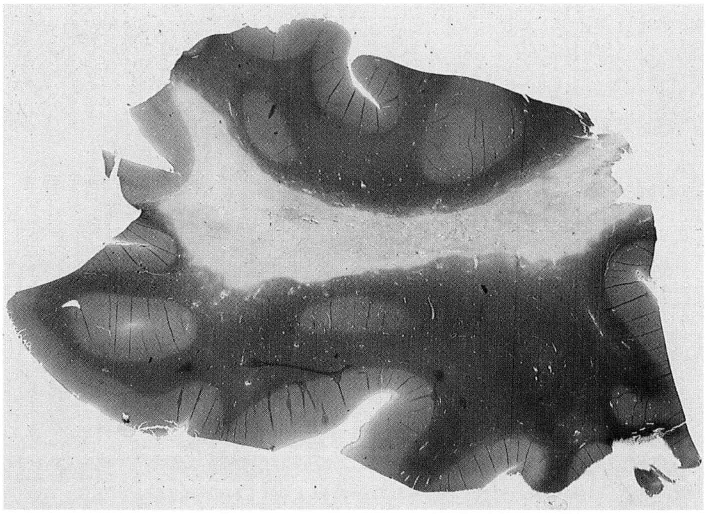

214 Chronic burnt-out sharply defined plaque with no residual axons. Phosphotungstic acid haematoxylin, × 2.

215

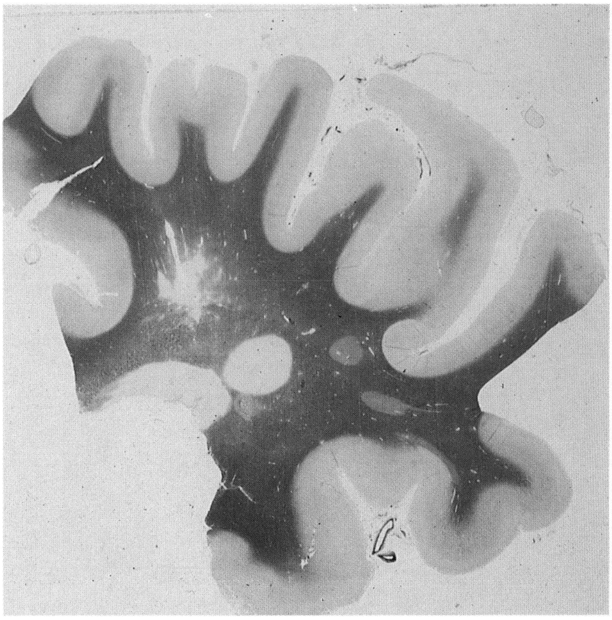

215 Chronic periventricular and adjacent circular plaque, with two shadow plaques and active star-like lesion in central white matter. Luxol fast blue, × 2.

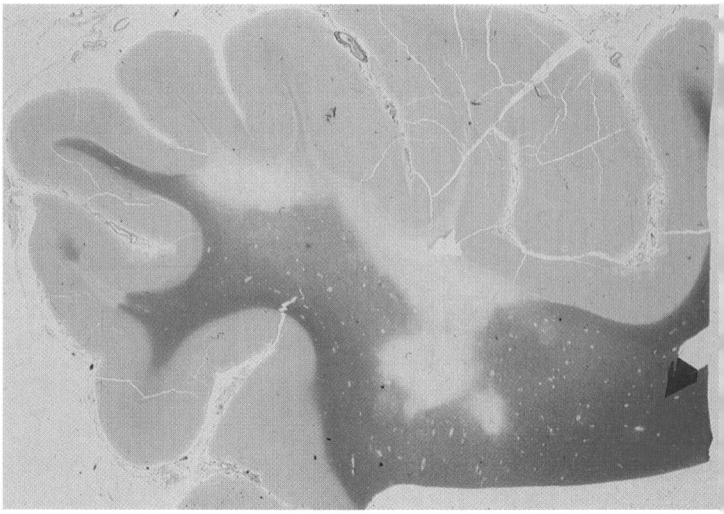

216 Chronic plaque extending into central white matter as a Dawson's 'fist'. Luxol fast blue-picric acid, × 2.

217 Optic neuritis, note sharply defined pale margin to right half of disc. *(Courtesy of Professor W.I. McDonald)*

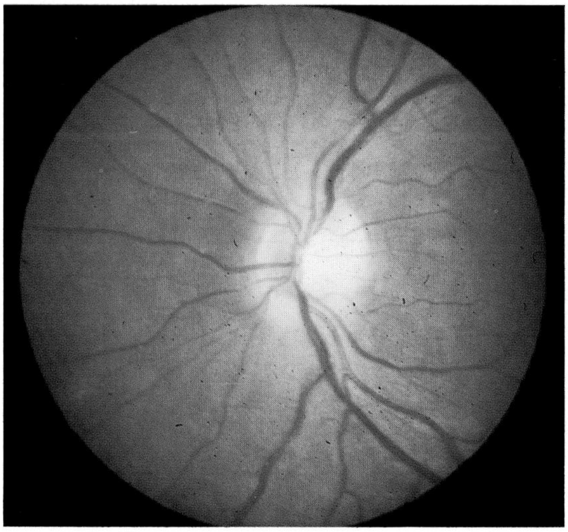

217

218 Visually evoked potentials. Left: normal conduction. Right: delayed conduction in right eye. (*Courtesy of Professor W.I. McDonald)*

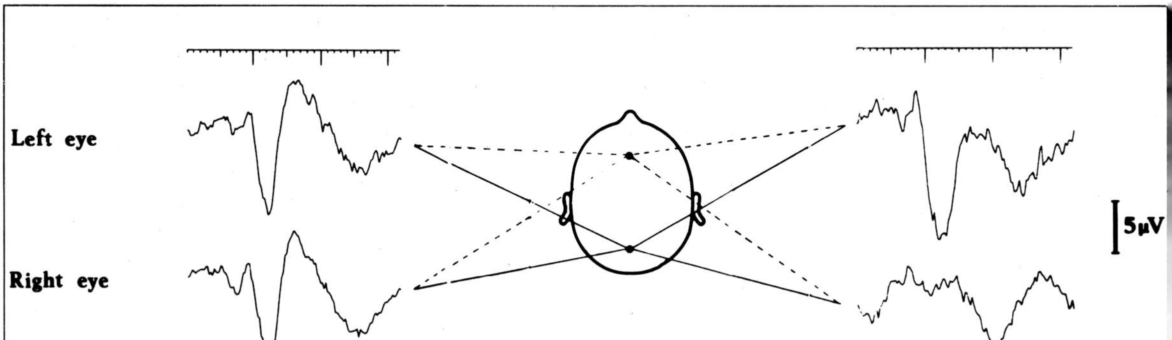

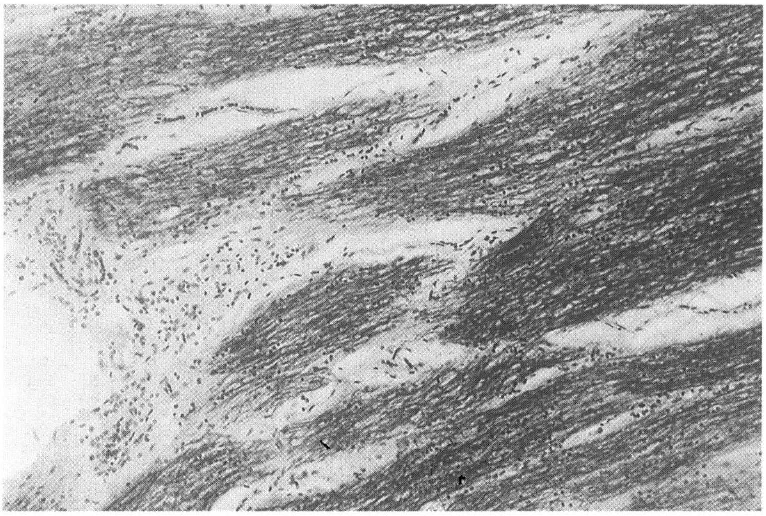
219

219 Small active plaque with inflammatory infiltrate (left) in optic chiasm. Luxol fast blue, cresyl violet, × 60.

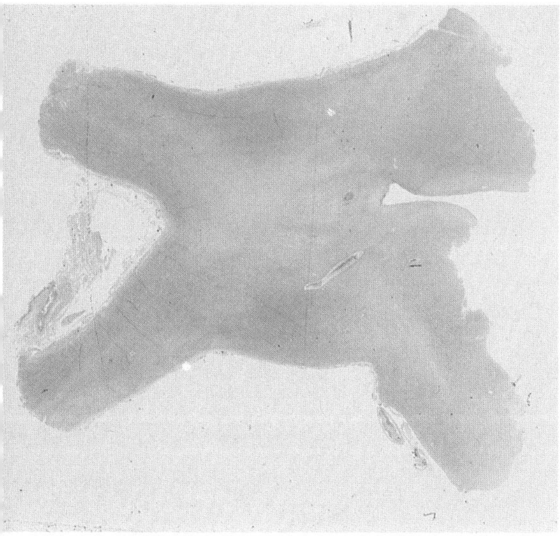
220

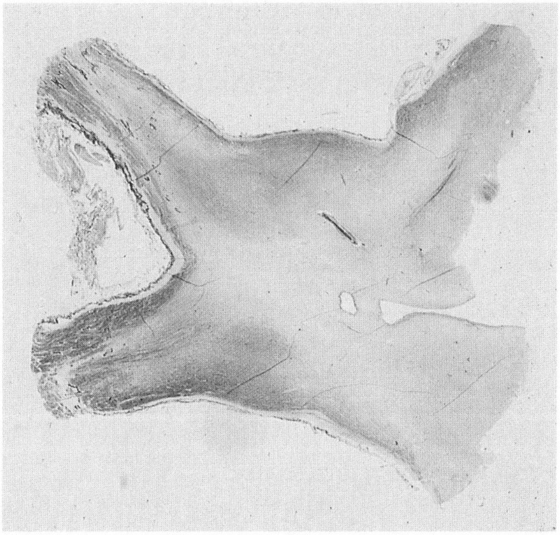
221

220 to **222 Optic chiasm 220** (haematoxylin-eosin); **221** (Luxol fast blue) and **222** (Palmgren silver). Chronic demyelinating plaque. The Palmgren stain shows considerable axonal loss, × 1.

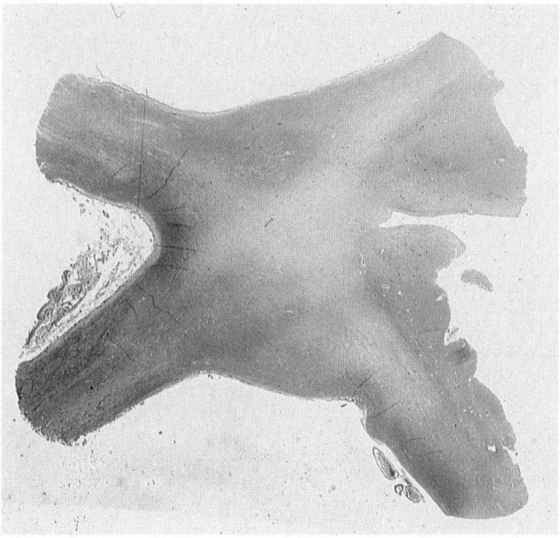
222

223

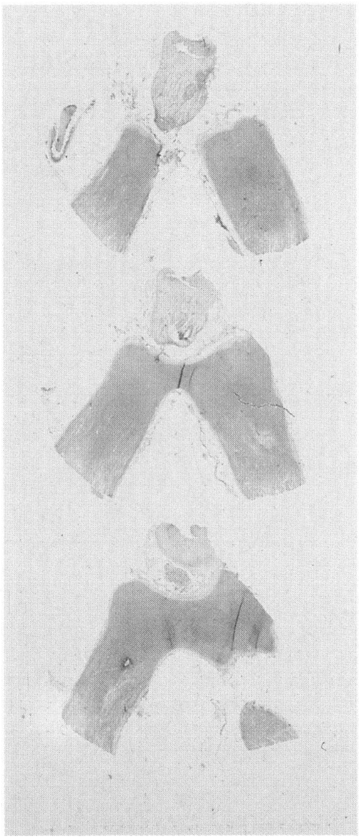

224

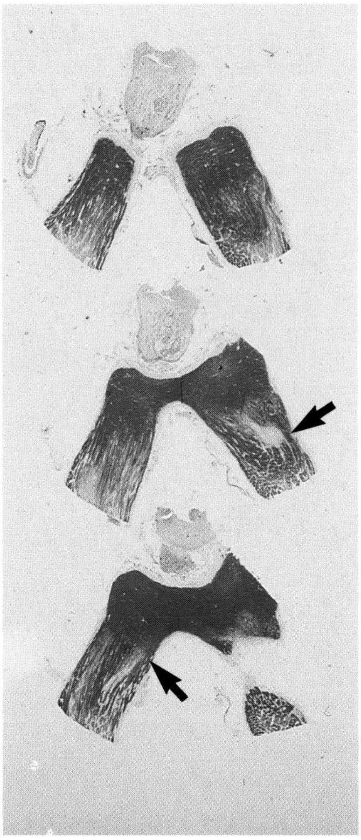

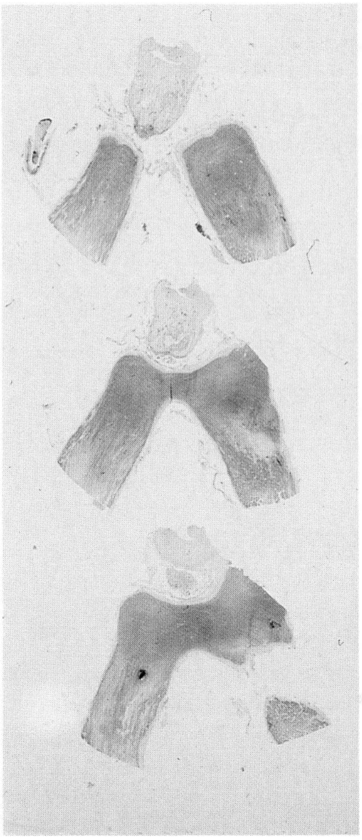

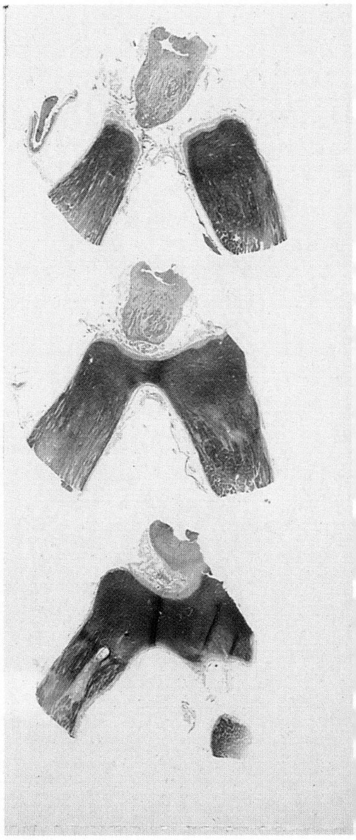

223 to **226** Optic nerve in old optic neuritis: **223** haematoxylin-eosin, **224** (Heidenhain), **225** (Luxol fast blue), and **226** (Weil-Davenport silver). Considerable loss of myelin in both optic nerves, but with less loss of axonal staining, × 2.

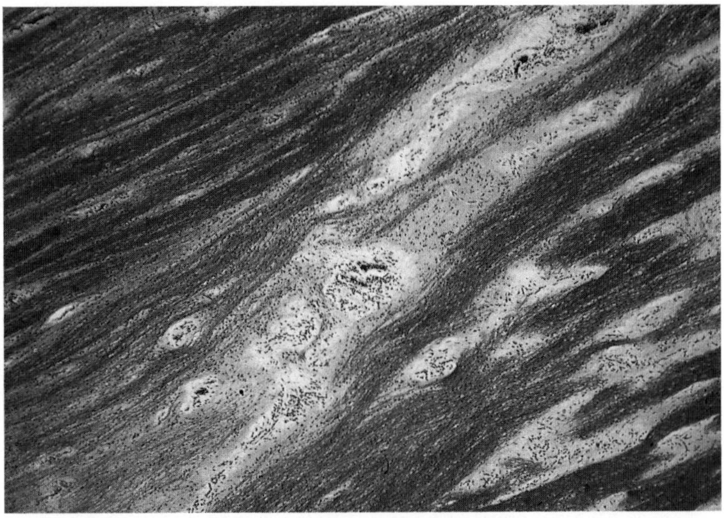
227

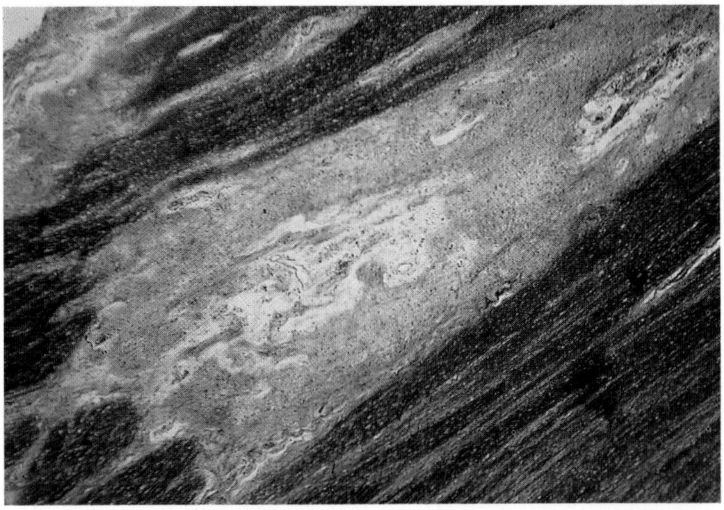
228

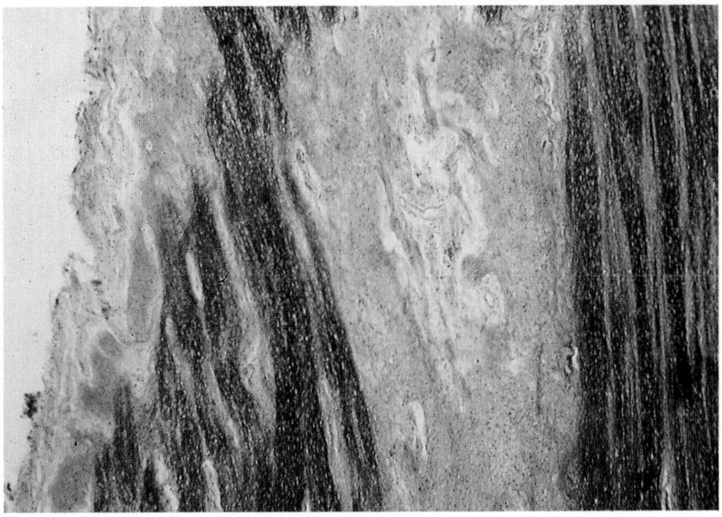
229

27 to 229 Optic nerve in old optic euritis: 227 (Luxol fast blue), **228** Heidenhain) and **229** (Weil-avenport). Chronic lesion with myelin oss and marked axonal loss, × 80.

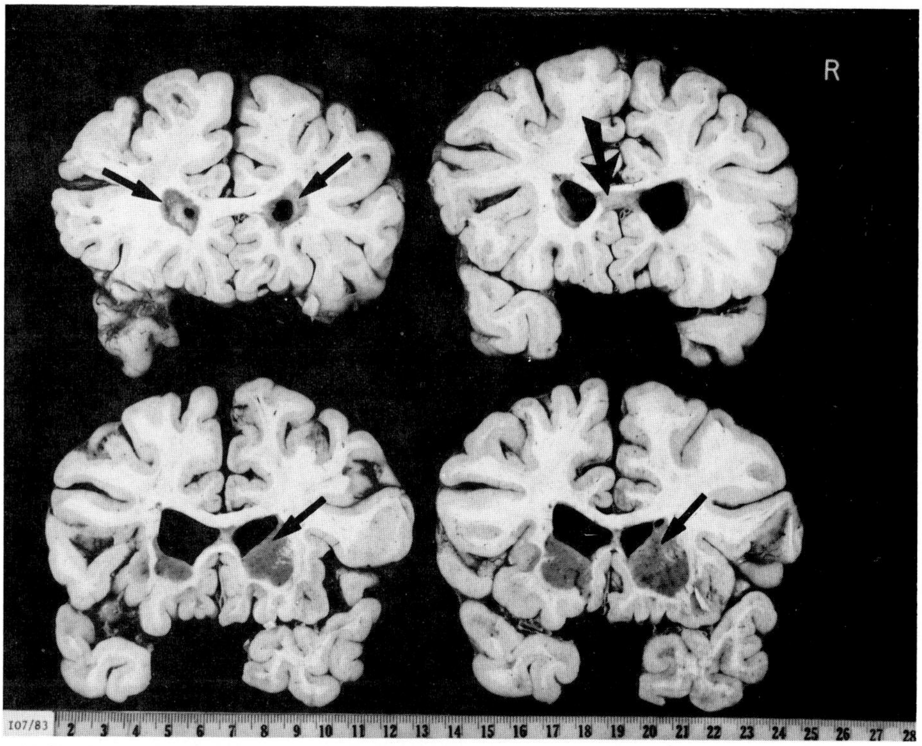

230 Periventricular lesions, a) at level of anterior commissure, b) in corpus callosum, c) and d) in floor of lateral ventricle and in septum pellucidum, × 1/4.

231 Large periventricular plaques around horns of lateral ventricle, same case as **230**, × 1/4.

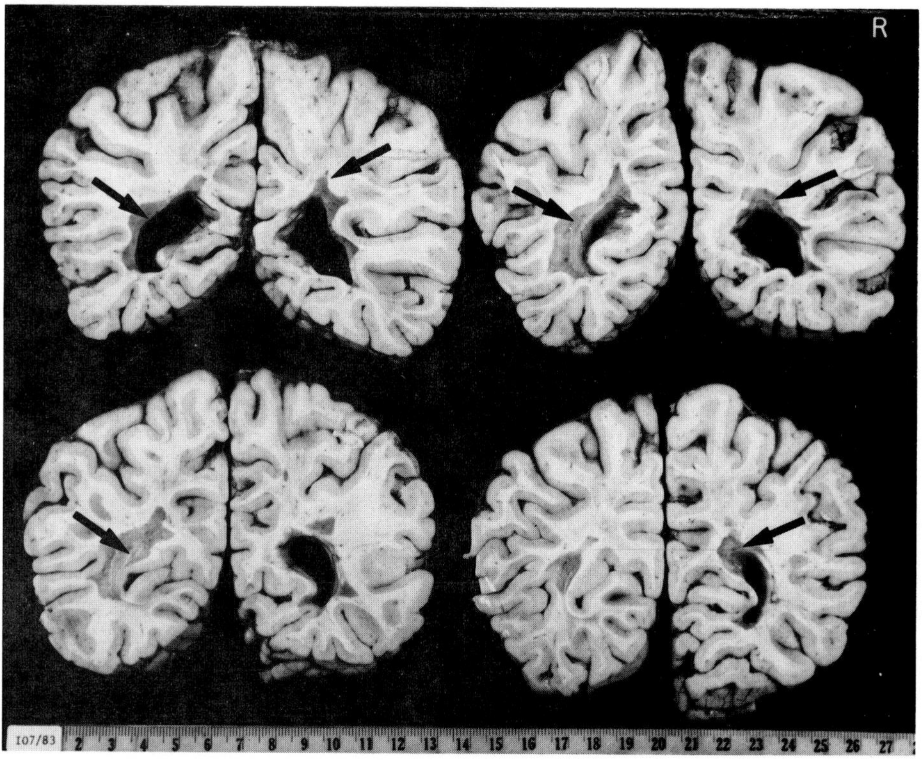

232

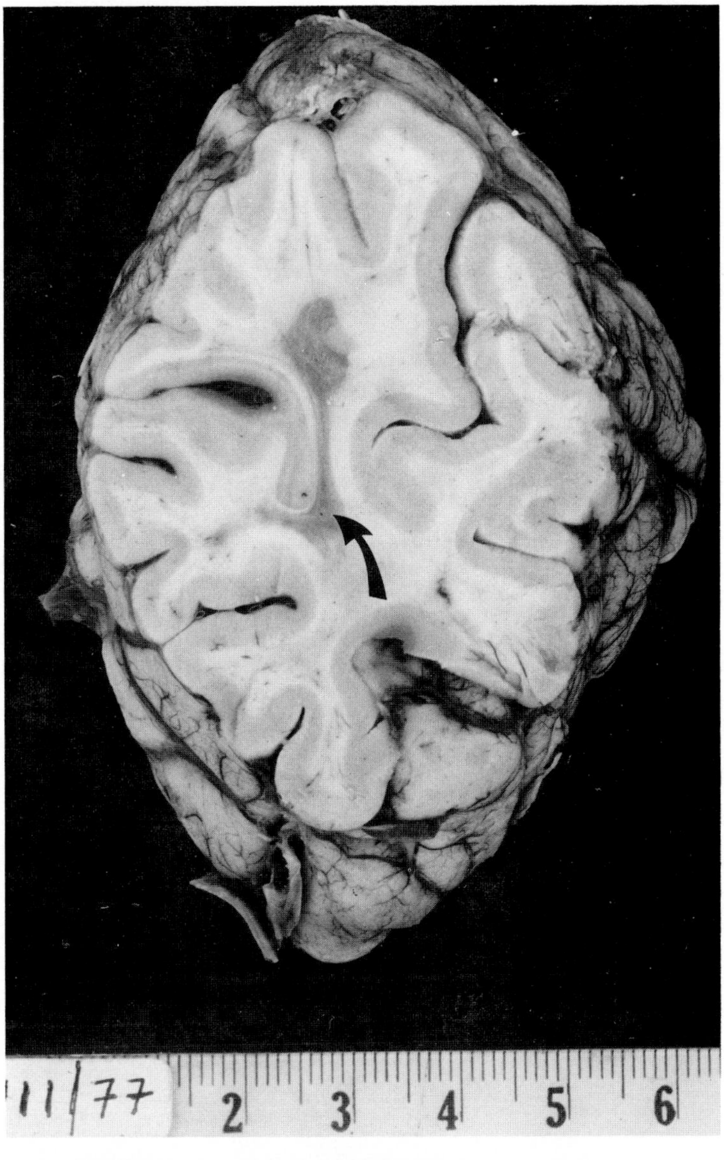

32 Plaque of multiple sclerosis in ntral white matter in continuity with teral ventricle, × 1.

233

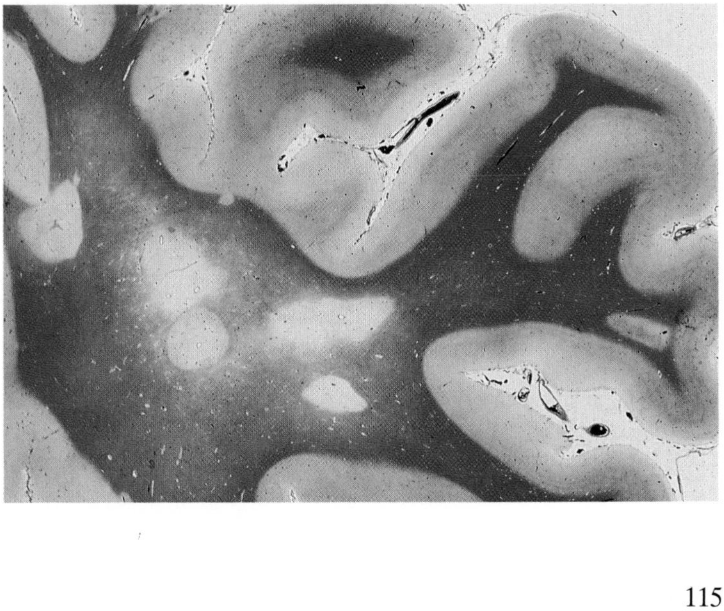

33 Periventricular plaque with urrounding extensions, some ctive with ragged edges and some active with sharp margins. hosphotungstic acid-haematoxylin, 2.

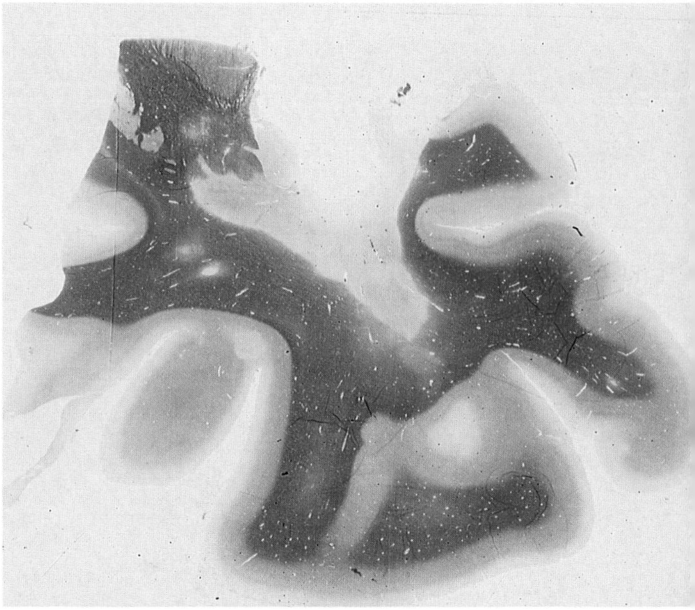

234 Multiple small mainly irregularly-edged active lesions in central white matter, apparently arising from periventricular plaque (lower central), × 1½.

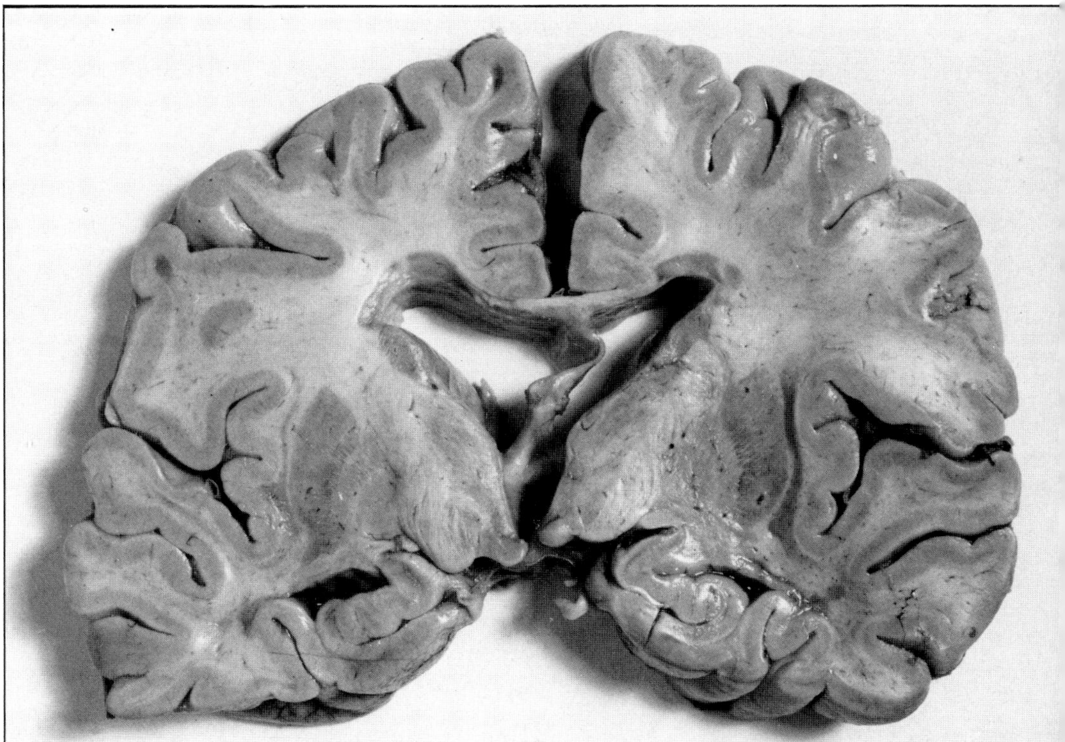

235 Ventricular dilatation and bilateral periventricular plaques. There is some overall loss of central white matter associated with ventricular dilatation, × 1.

236

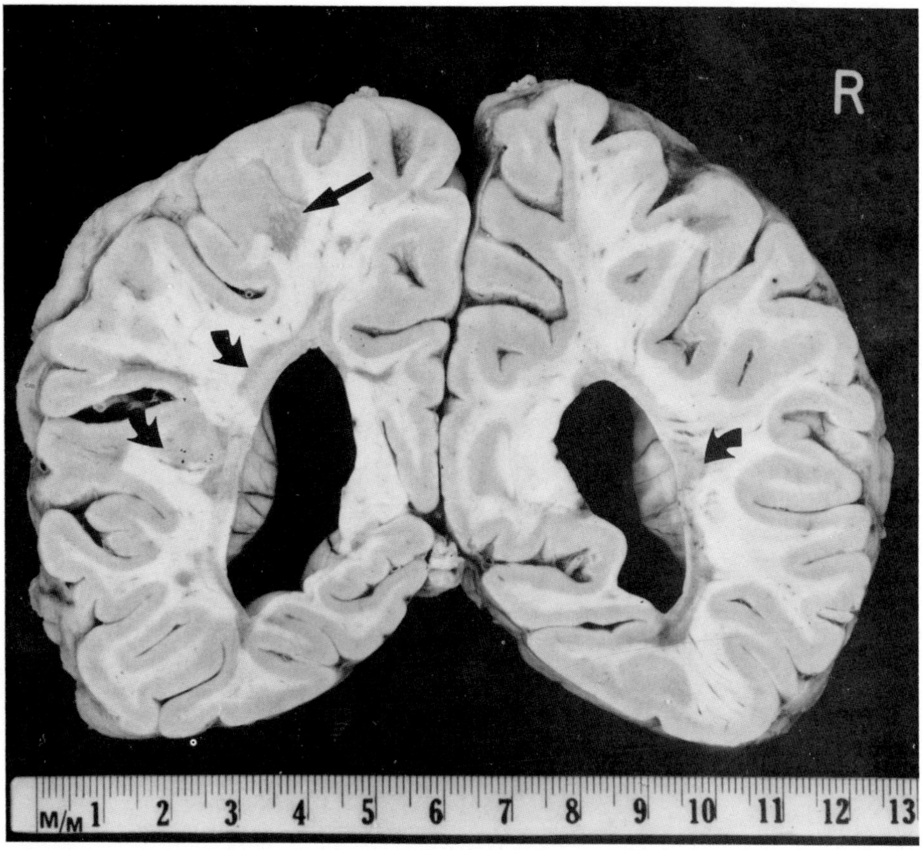

236 Plaques sited at cortico-medullary junction in central white matter and around lateral ventricles. Note ventricular dilatation, × 3/4.

237

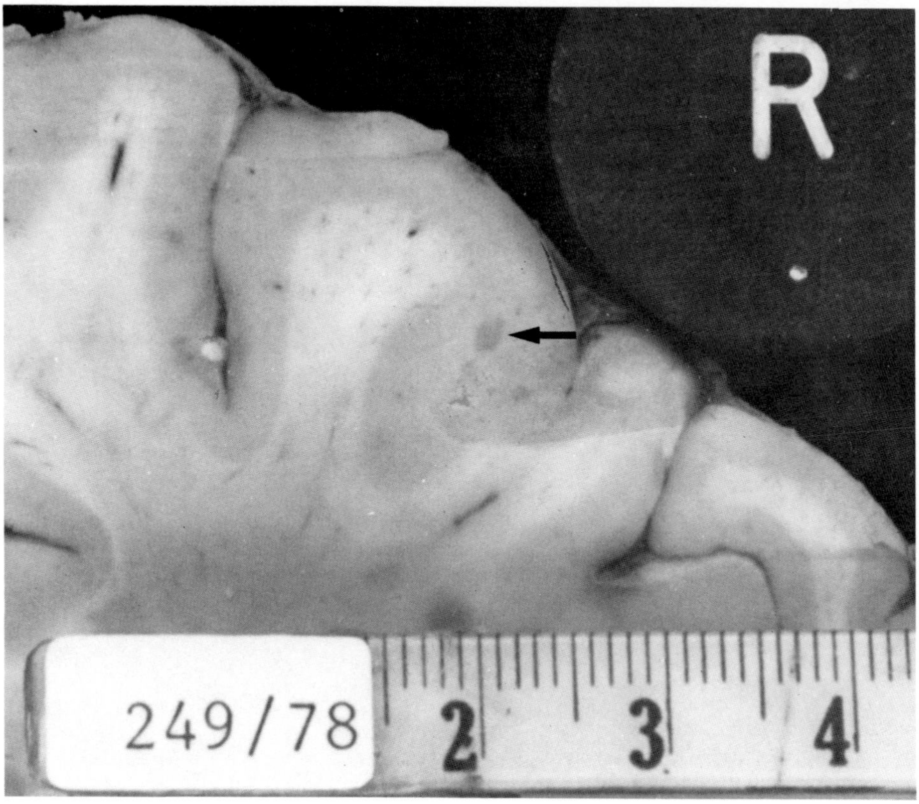

237 Plaque of multiple sclerosis in grey matter, × 4.

238
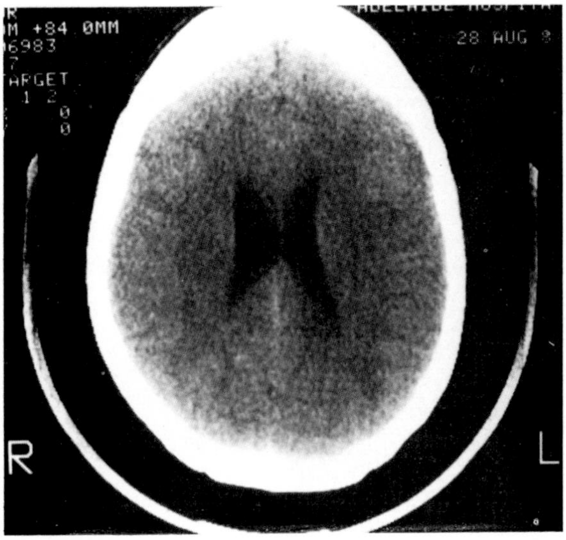

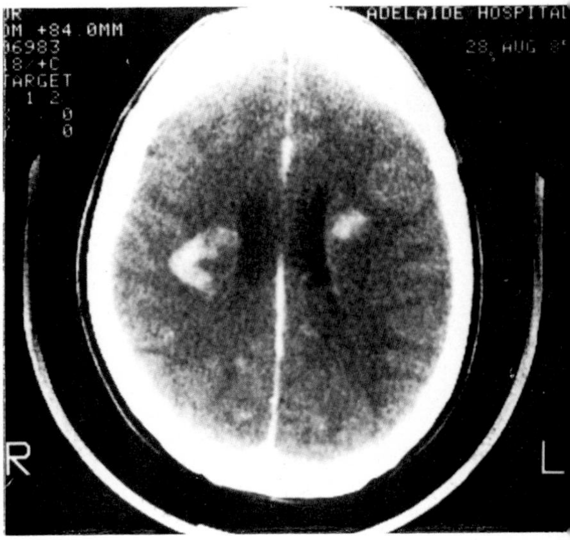

240
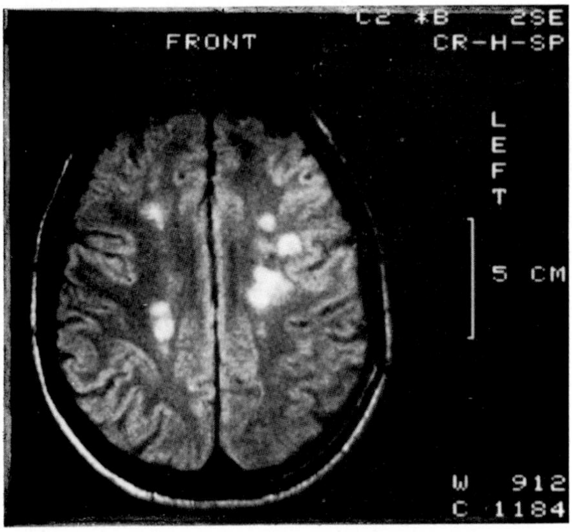

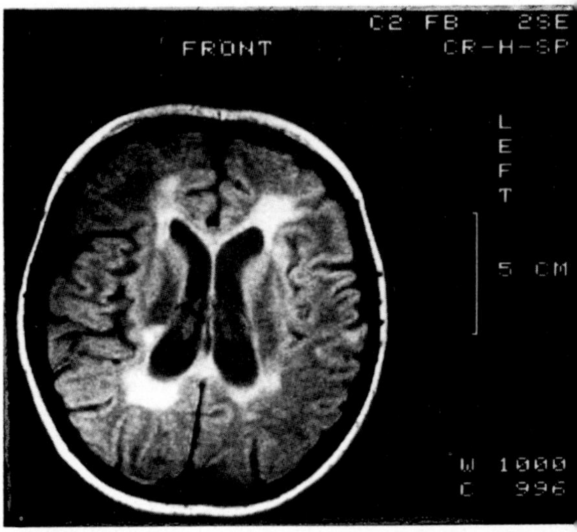

238 and **239** A 23-year-old female at initial diagnosis of MS. Xray CT before (**238**) and after (**239**) intravenous ionic contrast showing multiple areas of abnormal enhancement (BBB effects).

240 and **241** A 38-year-old, well-established progressive clinically definite MS. T2 – weighted MRI (short TE – 'proton density') images showing multiple 'high-signal' lesions in hemispherical white matter (**240**) and irregular periventricular changes confluent at the horns (**241**). 1.0 – Tesla superconductive Siemens magneton. *(Courtesy of Dr J. F. Hallpike and Addis Press Ltd; Hallpike, 1988)*

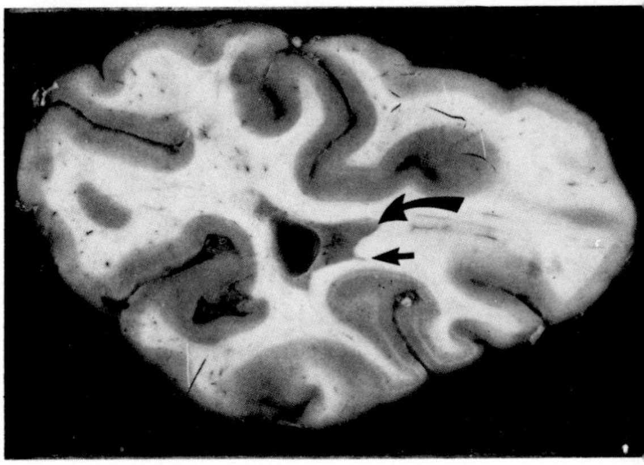

242 Two Dawson's fingers extending from plaque round lateral ventricle, × ¾.

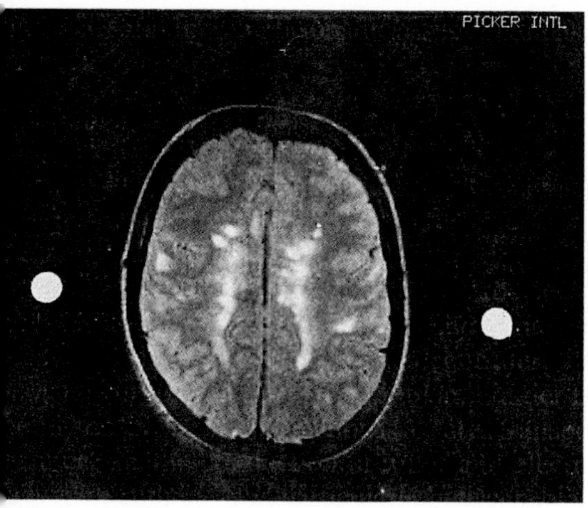

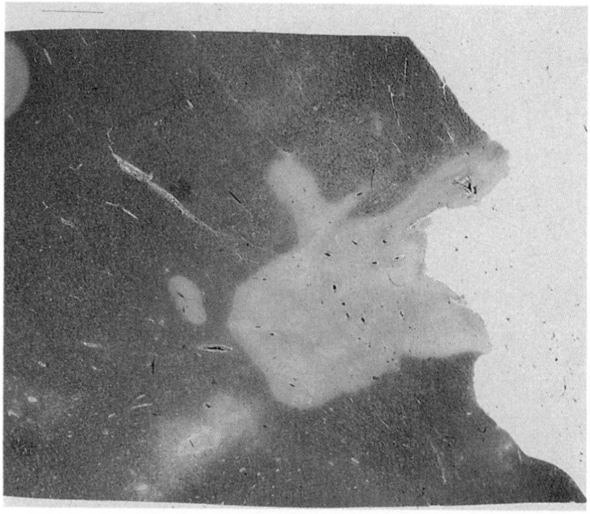

244

245

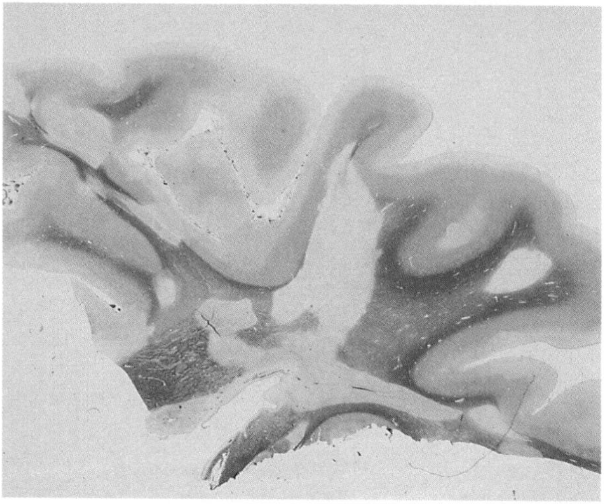

246

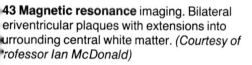

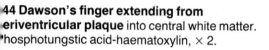

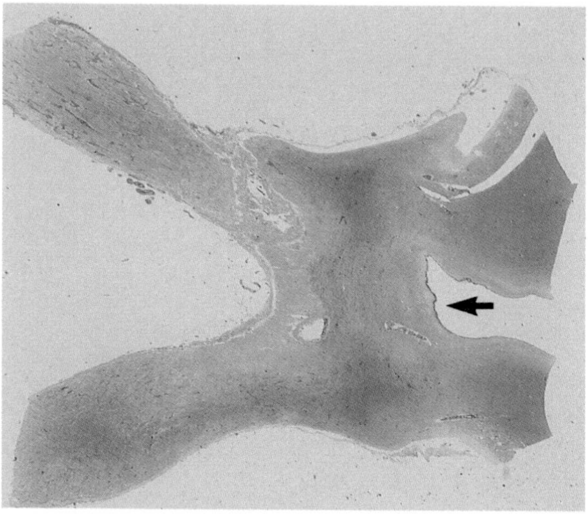

43 Magnetic resonance imaging. Bilateral eriventricular plaques with extensions into urrounding central white matter. *(Courtesy of 'rofessor Ian McDonald)*

44 Dawson's finger extending from eriventricular plaque into central white matter. 'hosphotungstic acid-haematoxylin, × 2.

45 Extension from periventricular plaque in ıe form of two claws. Luxol fast blue, × 1.

46 Extension of third ventricle (arrow) to osterior margin of optic chiasm. Haematoxylin-osin, × 2.

247

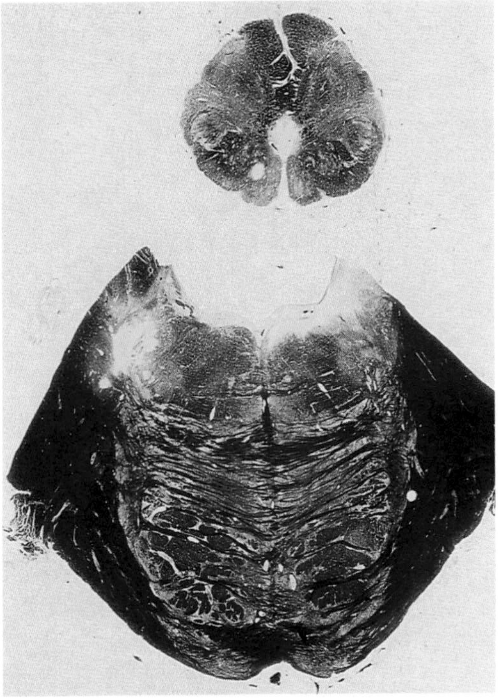

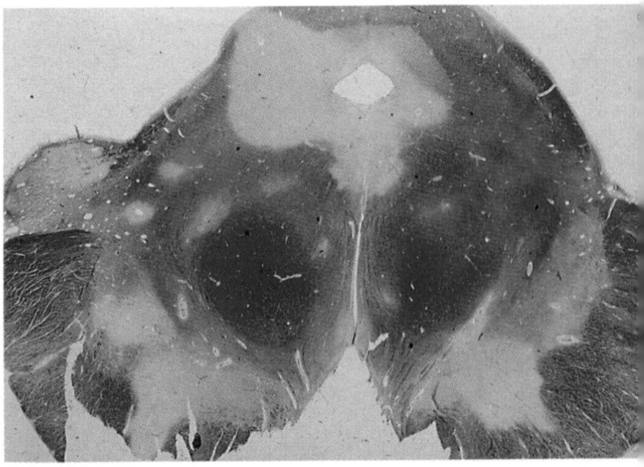

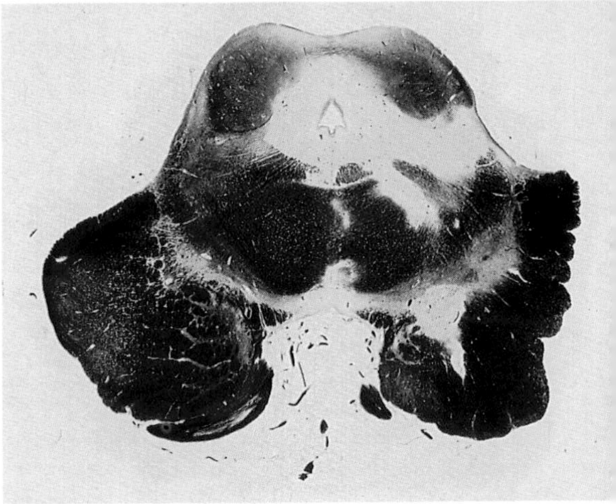

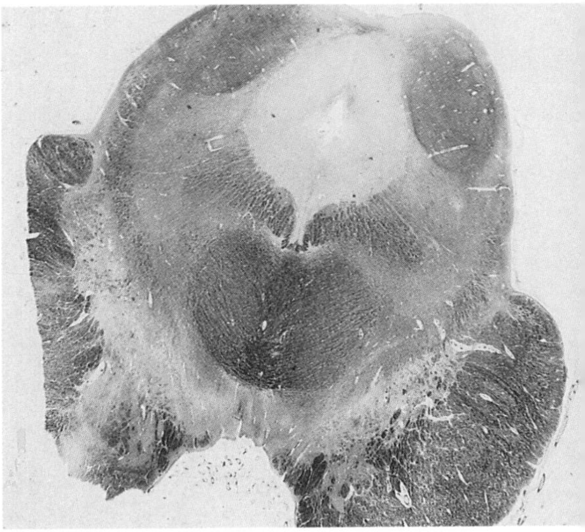

247 Plaques entending outwards from IVth ventricle towards reticular formation of pons. Small plaque in pyramid in lower medulla. Heidenhain, × 2.

248 Periaqueductal plaque with extension into tegmentum, substantia nigra and basis pedunculi. Luxol fast blue, × 2.

249 Periaqueductal plaque with extension into tegmentum and basis pedunculi. Heidenhain, × 2.

250 Normal midbrain for comparison with 248 and 249. Luxol fast blue-cresyl violet, × 2.

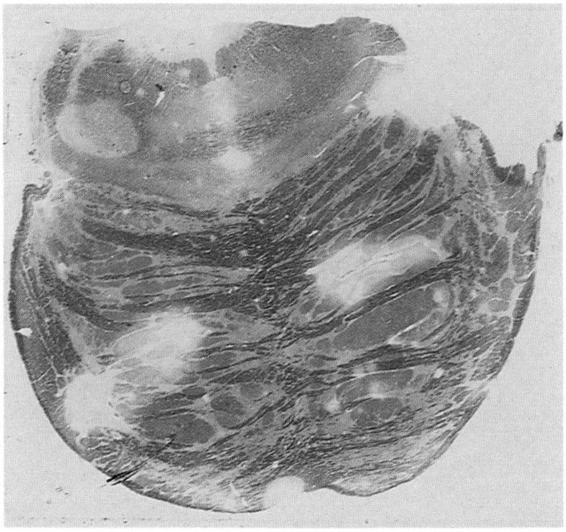

251

?51 Pons. Lesion around IVth
'entricle with small and large
extensions mainly in reticular
ormation. Luxol fast blue, × 2.

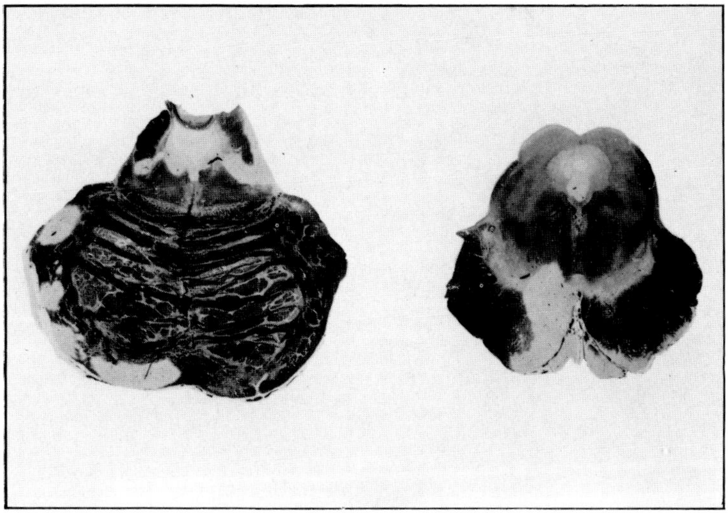

252

?52 Left: plaque extending
utwards from IVth ventricle with a
emi-circle of smaller plaques round
he outer margin of the pons. Right:
eriaquaductal plaque with large
extension into basis pedunculi.
Heidenhain, × 1.

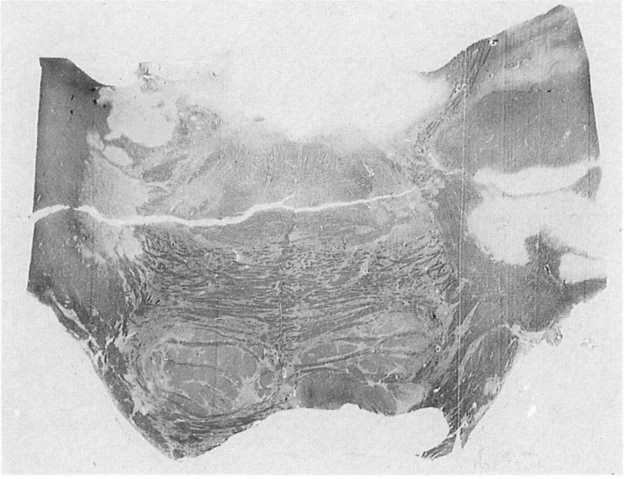

253

?53 Plaque at base of IVth ventricle
extending into middle cerebellar
eduncle. Luxol fast blue-cresyl
violet, × 2.

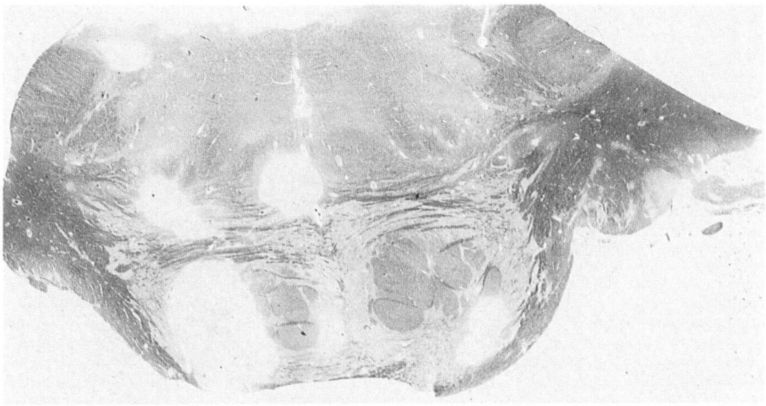

254 Chronic plaques of multiple sclerosis in reticular formation of pons. Luxol fast blue, × 2.

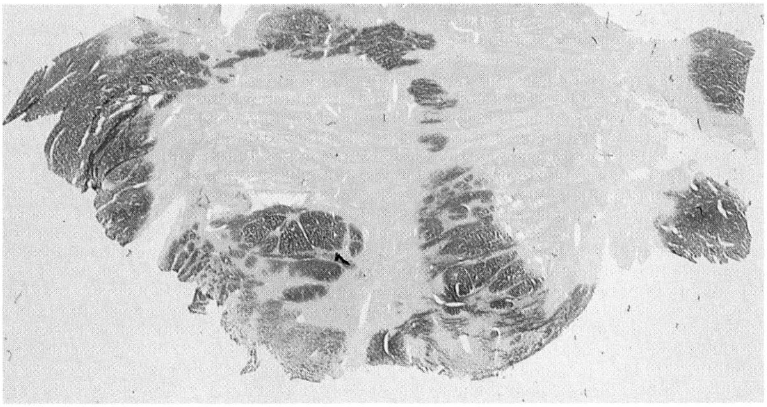

255 Gross demyelination of pons in chronic case of multiple sclerosis. Cryostat section, Sudan black, × 2.

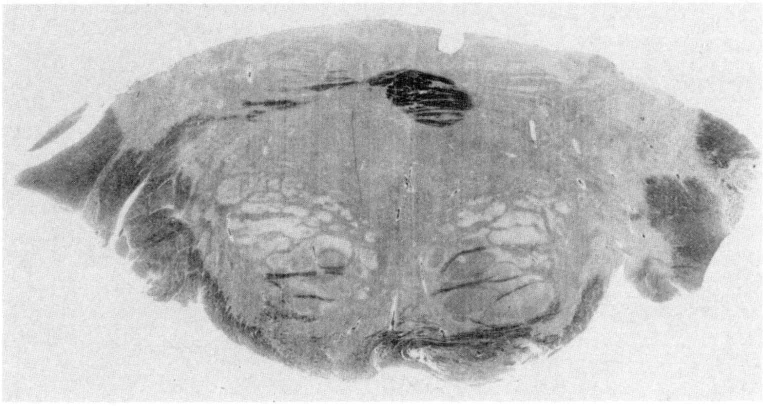

256 Another case of gross demyelination of pons with extension into both middle cerebellar peduncles. Cryostat section. Sudan black, × 2.

257

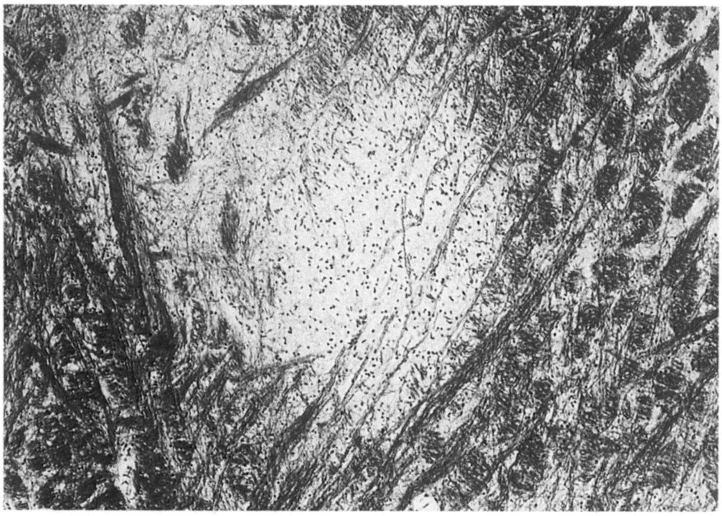

57 A patient with cerebellar ataxia ad this solitary demyelinating lesion in ne pons near the middle cerebellar eduncle. Luxol fast blue, × 2.

258

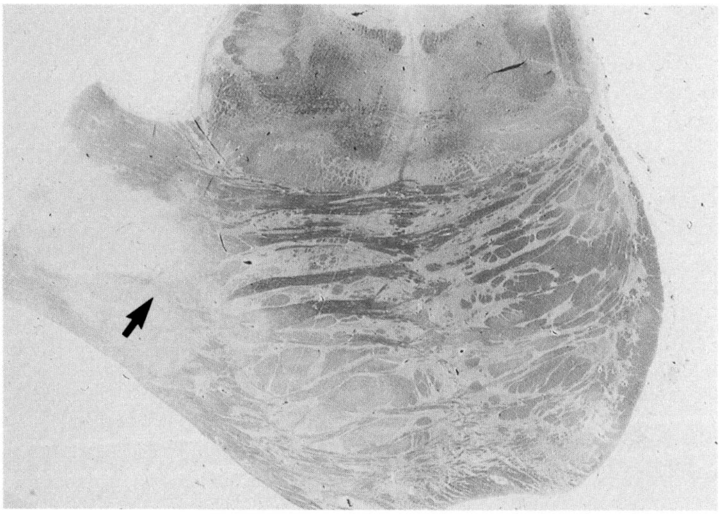

58 Demyelinating lesion in middle erebellar peduncle (brachium onjunctivum) at left. Luxol fast blue-resyl violet, × 2.

259

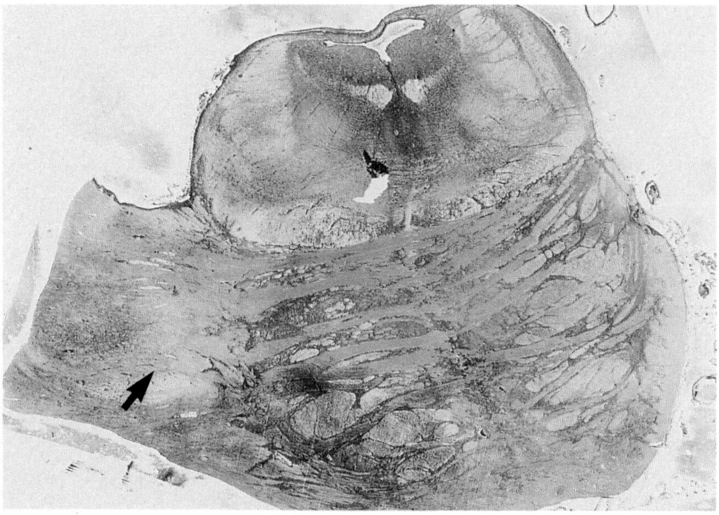

59 As for 258 but Glees and larsland silver stain to show loss f axons in brachium conjunctivum t left, × 2.

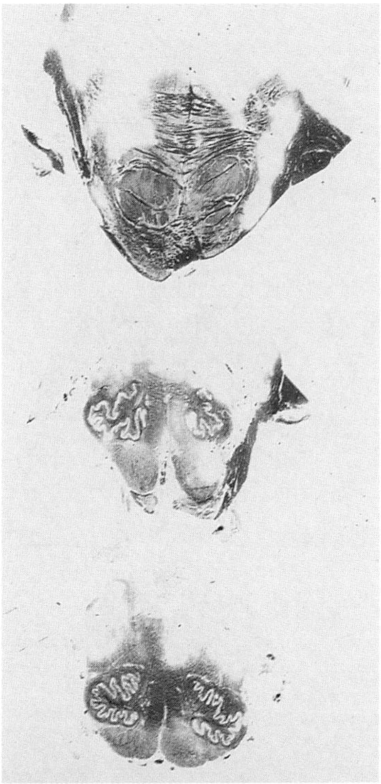

260

260 Medullary plaques of multiple sclerosis as extensions from a lesion round the IVth ventricle. Heidenhain, × 1.

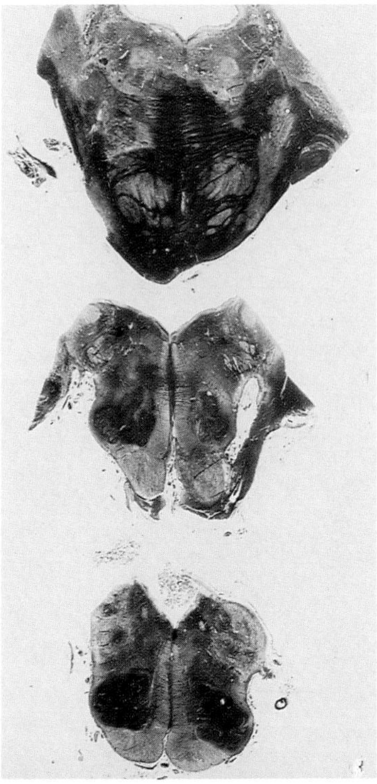

26

261 As for 259 but Weil-Davenport silver stain to show minimal loss of axons. Only the plaque to the right of the olive shows severe loss of silver staining, × 1.

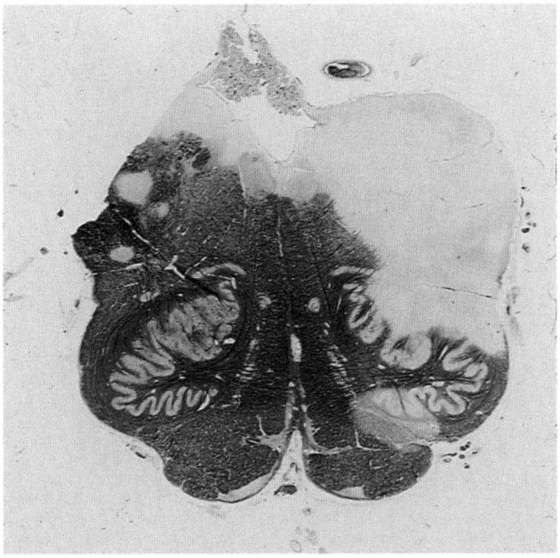

262

262 Rostral medulla with periventricular plaque extending into olive at right. Other smaller lesions in right olive and rest of medulla. Note choroid plexus in roof of IVth ventricle. Heidenhain, × 3.

26

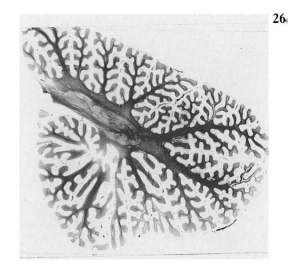

263 Normal appearance of dentate nucleus in cerebellar white matter. Luxol fast blue – cresyl violet, × 1.

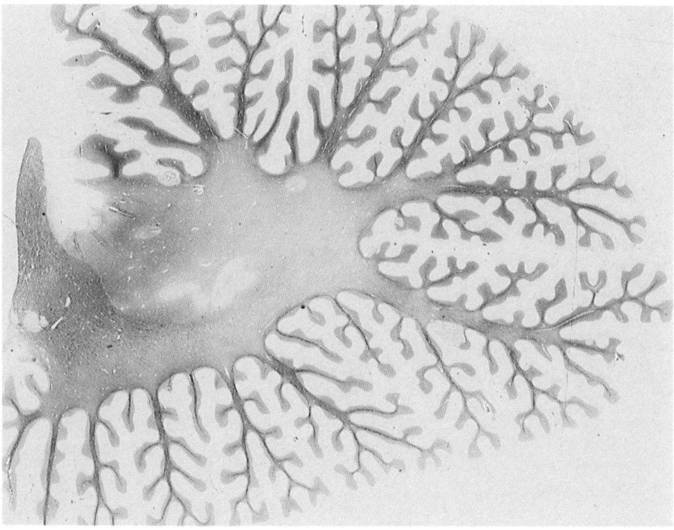

264

264 Four small plaques of multiple sclerosis and pallor of cerebellar white matter. Luxol fast blue-cresyl violet, × 1.

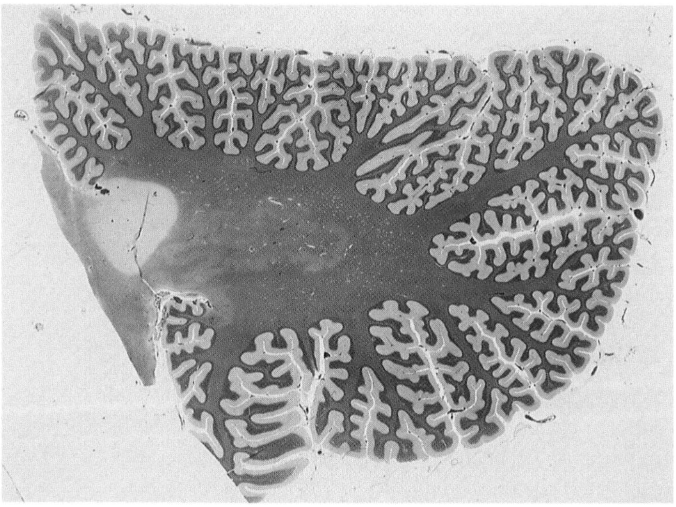

265

265 Medium-sized plaque in cerebellar white matter. Phosphotungstic acid haematoxylin, × 1.

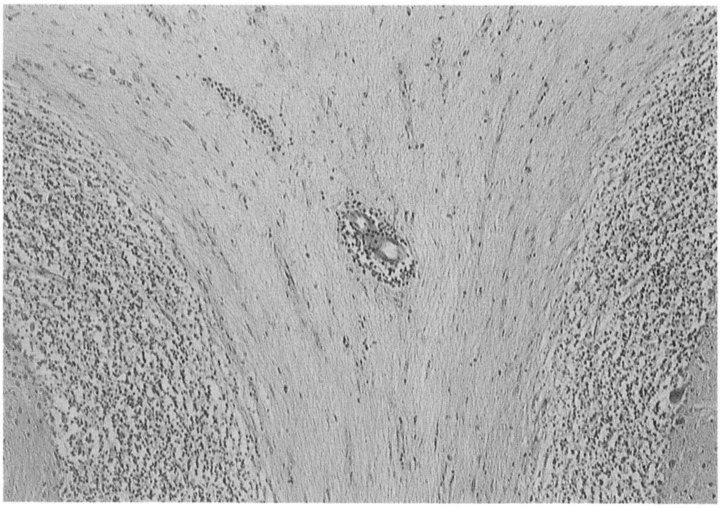

266

266 Perivenular lymphocytic infiltration at root of cerebellar medullary lamina. Van Gieson – elastic, × 40.

267

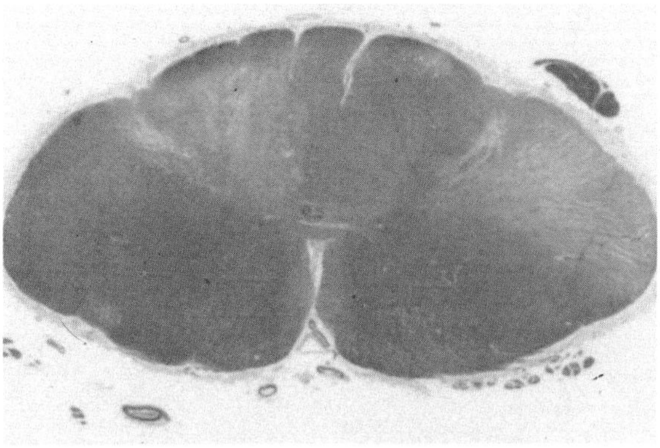

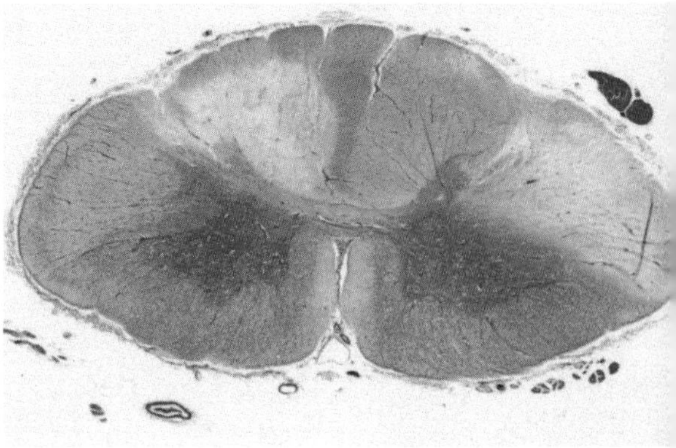

267 Chronic plaques of multiple sclerosis in lower cervical cord in multiple sclerosis. Haematoxylin-eosin, × 2.

268 Same as 267, but to show substantial loss of axons. Glees and Marsland, × 2.

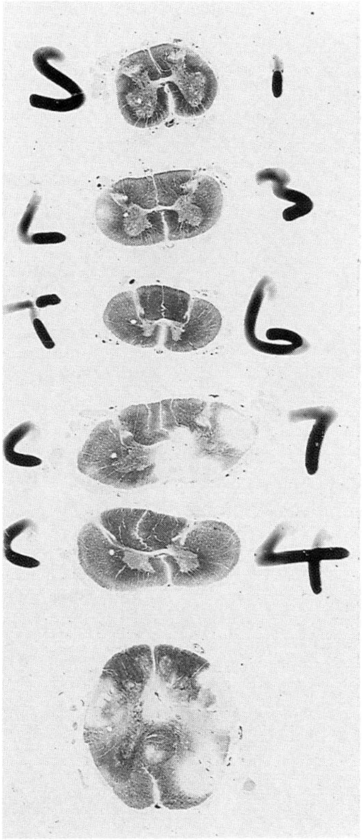

269

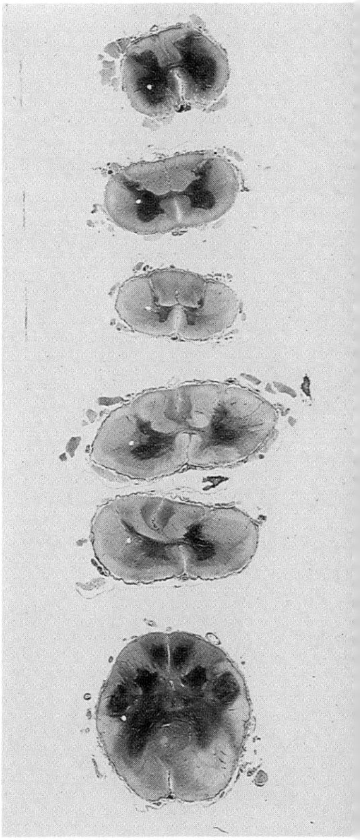

269 Plaques of multiple sclerosis in spinal cord. Note considerable involvement of cervical cord and medulla, but the rest of the cord only shows one small plaque in the lumbar region. Loyez, × 1.

270 As for 269 Glees and Marsland, × 1.

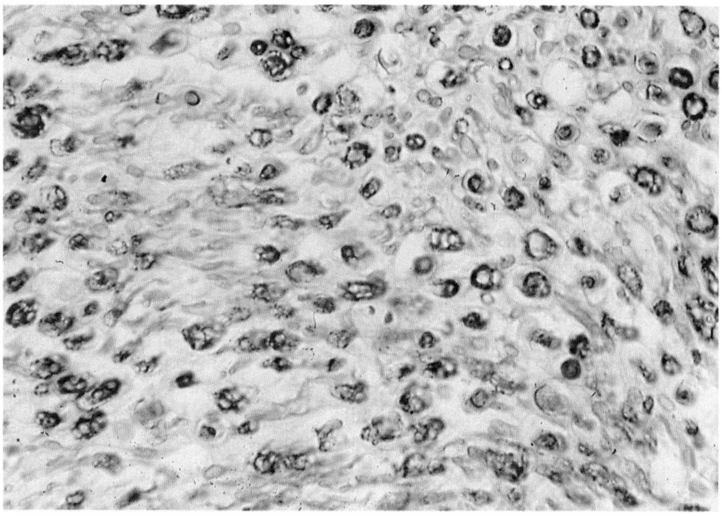

271

271 Modest demyelination in posterior columns in lower cervical cord. Luxol-picric acid-neutral red, × 250.

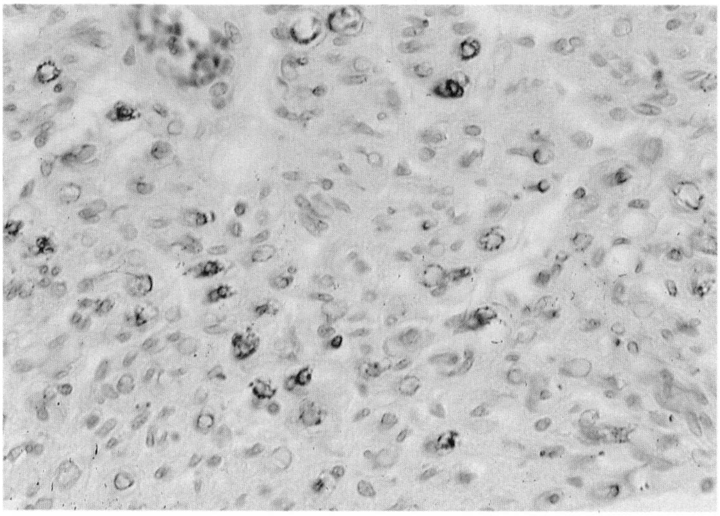

272

272 More severe demyelination as in 271.

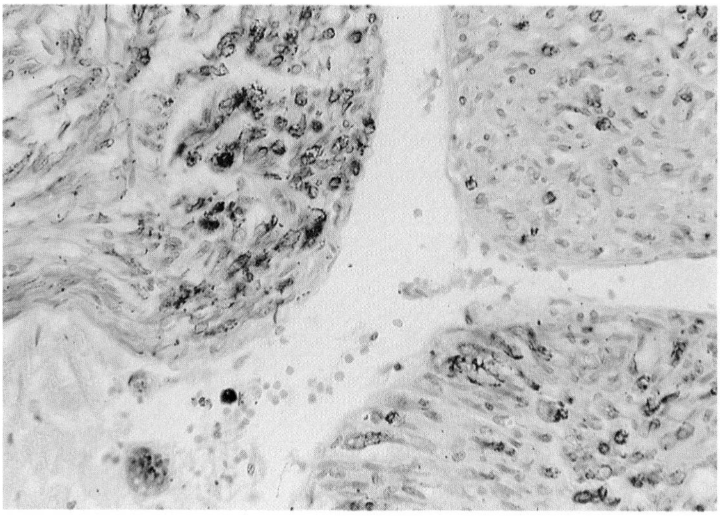

273

273 Probable Wallerian degeneration in sensory root of spinal cord in same case as **271** and **272.** Luxol-picric acid-neutral red, × 150.

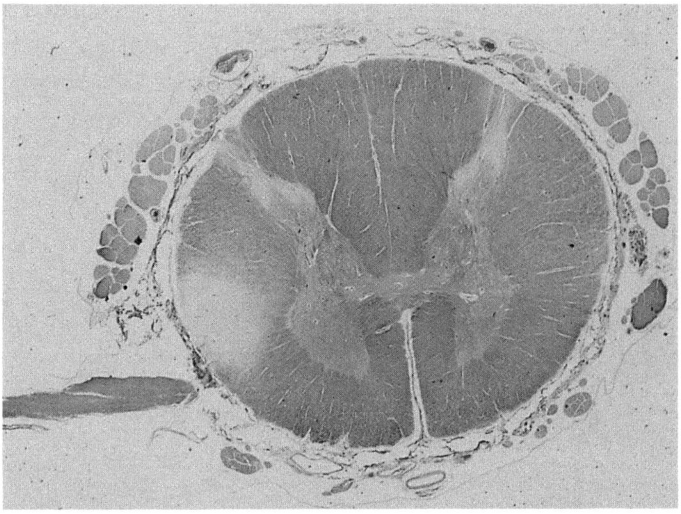

274 Plaque of multiple sclerosis in lateral column of lumbar cord with Wallerian degeneration in adjacent motor root (see **275**). Luxol fast blue – cresyl violet, × 4.

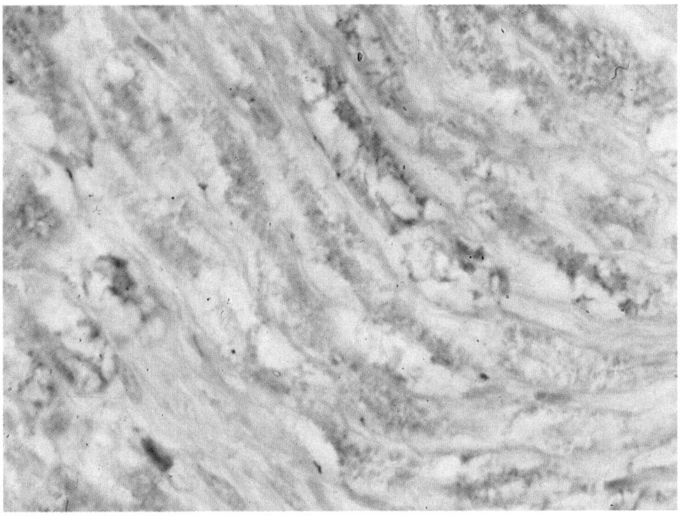

275 Wallerian degeneration with 'digestion chambers' in motor root adjacent to plaque in spinal cord (**274**). Luxol fast blue – cresyl violet, × 150.

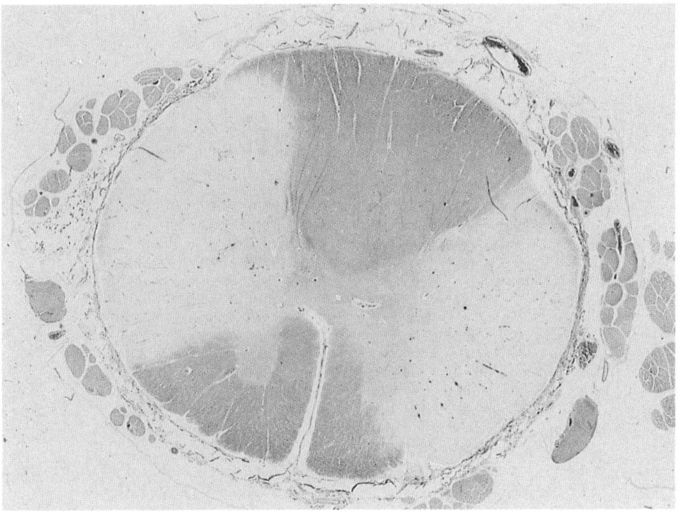

276 Symmetrical plaques of multiple sclerosis in upper cord. Luxol fast blue- cresyl violet, × 5.

277

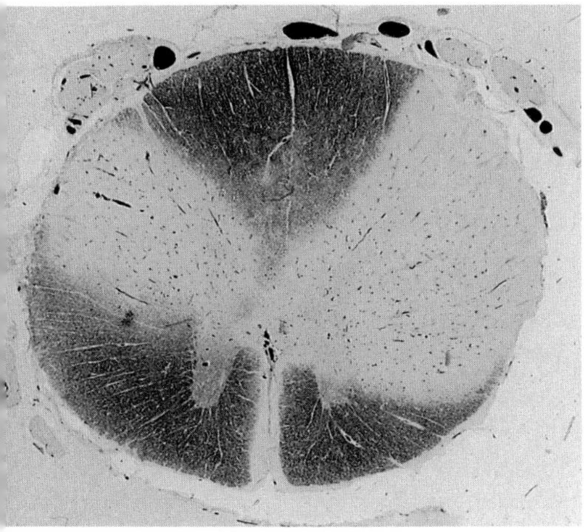

278

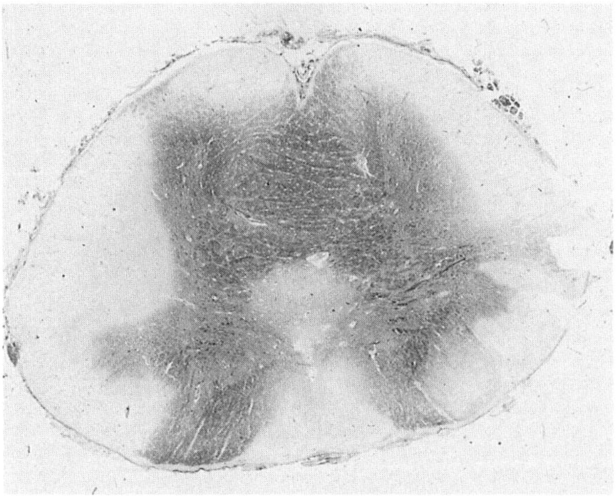

277 Nearly symmetrical plaques in upper cervical cord. Heidenhain, × 5.

278 Symmetrical plaques at junction of medulla and upper cervical cord. Luxol fast blue-cresyl violet, × 4.

279 Plaques in lateral columns of upper cervical cord (top); 'Kissing-plaques' in lower cervical cord (mid-right) and mid-thoracic cord (bottom left). Rapidly progressive acute multiple sclerosis. Heidenhain, × 2.

280 Devic's disease. Marked perivenular lymphocytic infiltration and inflammatory myelitis in cervical cord, but no necrosis. Haematoxylin-eosin, × 40.

279

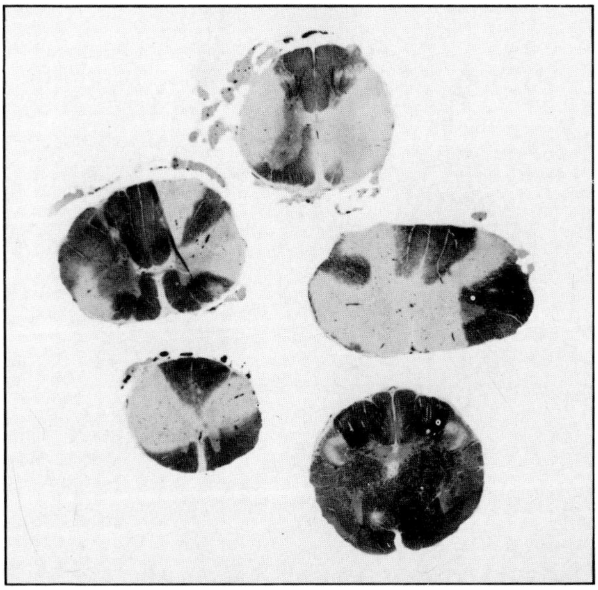

280

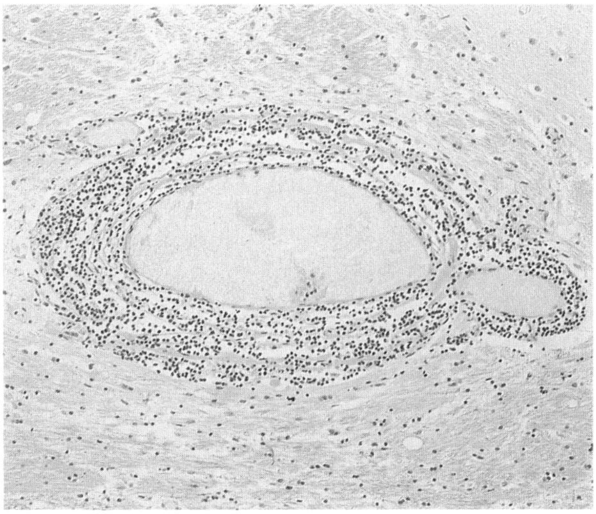

7 Histology and cellular features of multiple sclerosis

The characteristic feature of the recent MS plaque is the preservation of the axon but, as discussed in the Introduction to Chapter 2, axons in chronic lesions are frequently damaged and lost. Nevertheless, this initial preservation of the axon essentially distinguishes the demyelinating from a necrotic lesion.

The essential positive features of the 'classical' MS plaque is the loss of the myelin and its uptake and digestion by macrophages, or microglia. With the passage of time, astrocytic gliosis becomes prominent, the macrophages fully digest the myelin and, if the demyelinating process is arrested, the plaque becomes converted into a sharply circumscribed gliotic scar. The features of MS lesions in various phases of activity will be discussed and illustrated in the following pages.

Sometimes it is not always easy to determine whether an apparent plaque is in fact a chronic acellular plaque or just an area of grey matter dipping into white matter; this may be even more of a difficulty with a small plaque in the pons, due to the complexity of myelinated tracts in the reticular formation in this region. Figures **281** and **282** illustrate a useful distinction in that, at the edge of a plaque, parallel rows of myelinated tracts end fairly abruptly, whereas they merge in a more graduated and 'anatomical' manner at the junction of normal grey with normal white matter. When inflammatory, gliotic or reparative changes are evident, the distinction between plaque and an isolated rounded area of grey matter usually poses no difficulty.

Table 6. Indicators of activity in MS plaques

Grade of activity	Hyperactive	Active	Remyelination	Inactive
Edge of plaque	Indefinite or shadow	Shelving	Shadow	Usually punched-out
Lymphocyte cuffs:				
within plaque	Yes	Yes	Maybe	Slight
outside plaque	Maybe	Maybe	No	No
meningitis	Maybe	Maybe	No	No
Oedema or fibrin	Maybe	Maybe	No	No
Macrophages:				
blood origin	Yes	No	No	No
containing lipid-products and myelin	Yes	Yes	No	No
Oligodendrocytes:				
perinuclear oedema	Maybe	Maybe	No	No
proliferation	Maybe	Maybe	Yes	No
Hypercellularity	Yes	Yes	Yes, at edge	No
Astrocytes:				
activation	Maybe	Yes	Maybe	No
spider cells	No	No	Maybe	Yes
Veins:				
inflammation within wall	Maybe	Maybe	No	No
haemorrhage or iron	No	Maybe	No	Maybe
thrombosis/encrustation	No	No	No	Maybe
wall scarring	No	No	No	Maybe

see Table 7

Stages in plaque activity

The active lesion

Early lesions are small (**283** and **284**) and may be composed of multiple small perivenous components similar to those seen in acute disseminated encephalomyelitis (**285** and **286**). Some of these small lesions are analogous to Dawson's fingers discussed in the preceding chapter, and probably represent outward extensions from other plaques, and particularly from the draining veins around the ventricles. As mentioned above, axonal preservation is the rule in early lesions (**287**), but occasional active plaques may show intense damage resulting in a partly or frankly necrotic plaque (**288** and **289**). Necrosis may also occasionally be seen in more chronic lesions. These occasional necrotic plaques suggest that MS is not an obligatory demyelinating disease and that, if the process is sufficiently cytotoxic, a lesion focally resembling a necrotising encephalomyelitis may be encountered from time to time. MS causing Devic's disease could be cited as another example where necrosis may result (*see* Chapter 2). Another possibility to explain these necrotic lesions is that secondary thrombosis in vessels in or around a plaque may promote ischaemic necrosis.

Table 7. Characteristic staining for reticuloendothelial cells in acute and chronic MS lesions

	Recently recruited (haematogenous macrophage)	Longer-resident (haematogenous macrophage)	Microglia (endogenous)
Acid esterase	+	+/−	−
Acid phosphatase	+	+/−	−
Catalase/peroxidase	+	−	−
Muramidase (lysozyme)	+	−	−
RFD7	+	+/−	−
HAM 56	+	+/−	+/−
EBM11	+	+	+

(Derived from data by Esiri and McGee, 1986; Esiri and Reading, 1988; Adams *et al*., 1975; Adams *et al*., 1989)

Table 8. Cellular features of 16 acute cases of MS*

Length of clinical history	1-4 weeks	6-12 weeks	26-30 weeks
Lymphocytic cuffing	++ 8/8	++ 2/6 +4/6	++ 1/2 +1/2
Neuroglial proliferation (hypercellularity)	++ 5/8 + 3/8	++ 5/6 + 1/6	+ 2/2
Haematogenous macrophages** (lesion)	++ 3/7* + 2/7 − 2/7	++ 1/5* + 2/5 − 2/5	− 2/2
Macrophages** (perivenous)	++ 1/7 + 5/7 − 1/7	+ 5/5	+ 2/2

* In each category one tissue block unavailable

** Detached by immunocytochemical methods for blood macrophages (in collaboration with Dr R.N. Poston): Anti-lysozlyme, anti-α_1, antitrypsin, MAC and NSE. Because all these tissues were formalin-fixed, it was not possible to use pan-macrophage markers, such as EBM 11

A shadow plaque (**290** to **292**) may represent an early lesion, an acute ongoing lesion based on an older lesion (**293** and **294**), an aborted lesion or incomplete partial remyelination around a plaque (*see* Chapter 1; see Prineas and Connell, 1979; Ludwin, 1987). Some small plaques seem to have become arrested at an early stage (**295**; Lumsden, 1970). The significance of terms such as early, active and hyperactive is further discussed below.

Activity in a MS lesion is traditionally established by the presence of sudanophilic or osmiophilic lipid breakdown products within macrophages, gitter cells or microglia (**296** and **297**). These breakdown products are composed largely of cholesterol esters (see Chapter 2; Cumings, 1955), and are stained by osmium tetroxide, osmium tetroxide-chlorate (Marchi reagent), osmium tetroxide-α naphthylamine (OTAN; **298**) and by OT-resorcinol (**299**; Adams, 1958, 1959) for esterified cholesterol, and by perchloric acid naphthoquinone for free and esterified cholesterol (**300**; Adams, 1960). Unlike esterified cholesterol in atheroma (**301**), that in degenerating myelin does not usually give rise to Maltese-cross (liquid crystal) birefringence (anisotropism), probably because the cholesterol ester droplets and crystals within macrophages are not admixed with other lipids in a mesomorphic state. Normal myelin is paracrystalline and is birefringent in polarised light (**302**).

The cholesterol ester droplets within macrophages in an active lesion are birefringent, while the early 'myelinic' material (Petrescu 1969, 1982) within macrophages at the edge of the lesion or the surrounding white matter shows variable birefringence (**303** and **304**). Very acute demyelination, as in Schilder's disease, can sometimes give rise to birefringent cholesterol monohydrate crystals. However, the significance of myelin breakdown products *per se* in the brain and cord should not be overemphasised as they accumulate in a relatively late stage in the evolution of the demyelinating process. Furthermore, complete digestion of CNS myelin from the early 'myelinic bodies' to the formation of esterified cholesterol takes up to a year for completion, unlike the situation in the peripheral nerve where removal of lipid debris is virtually complete in various species within about 3-6 weeks (McCaman and Robins, 1959; Bignami and Rolston, 1969; Bignami and Eng, 1973; Perry *et al.*, 1987; present observations; see under macrophages below).

The histochemistry of early MS plaques shows increase of proteolytic enzyme activity (**185** and **186**) and loss of myelin basic protein (**305**), phosphoglycerides (**306**), phosphoglycerides and sphingolipids (**307**), cerebroside and cholesterol (Adams, 1968; Adams and Leibowitz, 1969; Hallpike *et al.*, 1970a). Myelin-associated glycoprotein (MAG) is also lost early and to a greater extent than other myelin proteins at the edge of the MS lesion (Johnson *et al.*, 1986).

A curious feature of some active MS brains is the presence of metachromatic birefringent lipid (**30** and **309**), probably partly within microglia, scattered throughout the brain (Bayliss and Adams, 1971). This material contains cholesterol and acidic galactolipid but its significance remains unexplained; it differs in appearance from both the grape-like bodies of Wolman (1960) and cerebral metachromatic bodies of MCB (Ibrahim and Levene, 1967).

The best criteria for recognising an active plaque are the presence of inflammatory oedema, perivenular infiltration by lymphocytes, similar lymphocytic cuffing outside the plaque and marked hypercellularity of the lesion (see Adams, 1980). The detailed features of active and chronic lesions are summarised in Tables 6 to 8. Previously, a shelving edge has been regarded as indicative of an active lesion, while chronic burnt-out plaques were held typically to show a sharp punched-out edge (**307**, Lumsden, 1970; Adams, 1980). This, however, cannot now be regarded as completely reliable because some chronic inactive lesions may also show an irregular shelving edge (**310** and **311**). Some lesions with shelving edges and thinly myelinated fibres probably represent abortive attempts at remyelination (**50**, **312**). However, not all the thinly myelinated fibres are necessarily remyelinating and some may be incompletely demyelinated (see Ludwin, 1987; Prineas *et al.*, 1984; Raine, 1983).

Inflammatory features and lymphocytes

The perivenular lymphocytic infiltration in active lesions ranges from a modest degree to as severe as that seen in an allergic arteritis, such as polyarteritis nodosa (**313** to **316**). In parenthesis, the inflammatory infiltrate in an acute viral disease such as poliomyelitis, may sometimes be quite modest (**317**). In general, the extent of lymphocytic infiltration in the perivascular region in MS correlates with disease activity. Many authors had previously expressed this as an opinion (or denied it), but more recent and larger studies have expressed this quantitatively (Adams, 1975, 1977; Guseo and Jellinger, 1975; Tanaka *et al.*, 1975). Mostly this inflammatory infiltrate in MS involves small veins but, occasionally, small arteries are also involved. The perivascular space (**313**) has been equated to a lymphatic channel by Prineas (1979), and would at least appear to be the functional equivalent of a lymphatic. In the earlier active phase the perivascular infiltrate is often nearly entirely lymphocytic (**316**), but an increasing content of macrophages is a characteristic of advanced lesions, particularly where there is abundance of myelin breakdown products (Symonds, 1924). As will be mentioned in Chapter 9 the T lymphocyte is predominant in the perivenular infiltrates. Only rather occasional T cells are found in the parenchyma and edge of MS plaques and, in light microscopy, they usually achieve a maximum of about one per high-power field (see Prineas, 1975; Hauser *et al.*, 1986; McCallum *et al.*, 1987; Adams *et al.*, 1989, Chapter 9).

Lymphocytes stain with the peroxidase method for anti-common leucocyte antigen (PD7/26), which reacts poorly with macrophages, and use of this reagent confirms the dominance of lymphocytes in the earlier stages of the lesion (**318**; also *see* Chapter 9). It should be emphasised that plasma cells are also seen in these lymphocytic infiltrates and in some cases, they may be very frequent (up to 9.5 per cent, Prineas and Wright, 1978), particularly in the established active lesion (**319** and **320**). Occasionally, these plasma cells contain Russell bodies (**320**), and these represent intracellular immunoglobulin storage as shown by staining with anti IgG peroxidase (Matthews, 1983). Another feature of activity is the occurrence of perivenular lymphocytic infiltrates outside plaques (Birley and Dudgeon, 1921; Adams, 1975, 1977; **321** to **324**). These may be interpreted as de-novo plaque formation or perivenular extensions of plaques into the surrounding white matter or a combination of both. Such centrifugal extensions are the early stages in the formation of Dawson's fingers, invasions of the demyelinating process into white matter (Chapter 6), superficially analogous to invasion by a carcinoma.

Lymphocytic meningitis is another feature of particularly active lesions. This may be manifest as a mainly perivenular meningeal infiltrate (**325**) or as a more diffuse generalised meningeal inflammation (**319** and **320**). An important deduction from the occurrence of meningitis in active MS is that, in some cases, most of the CNS lymphocytes may be concentrated in the meningeal inflammatory infiltrate. A lymphocyte count in the brains from our 10 most active cases indicated that these cells may be predominantly located in the subarachnoid space, particularly in the depths of the sulci (Adams, 1977; Table 9). It should be stressed that many active cases do not show significant meningitis, and it is not a feature of chronic lesions.

It is of considerable clinical and pathological interest that the occurrence of periphlebitis retinae (Engell and Andersen, 1982), an exudative lesion of the retina occurring during optic neuritis and with multiple sclerosis, correlates with active phases of the disease and, hence, appears to be a clinical correlate of cerebral perivenular exudates and cellular infiltrates (**328** and **329**; Engell, 1986; Engell *et al.*, 1984, 1986; Lightman *et al.*, 1987; see Fog, 1965). Chronic periphlebitis retinae shows a scanty infiltration of plasma cells and thick laminated collagenous repair, while acute lesions show lymphocytic cuffing (Shaw *et al.*, 1987).

The point of maximum emigration of lymphocytes into the perivascular space is at the venocapillary junction, the specialised area that allows lymphocytes to pass into the tissues (**326**). This explains the typical perivenular infiltrates seen in MS and viral diseases in general. In addition to this perivenous lymphocytic infiltration further evidence of the inflammatory nature of MS is provided by the intense oedema (**327**), fibrinous exudation (**330** to **333**), and IgG and complement deposition seen in some cases (**334** and **335**; see Esiri, 1977, 1980; Adams *et al.*, 1985, 1987). Oedema and fibrinous exudation are, of course, cardinal features of inflammation, and together are the pathological counterpart of the increased permeability around active lesions detected postmortem by Broman (1947, 1964) and in vivo by computerised axial tomography, magnetic resonance imaging (Simon *et al.*, 1986; Gonzales-Scarano *et al.*, 1987; Stewart *et al.*, 1987), brain scintigraphy (Engell *et al.*, 1984) and by retinal fluorophotometry (Engell *et al.*, 1986; Lightman *et al.*, 1987). However, it must be stressed that, although oedema is frequent, fibrinous exudation is not always present and is not an invariable diagnostic histological feature of active MS.

Oedema

Some cases of acute multiple sclerosis show a widespread vesicular form of oedema (Kirk, 1979). A coarse vacuolar oedema ('spongiform degeneration') may also be found in the central white matter in MS (**336**), as well as a finer oedematous vacuolation around both inflamed and otherwise normal veins. Vesicular myelin is also seen in Wallerian degeneration, EAE and the lysolecithin lesion (*see* Chapter 4), and seems to be an early or initial phase in myelin breakdown. However, vesicular myelin leads on to massive intramyelin vacuolation (**196**); this differs from the intramyelin oedema caused by triethyltin intoxication which is usually a series of single large vacuoles within the myelin sheath (**197** and **198**). These two types of oedema probably represent intramyelin water accumulation at different sites and at different stages of metabolic damage.

Myelin oedema has frequently been regarded as a cause of demyelination, for example the myelin pallor, oedema and early or partial demyelination around intracranial tumours (Greenfield, 1939). Severe hypertension is known to promote both cerebral oedema and demyelination, as in Binswanger's disease (Table 3). Feigin and Budzilovich (1980) consider that oedema and ring haemorrhages in severe hypertension result from a failure in astrocyte control of water metabolism, so that the ground substance swells and becomes oedematous and demyelination commences. The relationship of oedema to demyelination is a problem that requires much further thought and observations. The role of perivascular mast cells in cerebral oedema, see 'cerebral urticaria' and multiple sclerosis, also requires further exploration (Ibrahim, 1974). Recently, it has been suggested that mast cells release proteases in demyelination (Johnson *et al.*, 1988).

Neuroglia

The increased cellularity in the active plaque is due to proliferating neuroglia and macrophages. Small supposedly early plaques show proliferating glia throughout the lesion (**337**), whereas in larger more advanced plaques hypercellularity is more prominent as a peripheral rim to the lesion (Rindfleisch, 1873; **338**).

Oligodendroglia

As discussed in Chapter 1, the oligodendroglia are directly concerned in the synthesis and maintenance of myelin, and they act as nurse cells for certain 'ganglionic' neurones, where they are known as satellite cells. A number of immuno-staining 'markers' have recently been introduced to display these cells in brain sections and in culture. Many further advances can be expected in our understanding of oligodendroglia based on their use. These immunocytochemical methods include the use of an antigalactolipid antibody (**339**; Raff *et al.*, 1979), an anticarbonic anhydrase antibody (**340** and **341**; N. A. Gregson, unpublished), anti-transferrin (Connor and Fine, 1987; Koeppen *et al.*, 1988), an antibody prepared against oligodendroglia in culture (**342**; Newcombe and M. L. Cuzner, to be published) and histoenzymic staining for butyryl (non-specific) thiocholinesterase. Other immunocytochemical methods display oligodendroglia during myelination, for example, anti-myelin basic protein (*see* Chapter 1).

The view had previously been expressed that oligodendroglia are damaged in multiple sclerosis and disappear abruptly at the edge of the lesion (Lumsden 1951, 1970). Pseudocholinesterase, an enzyme concentrated in oligodendroglia, is lost from the centre of chronic plaques (Barron and Bernsohn, 1965; Roessmann and Friede, 1966; Wender and Kozik, 1969). It is true that oligodendroglia 'disappear' abruptly at the edge of the chronic inactive plaque (**343**), but it is hardly surprising that this should occur at the well-defined boundary between normal white matter and demyelinated tissue in the chronic plaque. The active plaque, however, presents a very different picture (Ibrahim and Adams, 1963, 1965), where a rim of persisting oligodendroglia at the edge of active lesions (**344** to **348**) sometimes show evidence of reactivity, such as perinuclear oedema (**349** and **350**; Cone, 1928), increased oxidative activity (**351** and **352**; Table 10), proliferation (hyperplasia; **344** to **346**, Table 6) and enlargement (hypertrophy; **351** and **353**). Electron microscopy confirms the persistence and proliferation of oligodendroglia at the demyelinating edge (**354**; Raine *et al.*, 1981; Raine, 1983). This rim of oligodendroglial cells at the periphery of the active plaque (**337, 338, 344** to **346**) has for many years been considered by some as a hyperplastic response associated with remyelination. As discussed above, thin remyelinating sheaths may on occasion be seen at the edge of plaques (Prineas and Connell, 1979; Prineas *et al.*, 1984; Ludwin, 1987).

It is likely that new oligodendroglia can be recruited from a glial progenitor cell, capable of giving rise either to astrocytes or oligodendroglia (Raff *et al.*, 1983; Chou, 1986). A feedback mechanism is also involved, whereby interleukin 2 stimulates proliferation of oligodendroglia, and interleukin 1 stimulates astrocytic proliferation (Beneveniste and Merrill, 1986). Interleukin 2 is bound by receptors on the surface of the lymphocyte, so that the activated lymphocyte in MS would stimulate oligodendroglial proliferation.

In summary, a variety of proposals have been put forward for the fate of oligodendroglia in MS: (a) the oligodendrocytes are killed outright and, because they control myelin maintenance, demyelination nsues; (b) the cells initially respond by hyperplasia nd activation, but subsequently die as the myelin is estroyed by the direct or indirect effect of the ausative agent; (c) the cells proliferate and activate n an attempt to remyelinate the plaque. A mixture of actors (b) and (c) is a reasonable assessment based n available evidence.

strocytes

'he astroglia can be demonstrated with Cajal's gold ublimate and by their possession of the cytoskeletal bres glial fibrillary acid protein (GFAP, **355** to **357** nd **365**) and vimentin (**363** and **364**). Astrocytes are ormally located throughout the central nervous ystem, and are particularly concentrated immediately under the pia mater (**356**) and under the pendyma (**357**). Their function is to act as transport hannels for the conduction of water and electroytes within the CNS, particularly between blood essel and neurone (**358** and **359**). They also possess hagocytic activity, as shown by their uptake of debris nd waste material, such as immunoglobulin (see **51** and **452**). Astrocytes subserve the function of esenchyme within the CNS. Thus, fibrillary astroytes secrete glial fibres which are, in part, analogous collagen fibres elsewhere in the body.

Astrocytic activation is not a feature of the very arliest stage of multiple sclerosis (see Table 6), but active astrocytes are seen soon afterwards. The nction of astrocytes in MS is to respond to the dema and inflammatory changes that accompany e active stage of the disease. In view of their ansport role within the CNS, they would be pected to activate in response to permeability anges. Astrocytic activity is revealed by nuclear nlargement, binucleate or polyploid forms, enrgement of the cell-body (**360** to **362**), increased xidative enzyme activity (**360** and **361**), proliferaon (**362** to **365**) and astroglial fibre production (**362** **365**). A primary role for astrocytes in MS has been roposed by several workers (Field, 1967; Arstila *et* ., 1973): diffuse activation of astrocytes – as shown y increased lysosomal enzyme activity – has also een proposed as a primary feature of MS McKeown and Allen, 1978; Allen and McKeown, 979; Allen *et al.*, 1979a). The proliferating rim of nzymatically active neuroglial cells at the edge of me active MS plaques has been attributed to troglia (Friede, 196l, 1965) but, if oligodendroia arise from astrocyte-like stem cells (see above), en this view could be compatible with observations at these proliferating cells are mainly oliodendroglia (Ibrahim and Adams, 1963; 1965; Raine *et al.*, 1981; Raine, 1983).

The fibrillary activity of astrocytes (**362** to **365**) leads to the repair of MS plaques by fibrillary gliosis (**366** to **371**), which leads on to a dense 'scar' composed of parallel rows of isomorphic astroglial fibres (**372**). This is the end-stage of repair of the burnt-out chronic lesion – electron microscopy of chronic lesions reveals demyelinated axons surrounded by astrocytic processes (**373**).

In areas of intense and prolonged astrocytic activity, degenerate forms of astrocytes can sometimes be seen in the form of bizarre rounded bodies or clubs or elongated structures known as Rosenthal fibres (**374**; Herndon *et al.*, 1970). These show all the classic staining characteristics of astrocytes, namely staining with PTAH (**375**), Holzer (**376**), Bielschowsky (**377**) and with Heidenhain (**378**). However, anti-GFAP stains only the periphery of some and not all fibres (**379**), while anti-vimentin peroxidase fails to stain them at all (**380**). Herndon *et al.*, (1970) suggested that hyaline bodies within astrocytes give rise to Rosenthal fibres, and that long-continued astroglial activity and gliosis are the circumstances that promote the formation of these fibres. Rosenthal fibres are also seen in Alexander's disease (Chapter 2).

Macrophages

The reticuloendothelial response in MS seems to be initially mediated by blood monocytes, which can be seen emigrating from small veins in active lesions (**381**). The immuno-staining of foam cells in early lesions is summarised in Table 7. The immunocytochemical and enzyme histochemical markers used for blood-recruited monocytes are anti-lysozyme (muramidase; **381** to **383**), anti-α_1, antitrypsin the monoclonals MAC (**384**), HAM 56, LeuM1 and anti-vimentin (**385**), and E600-resistant non-specific esterase (**386** and **387**). The latter includes E600 – resistant α-naphthyl acetate esterase and 'acid' esterase. Likewise, acid phosphatase activity is prominent in macrophages in active lesions (**388**). Acid esterase, acid phosphatase and lysozyme are all known lysosomal enzymes. Peroxidases, catalase and cytochrome oxidase are additional histoenzymic markers of blood-recruited macrophages (Adams *et al.*, 1975).

Although the foam cells in early lesions react with these monocyte markers, those plaques from cases with a history of more than a month show few such haematogenous cells (Table 8), and foam cells in

Table 9. Lymphocyte distribution in CNS in multiple sclerosis (after Adams, 1977)

	Total lymphocytes in CNS
Perivenous cuffs	1.02×10^8
Cerebral meninges	4.74×10^8
CSF (assumed maximum in 125 ml)	0.07×10^8
Total	5.83×10^8

These data are derived by extrapolation to the whole CNS from counts on tissue sections. The sections were obtained from 10 active cases, selected for high lymphocyte counts, out of 64 cases of MS

later lesions seem to stain better with a pan-macrophage marker, such as EBM11 (**389** and **454**; Esiri and McGee, 1986) or HAM56, Adams *et al.*, 1989. RFD7 is intermediate in this respect (Esiri and Reading, 1987). Possible explanations are that the blood monocyte dedifferentiates as regards its marker antigens and enzymes after passage of time in the tissues, or that the foam cells in later lesions are derived from the endogenous microglia. The latter explanation, however, is unlikely, because the macrophages in later plaques are 'esterase' positive (acid esterase and E600-resistant α-naphthylacetate esterase; **386** and **387**), whereas the endogenous microglia are not. This is consistent with the conclusion that cerebral macrophages are recruited from monocytes and never from microglia (Schelper and Adrian, 1986). These conclusions are summarised in Table 7.

Macrophages in active lesions seem to pick up myelin in the form of globules (myelinic bodies) which stain with the blue oxazine component of Nile blue sulphate, implying that the material contains phospholipid or free fatty acid (**390**; Dragenescu *et al.*, 1961; Petrescu, 1966; 1969; 1981; 1982). These early myelin granules within macrophages can also be stained with solochrome cyanin-oil red O (**391** and **392**), and are variably birefringent in polarised light (**303**). With the solochrome sequence phospholipids are blue and the esterified cholesterol is red. These granules are probably similar to the ultrastructural myelin bodies identified in macrophages in acute multiple sclerosis by Prineas (1975). Subsequently, the myelin lipids are slowly degraded to esterified cholesterol (*see* Chapter 1), which process is a major function of the macrophages of the reticuloendothelial system (Day, 1964). The esterified cholesterol formed by macrophages can be identified by its pink reaction with the oxazone of Nile blue (**390**).

A controversial question about the macrophage i the active MS plaque is whether or not it is concerne in the initial attack on myelin, such as that observe by Lampert (1969, 1983) in Wallerian degeneratio EAN and Guillain-Barré disease. The ter 'myelin'-stripping, used in respect of macrophage phagocytosing myelin begs the question. Indee Schröder and Krücke (1970) observed that myeli lesions in EAN were not always in contact wit macrophages.

Immunoglobulin-capping of macrophages ha been noted in active lesions (Prineas and Graham 1981; Prineas, 1985). This immuno-activation c arming of macrophages indicates a positive im munological function for these cells, but is th function a direct attack on the myelin sheath or a inflammatory and reparative response to the pre viously damaged myelin? The release of prostaglan din PGE by macrophages is increased early in relapse of MS (Dore-Duffy *et al.*, 1986), but is th just a general response in an inflammatory proces There is no firm evidence to decide the importa issue of whether macrophage activation is post hoc c propter hoc.

Reports on active 'acute' plaques (reviewed b Prineas, 1985) and our 16 acute cases (Table 8) i general show that such plaques are hypercellul and, in the early stages, are infiltrated with a numb of blood-recruited macrophages. The lipid-lade sudanophilic foam cells in some moderately activ plaques tend to lie at a distance from the demyelina ing edge and, thus, seem to be mainly concerned i the secondary task of removing lipid debris (se Petrescu, 1981). However, macrophages in activ lesions are sometimes seen in more direct conta with the demyelinating edge **390** to **395**, **397** an **398**), and in the white matter immediately outside th lesion (**303**). Such macrophages often contai myelin' debris (**303, 391** and **392**) stained by phospholipid methods (for example, Nile blue, Solochrome cyanin, Sudan black B, Luxol fast blue and acid haematin; see Petrescu, 1969, 1981, 1982). Nevertheless, such macrophage activity at the demyelinating edge still does not indicate whether this is a primary immune-directed attack on the myelin sheath or a scavenger response to myelin already damaged in some other way.

Figure **396** shows macrophages involved in digesting cholesterol crystals in a human atherosclerotic lesion: this is a purely scavenger function, and results in the formation of esterified cholesterol from the crystals of free cholesterol. The blue staining material is a mixture of free and polymerised fatty acids which could be a precursor for the cholesterol ester synthetase (acyl-cholesterol: acyl transferase; ACAT) reaction involved in cholesterol esterification. It could be that the formation of esterified cholesterol in demyelination is another example of this function of macrophages (see above). In summary, the important question is still unresolved, whether macrophages in MS are directly attacking myelin or whether they are simply exerting their well-established scavenging and lipid catabolic functions.

Acute, early and hyperactive lesions

The term *active* used previously in this text does not require elaborate explanation in that the cellular features of the active plaque (immuno-inflammatory cells, inflammatory exudation, phagocytic and repair cells) are indeed self-evident. The *hyperactive* lesion is, likewise, not difficult to delineate; it is simply that all or some of the features of the active plaque are more pronounced (**296** to **299**, **303** to **306**, **313** to **316**, **321** to **325**, **381** to **395**). However, the terms *acute* and *early* are more difficult to establish, they are not synonymous and it cannot be concluded that all active plaques are necessarily acute or early. Also the converse cannot be assumed that all early plaques are active, because some early lesions seem to abort (**399**) and one type of shadow plaque (**400**) may also come into this category. Lumsden (1970) considered that the development of the lesion was cut short and the pathology appears incomplete.

The term *acute* is usually taken to mean that the lesion is both early and hyperactive. It depends on establishing that the lesion is indeed early. This is a rare situation and depends on being able to date the onset of disease or the onset of a well-defined complication or exacerbation. Table 8 gives details of 16 cases of MS, where the onset of disease occurred within a year of death or where death followed a exacerbation involving a new anatomical area. Eight of these cases were new onset of MS within a month, and were culled from a previous total of 193 cases within our bank. These acute cases were mainly identified by early involvement of the pons/medulla and the rapid course of their disease must be attributed to the consequent early involvement of medullary centres and cranial nerve nuclei, controlling respiration and swallowing. Rindfleisch (1873) recorded that acute grey degeneration (multiple sclerosis) in the medulla is associated with 'masticatory spasm'. All of our cases were clearly MS, and not acute diffuse encephalomyelitis. However, it must be recognised that the pathology in these early cases was possibly of longer duration than the length of the clinical history but, nevertheless, were clearly of recent origin.

The pathological features of acute lesions are summarised in Tables 6 and 8. Lymphocyte cuffing is present in every case, and is usually pronounced. Hypercellularity *throughout* the lesion is characteristic, a proportion of such cells being macrophages. Where the clinical age is less than 1 month, some of these macrophages are usually stained by immunological markers for monocytes, indicating their recent recruitment from the blood (see under *macrophages* above). With a clinical age of up to 3 months, a proportion of macrophages may still stain with monocyte markers. Occasionally, blood monocytes may be seen in process of emigrating through the venule wall (**381**). Some of the lesions in acute cases show macrophages at or outside the demyelinating edge and these cells contain the myelinic bodies described by Petrescu (1969, 1981). These myelinic bodies are stained by phospholipid stains (**303**, **390** to **391**; Solochrome cyanin and Nile blue) and, hence, appear to be phagocytosed myelin debris.

The chronic lesion

The plaque may continue to be active at its periphery (**401**) or by focal extension outwards as Dawson's fingers (*see* Chapter 6). The degree of activity may be only modest, as shown by a residual modest infiltrate of lymphocytoid cells (**402**), or occasional foam cells at the periphery of the lesion. Perivascular foam cells

Table 10. Correlation between dehydrogenase activity and oligodendroglial proliferation at edge of eleven active plaques of multiple sclerosis (after Ibrahim and Adams, 1965)

Dehydrogenase activity at edge of plaque	Oligodendroglia % counts at edge of plaques
Slight just detectable increase	100
	118
	121
	128
Clearcut increase	131
	137
	182
	202
Marked increase	187
	206
	271

(**403**) are converted in the chronic or burnt out lesion into pigmented lipofuscin (**404**). Such peroxidised lipid acts as a tombstone for a long-past episode of demyelination. This pigment was described by Rindfleisch (1873) as characteristic of grey degeneration (an old term for MS), but is often seen commemorating some other past disorder in the brain.

The chronic lesion shows an abundance of astrocytes or spider cells (**405**). These cells subserve the function of repair cells, as well as controlling water movement in the brain, and acting as additional phagocytes (see Astrocytes, above).

Many chronic plaques enter a stage of complete inactivity. The fully burnt-out plaque represents the termination of the pathological process akin to the scarred end stage of other chronic progressive inflammatory processes, such as pulmonary tuberculosis or chronic glomerulonephritis. It is not certain whether the burnt-out plaque can be reactivated, yet there is no evidence to suggest that it does. Probably the marked gliosis would impede a further immuno-inflammatory response.

The astrocytes that proliferate within the chronic lesion become fibrillary by nature (**362** and **364**) and proceed to lay down parallel rows of astrocytic fibres, which eventually become arranged in packed parallel rows, known as isomorphic gliosis (**372**). Occasionally, astrocyte cell bodies in chronic lesions degenerate and form rounded or elongated bizarre bodies known as Rosenthal fibres (see under Astrocytes above, **374** to **380**). Corpora amylacea may also bear some relationship to astrocytes. These rounde degenerative bodies (**406**) are commonly found i the ageing brain, but also are unusually frequent i some cases of MS (see also Rindfleisch, 1873 Moxon, 1875).

In chronic lesions the vein wall becomes thickened and collagenised, often in a concentric onion-skin fashion. Sometimes organising thrombi ar observed on the walls of veins (see Table 6). Thes matters are further discussed in Chapter 8.

Another feature of chronic MS is the development of granular ependymitis in the ventricula system (Ziegler, 1886; Adams *et al.*, 1987). Thes areas of chronic focal dome-shaped inflammatio (**407** and **408**) may be seen on the ependymal surfac in the IIIrd, lateral and IVth ventricles and in th aqueduct (**409**), but most commonly they are foun in the lateral ventricles opposite the septum pelluci-dum (**407**). Granular ependymitis in MS probabl reflects the involvement of the ependyma (**410** an **411**) in inflammatory, healing or sclerotic processe in the plaque, but it is a non-specific process that i particularly encountered in focal chronic inflamma tory disease, meningitis or in ventricular dilatatio (including hydrocephalus). It is common in all sub jects over 70 years, when it probably reflects com pensatory ventricular dilation accompanying senil and arteriosclerotic changes in the brain. The loca pathogenesis is probably due to failure of the astro cyte-derived ependymal cell to repair by prolifera tion after either injury or splits induced by ventricula dilatation: the resulting gap is filled with a glia nodule composed of astrocytes and packed glial fibres (**412** to **415**). Sclerosis and shrinkage around a periventricular plaque of MS might induce local ventricular dilatation, splits in the ependyma and, hence, granular ependymitis. It must be stressed that neither granular ependymitis nor multiple sclerosis are in any sense specific granulomatous inflammations in that they are never populated by epithelioid cells. Furthermore, granular ependymitis is a chronic low-grade reparative process with minimal inflammatory cells, and differs completely from the acute inflammatory ependymitis (**416** and **417**) that somewhat rarely accompanies acute meningitis.

The ependymal 'granulation' in chronic MS may act as a portal of entry for IgG and other immune agents (Adams *et al.*, 1987). Thus, the granulation may constitute an important channel for CSF components to enter the brain or for plaque components to enter the CSF, but it is emphasised that such entry would only occur in the chronic lesion because granular ependymitis is not characteristic of the early MS lesion.

Conclusions

A perivenular inflammatory infiltrate of lymphocytes together with some plasma cells and macrophage is characteristic of the active MS lesion. Early lesions contain a greater predominance of lymphocytes. Adams and Kubik (1952) made the penetrating remark that this infiltrate in MS is not a secondary response to myelin breakdown, as it does not regularly accompany other conditions where myelin is destroyed. Likewise, Lightman *et al.*, 1987 make the point that periphlebitis retinae in multiple sclerosis occurs in the absence of surrounding myelinated fibres. There is an approaching consensus that this perivenular inflammatory process is an autoimmune response to some non-specific viral or traumatic injury.

There is little evidence to inculpate oligodendroglia in the direct pathogenesis of MS: the evidence is that they survive at the edge of the lesion and sometimes proliferate there in partial or abortive attempts at remyelination. The role of astrocytes in MS would seem to be limited to controlling oedema, to phagocytic/lysosomal activity and to fibrillary repair. The role of the macrophage in the MS plaque remains a controversial issue: the question is whether it directly causes demyelination by attacking myelin under instruction from T helper cells or whether it is merely subserving its general function as a scavenger cell in removing myelin already damaged by an immune or other inflammatory reaction. Although there is no doubt that some areas of active demyelination in MS show macrophages phagocytosing myelin, yet other active areas do not seem to be under a macrophage 'attack'. Even if this statement is wrong, it is difficult to see how (in morphological terms) the primacy of a macrophage attack in MS can be established. At the risk of stating the obvious, the hypothesis now requires to be tested in an experimental-immunological rather than in an observational-morphological system.

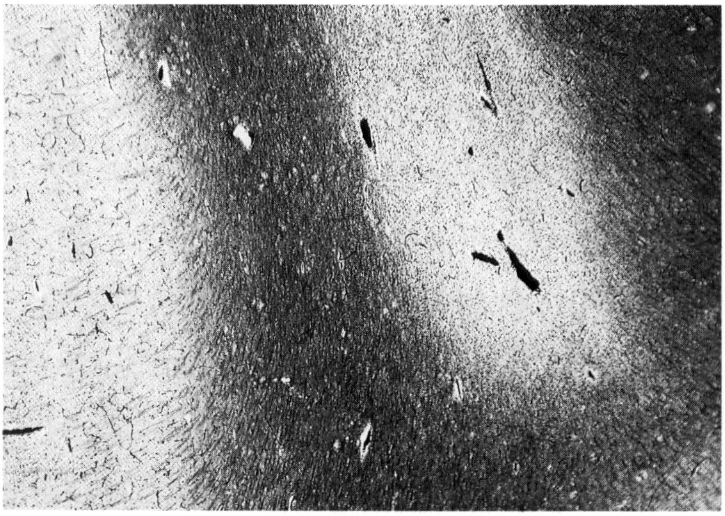

281 Left: isolated focus of grey matter, which can sometimes resemble plaque. Note gradual transition from white matter to cortex. Right: small chronic plaque of multiple sclerosis. Note more abrupt transition. Loyez, × 10.

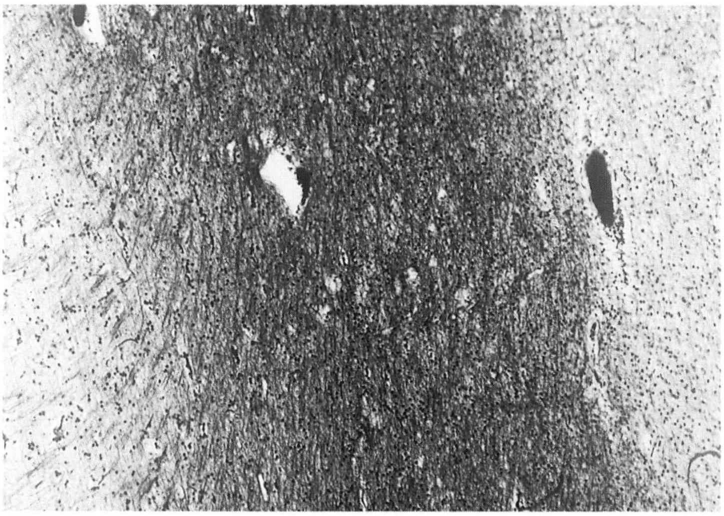

282 As for 281, but × 25. Note small focus of modest perivenular infiltration in plaque at right centre. The abrupt edge of the plaque (right) is compared with the normal grey/white margin (left).

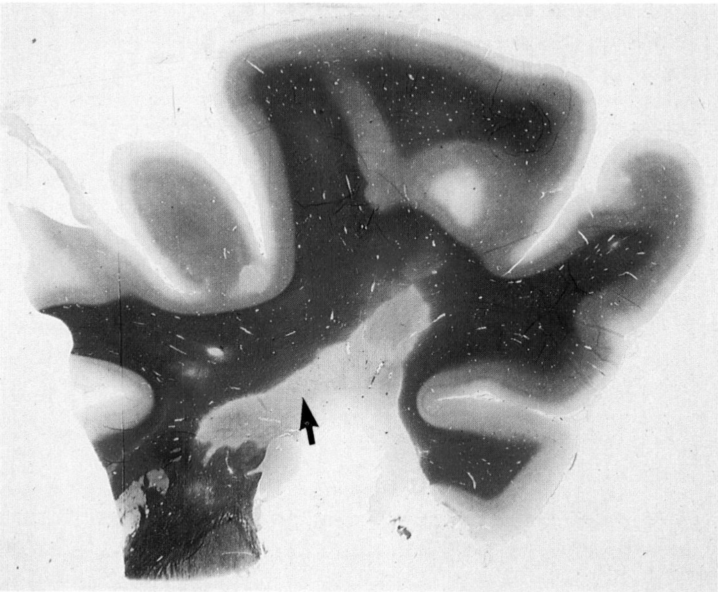

283 Multiple sclerosis. Small early lesions in central white matter; these are probably extensions from the adjacent chronic periventricular plaque (arrow). Loyez, × 2.

284

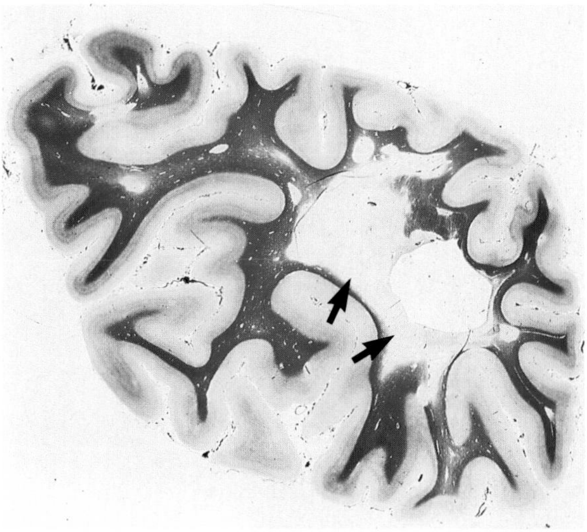

284 Multiple sclerosis. Small early lesions in subcortical white matter at left, with massive old chronic periventricular plaque at right (arrows). Heidenhain, × 1.

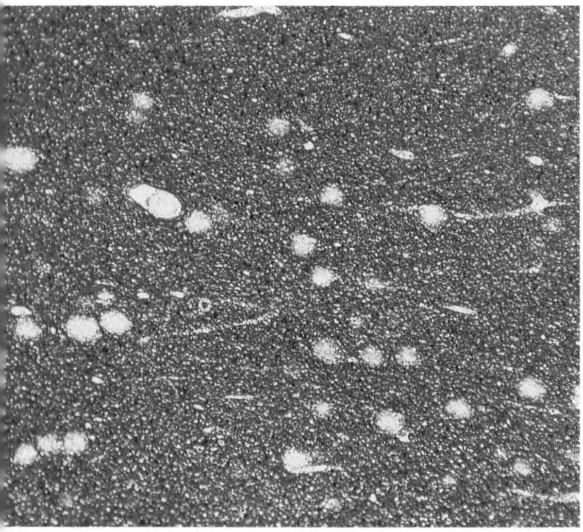

286

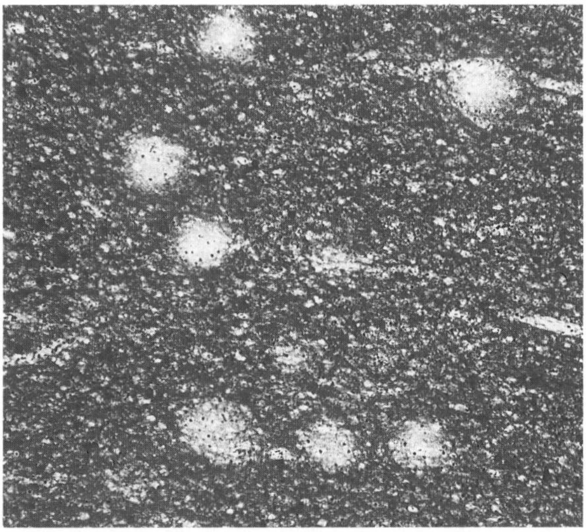

285 Small multiple, perivenular demyelinating lesions in multiple sclerosis. Note relationship to longitudinally orientated venules. The lesions resemble acute disseminated encephalomyelitis. Heidenhain, × 20.

286 Perivenular demyelination in MS. As for **285**, but × 60.

287

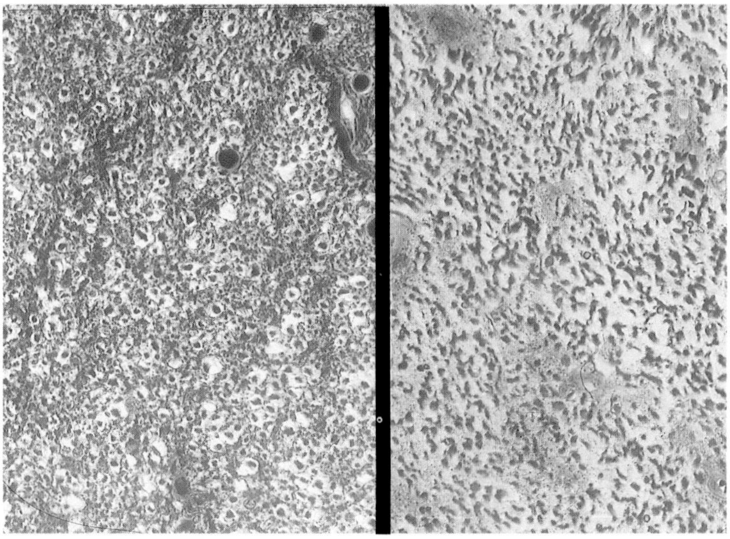

287 Preservation of axons in demyelinating non-necrotic plaques of multiple sclerosis. Palmgren silver, × 200.

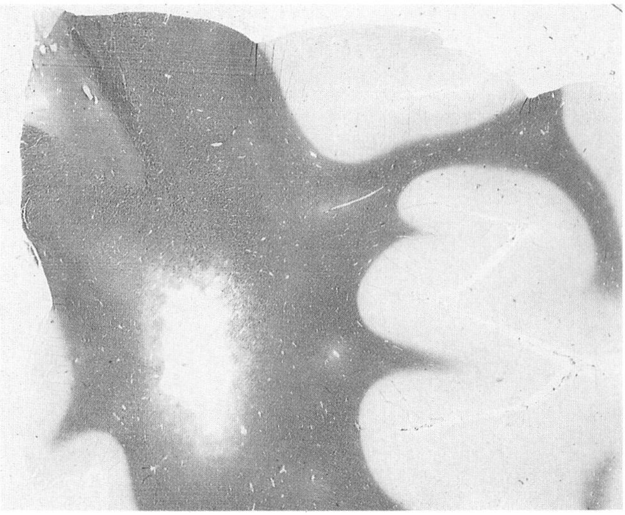
288

288 Necrotic lesion with ragged edges in multiple sclerosis. Luxol fast blue, × 2.

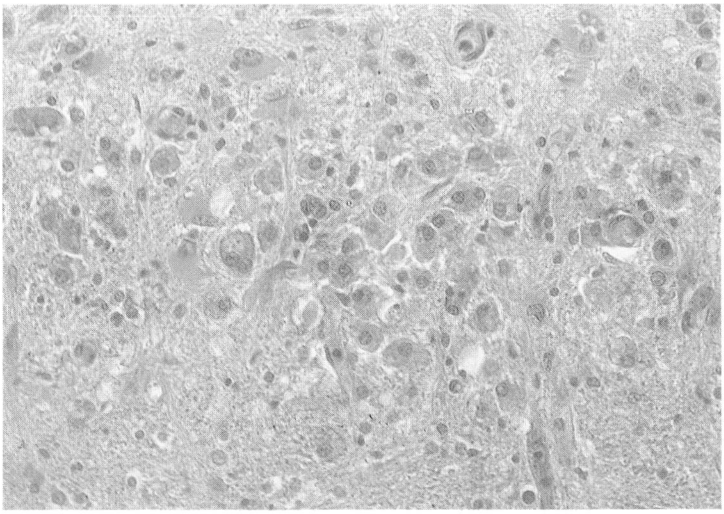
28

289 Necrotic lesion with marked macrophage infiltration at edge. Haematoxylin and eosin, × 150.

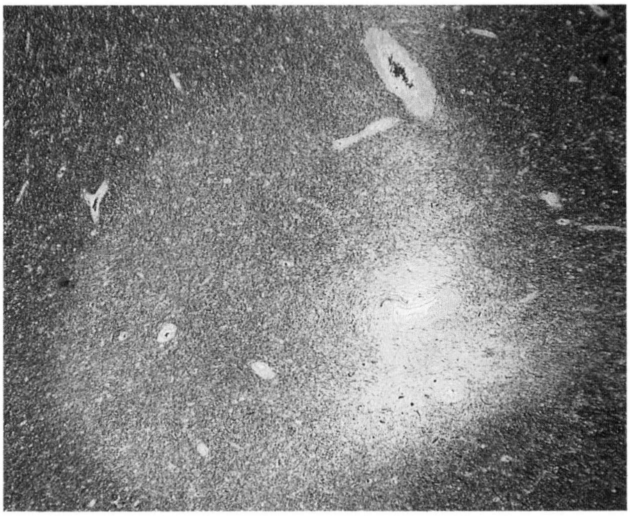
290

290 Shadow plaque with older and more recent components. Heidenhain, × 30.

291

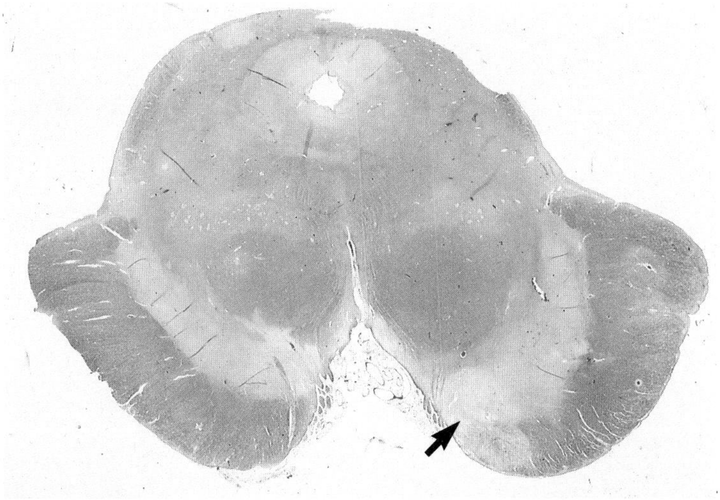

291 **Shadow plaques in basis pedunculi of midbrain.** The plaque extends into the substantia nigra (arrow). Phosphotungstic acid-haematoxylin, × 3.

292

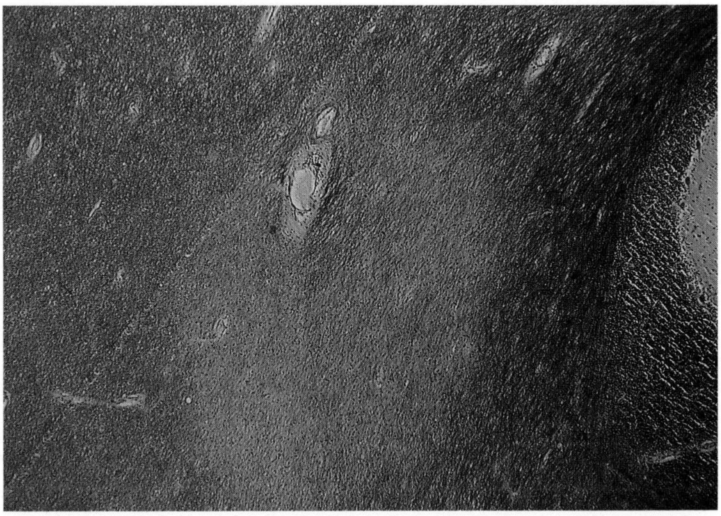

292 **Shadow plaque around a venule with surrounding perivascular infiltration and sclerosis.** Heidenhain, × 30.

293

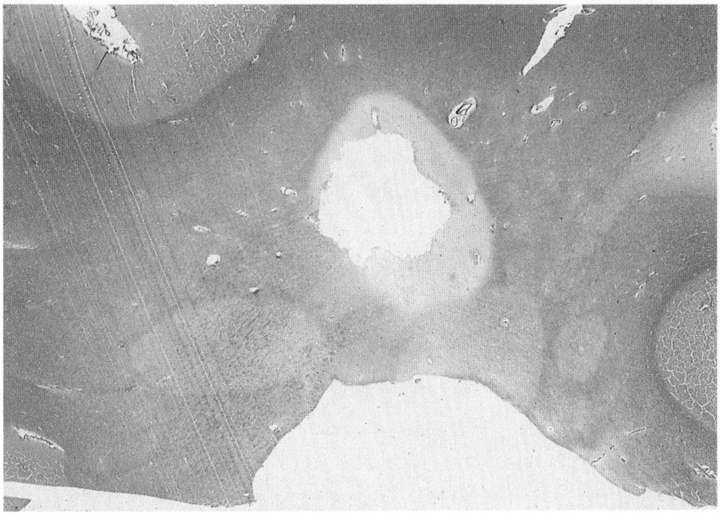

293 **Shadow plaques in periventricular white matter with old plaque encircling lateral ventricle.** Haematoxylin-eosin, × 3.

294

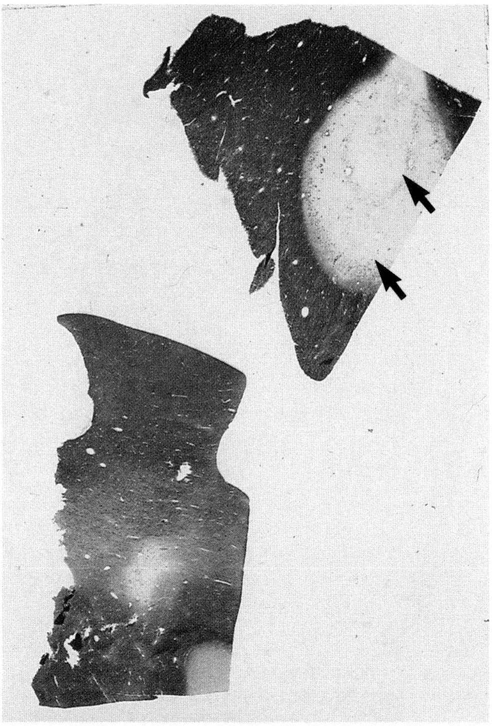

294 Shadow plaques. Bottom: area of complete demyelination within shadow plaque. Top: two zones of remyelination within plaque (arrows). Heidenhain, × 2.

295

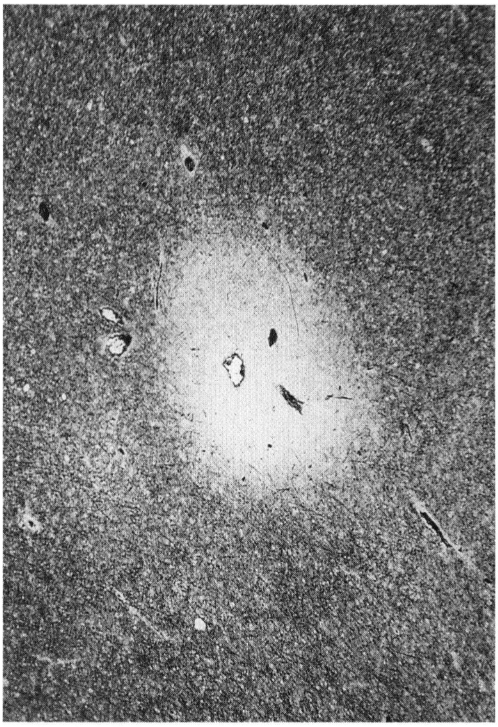

295 Small aborted lesion in multiple sclerosis. No products of demyelination are present. Heidenhain, × 30.

296

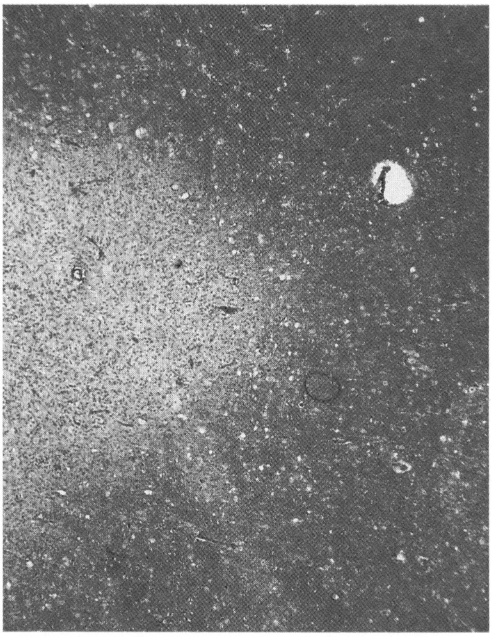

296 Active demyelinating lesion in acute multiple sclerosis with intense uptake of sudanophilic lipid by macrophages. This patient died in the bath, probably an example of the Uhthoff syndrome (impaired nerve conduction with increase in temperature). Oil red O, × 30.

297

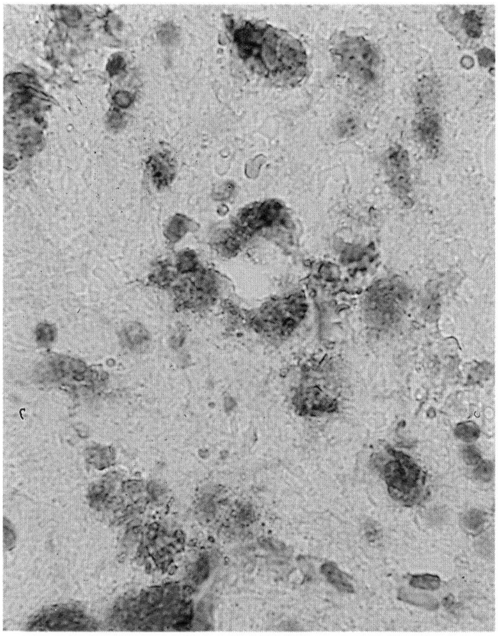

297 Active plaque with macrophages containing sudanophilic lipid (esterified cholesterol) lining edge of plaque. Oil red O, × 100.

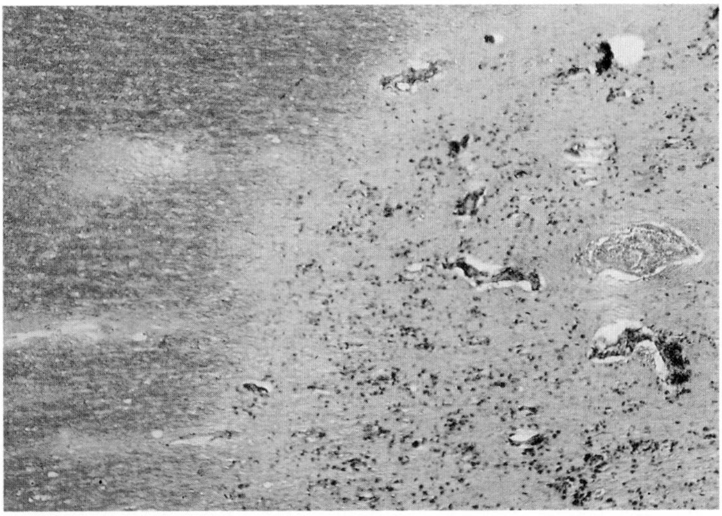

298

298 Active MS plaque stained with osmium tetroxide-α naphthylamine (OTAN); esterified cholesterol (black) within macrophages, × 30.

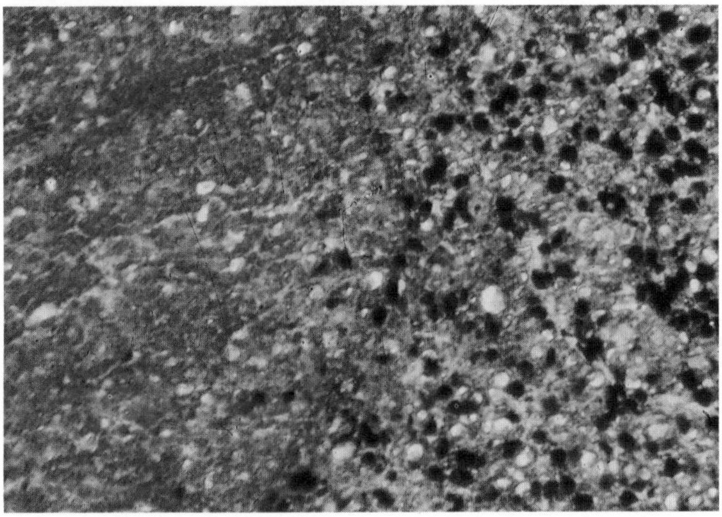

299

299 Edge of active demyelinating plaque stained with osmium tetroxide-resorcinol. Esterified cholesterol is black, normal myelin is purple, × 100.

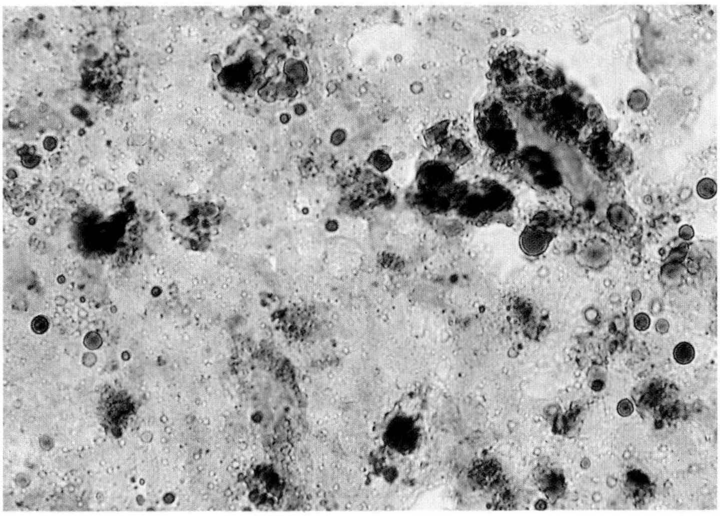

300

300 Blue-black staining of free cholesterol and/or ester cholesterol in myelin breakdown products in active MS plaque, perchloric acid-naphthoquinone, × 100.

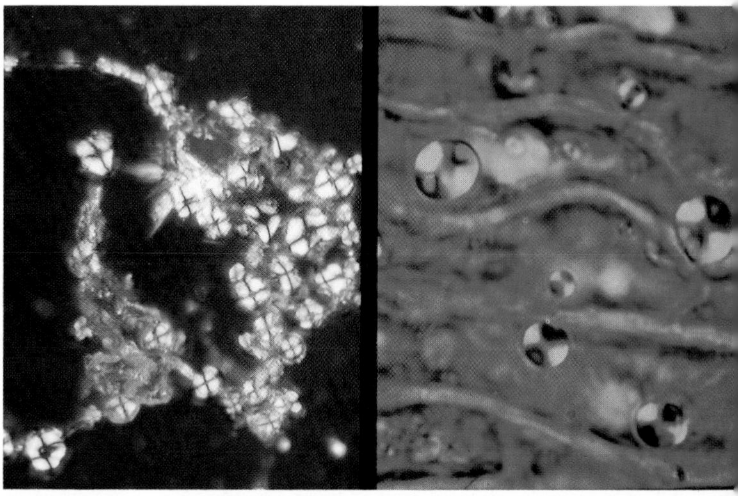

301 Maltese cross formation; esterified cholesterol in atheroma viewed in polarised light. Left: simple polarisation, × 100. Right: with retardation plate, × 300. *(Right illustration, courtesy of Professor R.O. Weller)*

302

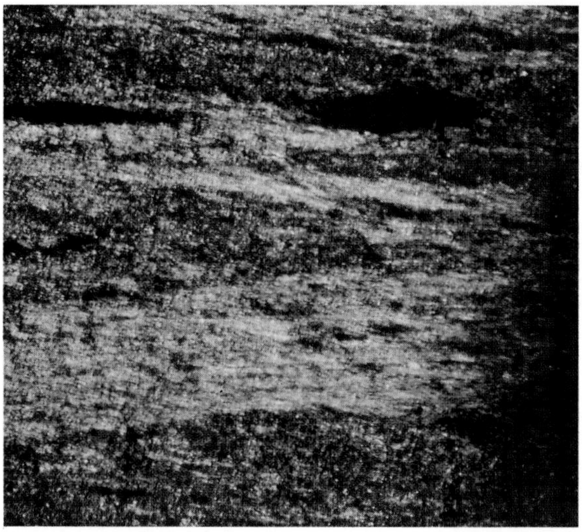

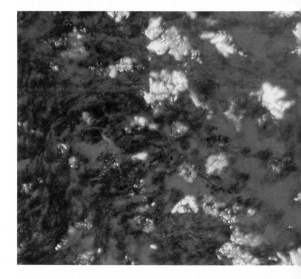

302 Birefringent myelinated tracts terminating at edge of inactive plaque of multiple sclerosis. Polarised light, × 30.

303 Acute MS. Birefringent lipid in macrophages at centre of lesion at right. Variably birefrigent lipid in 'myelinic' macrophages in demyelinating edge of plaque at left. Oil red O – polarised light, × 280.

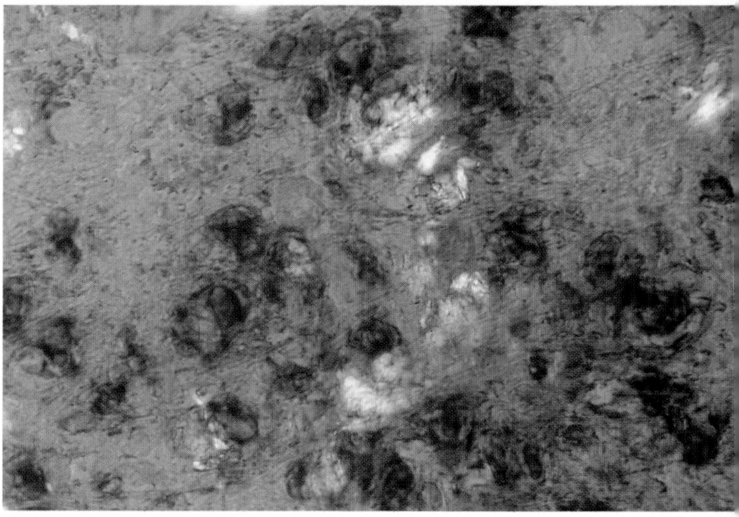

304 Anisotropic (birefringent) sudanophilic cholesterol ester droplets and crystals within macrophages in active MS lesion. The demyelinating edge shows isotropic blue-staining 'myelinic' (non-birefringent) lipid within macrophages. Solochrome cyanin – oil red O, × 250.

305

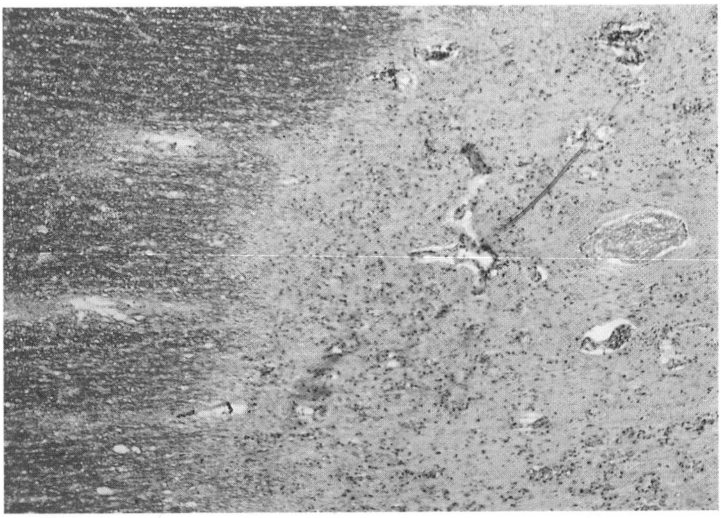

305 Active plaque to show loss of myelin basic protein. Trypan blue, × 50.

306

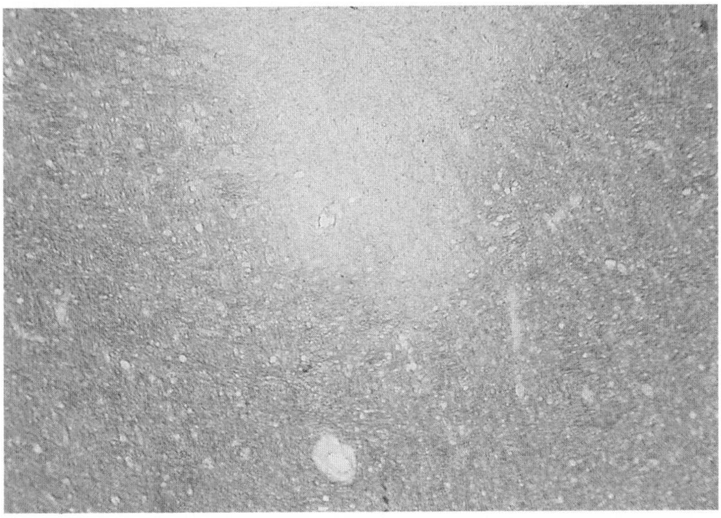

306 Active plaque to show loss of myelin phospholipids. Gold hydroxamic acid method for phosphoglycerides, × 30.

307

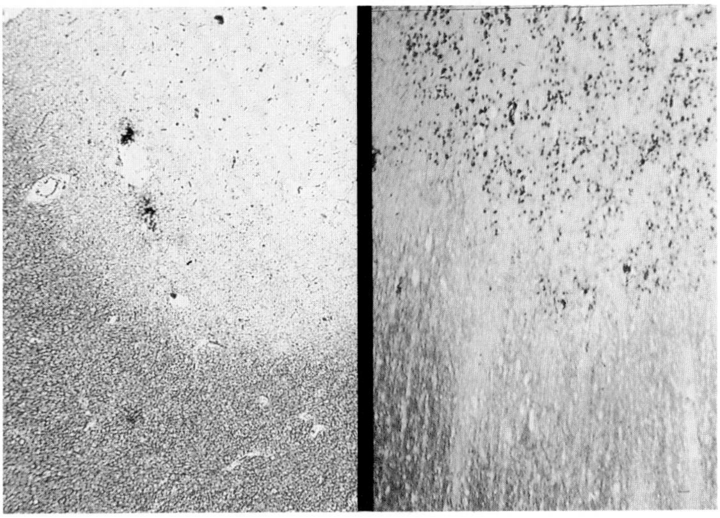

307 Left: chronic burnt-out plaque of multiple sclerosis. Note sharp edge to lesion, little lipid in macrophages except around blood vessels. Right: active plaque showing shelving edge and abundant lipid containing macrophages. The phospholipids in normal myelin are stained, reddish brown. OTAN, × 30.

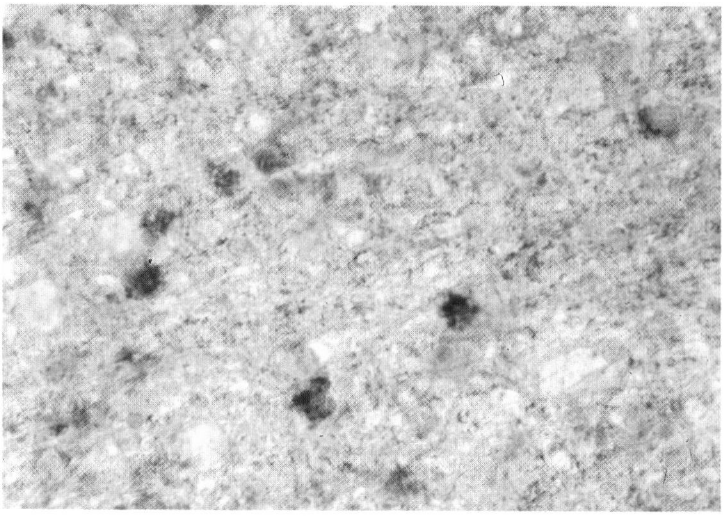

308 Metachromatic material probably within neuroglia of white matter in multiple sclerosis. Acidic lipid stained with Nile blue oxazine, × 150.

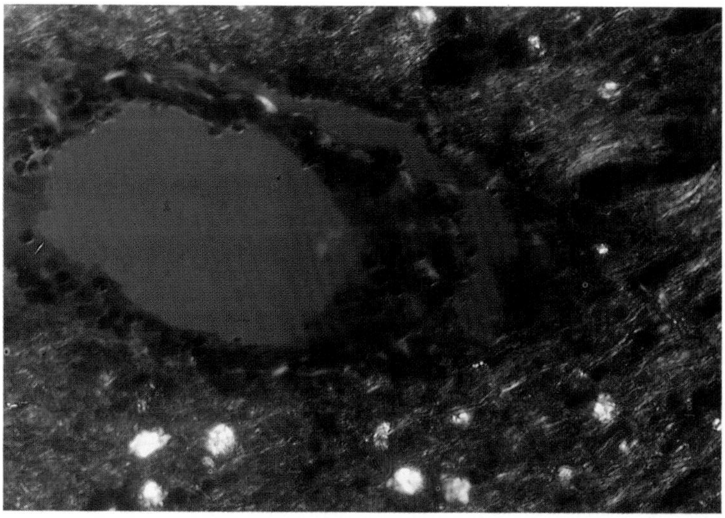

309 The material shown in 308 is also birefringent in polarised light, × 120.

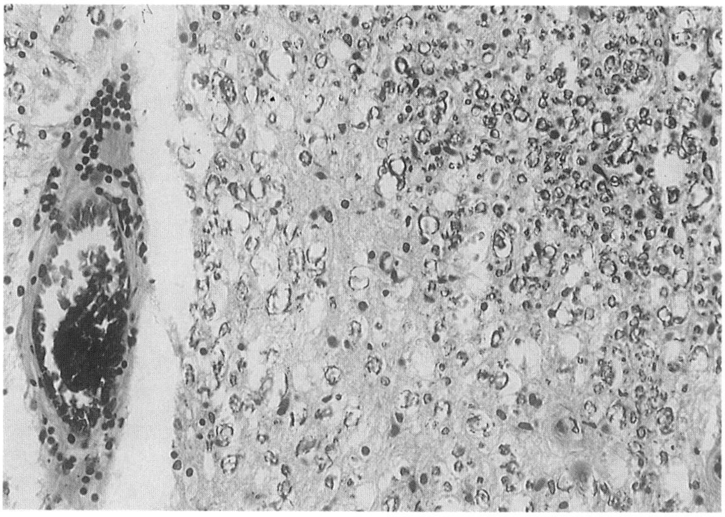

310 Thinly myelinated but irregular fibres at edge of chronic progressive plaque of multiple sclerosis in spinal cord. These fibres are probably slowly demyelinating rather than remyelinating. Luxol fast blue, × 200.

311 Area of unaffected myelin from spinal cord in the same case as **310**. Luxol fast blue, × 200.

311

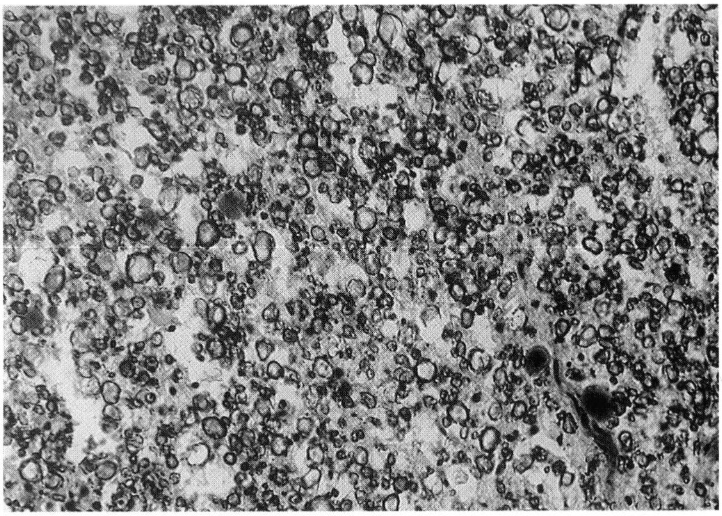

312 Chronic plaque of multiple sclerosis, showing demyelinated and thinly myelinated fibres. Where the axon appears normal, these thinly myelinated fibres may be in the process of remyelination, × 7,200. *(Courtesy of Professor C.S. Raine)*

312

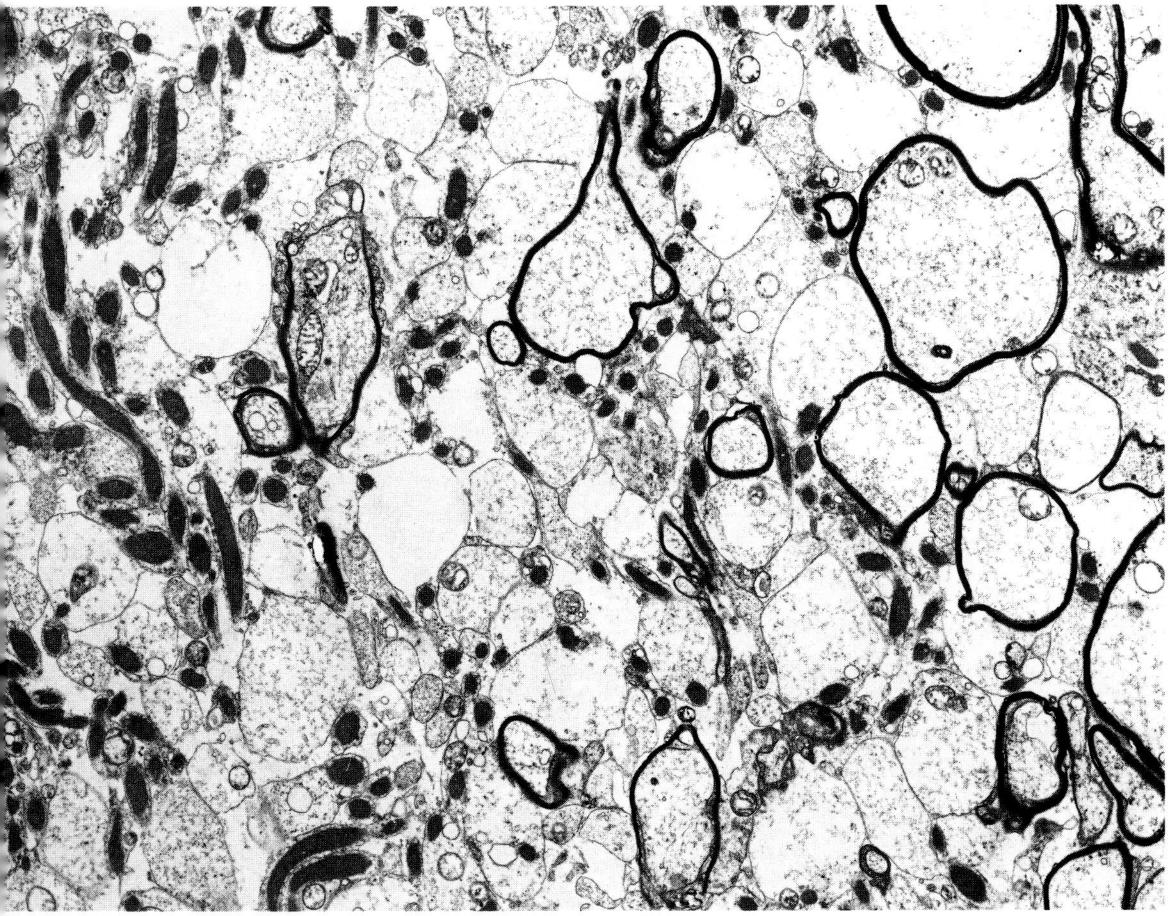

31

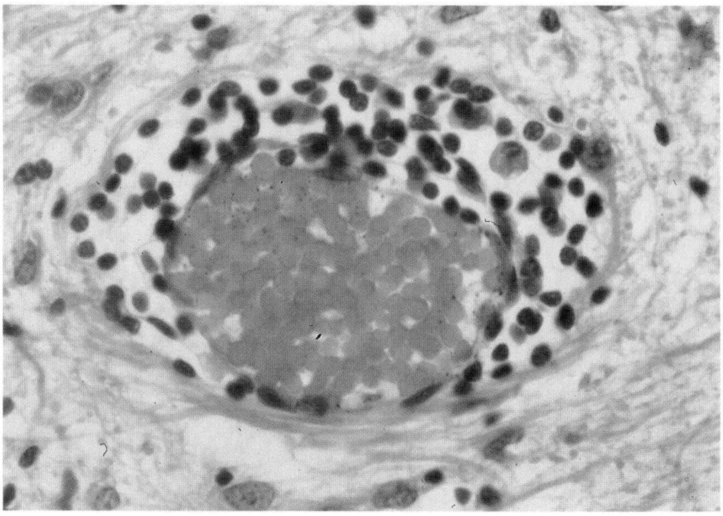

313 Perivenular infiltrate of lymphocytes and plasma cells in active plaque of multiple sclerosis. Haematoxylin-eosin, × 300.

31

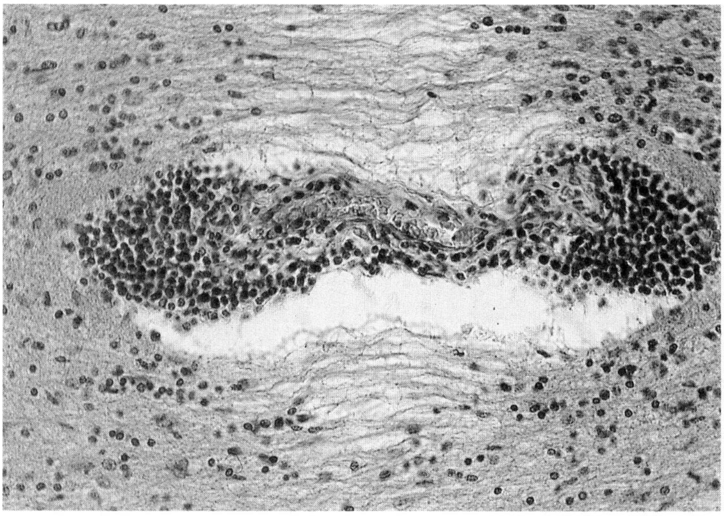

314 Perivenous lymphocytic infiltrate in white matter outside plaque in active multiple sclerosis. Haematoxylin-eosin, × 100.

31

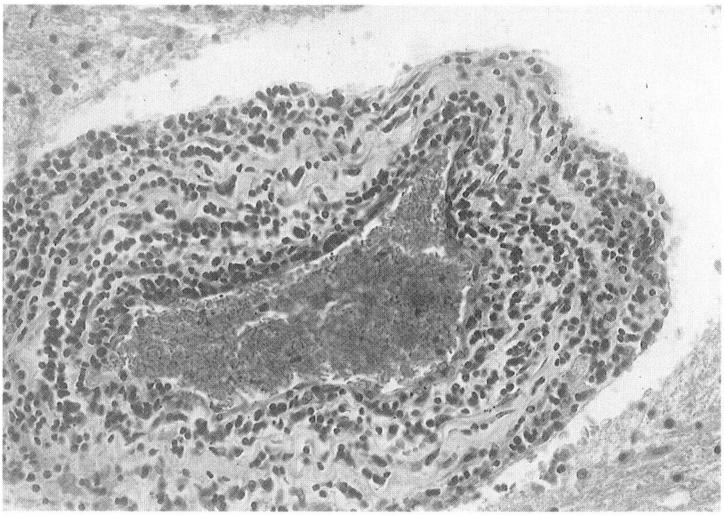

315 Perivenous inflammatory infiltrate involving wall of vein. Haematoxylin-eosin, × 150.

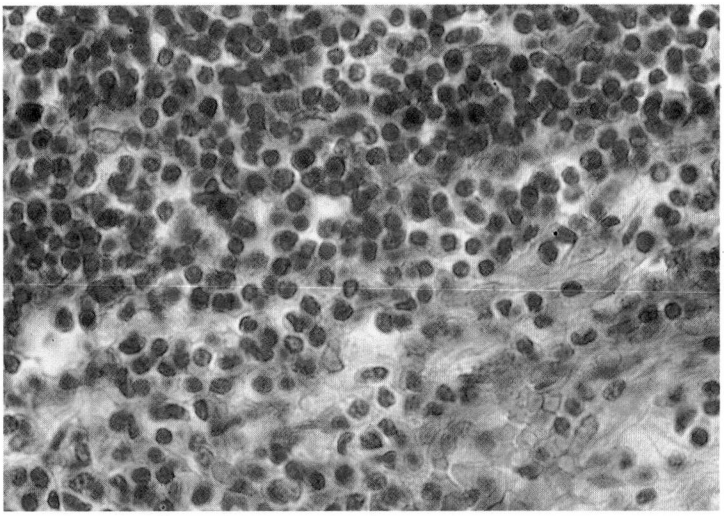

316

·16 **Predominantly perivenular ymphocytic infiltrate**, with ccasional plasma cells in ıflammatory infiltrate in acute multiple clerosis. Phosphotungstic acid-aematoxylin, × 300.

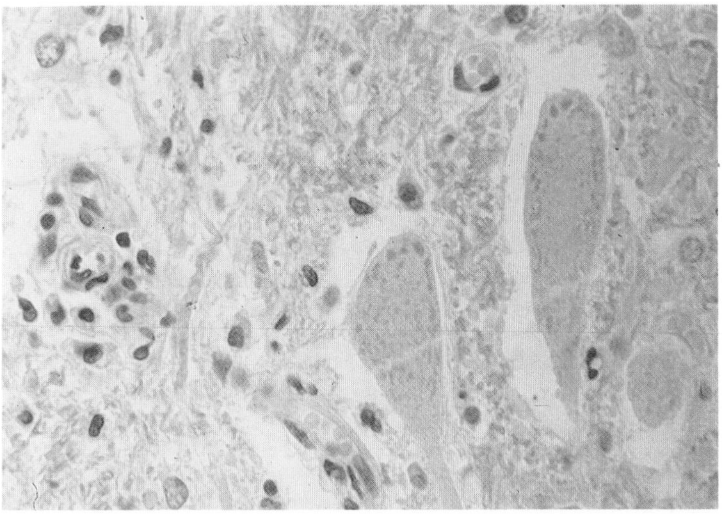

317

17 **Anterior poliomyelitis.** Margination of chromatin in hromatolysis of anterior horn cells of pinal cord. Note absence of ıflammatory infiltrate apart from euronophagia at left. Haematoxylin-osin, × 200.

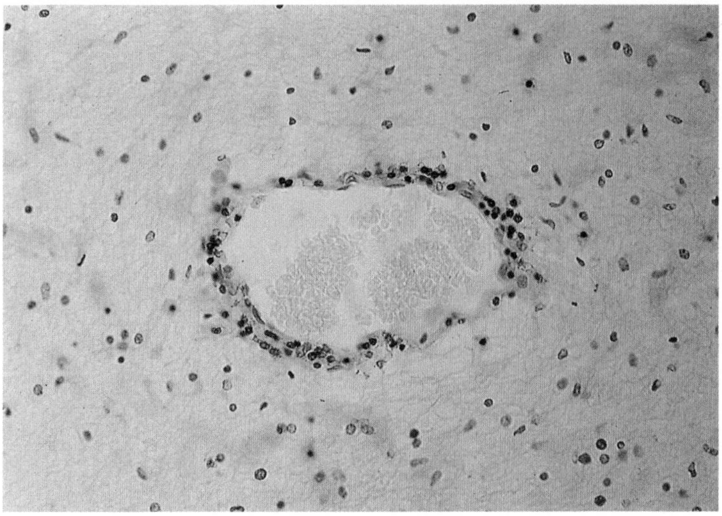

318

18 **Lymphocytes around vein in ıultiple sclerosis.** PD7/26-eroxidase (common leucocyte ntigen), × 100.

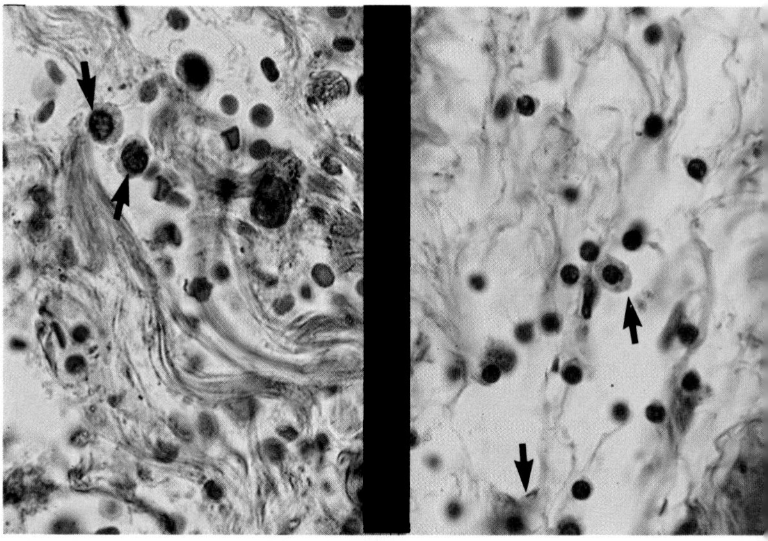

319 Plasma cells (PC) in multiple sclerosis.
Left: PC in perivenous infiltrate (arrows), Bielschowsky, × 300. Right: PC in subacute meningitis (arrows). Haematoxylin-eosin, × 300.

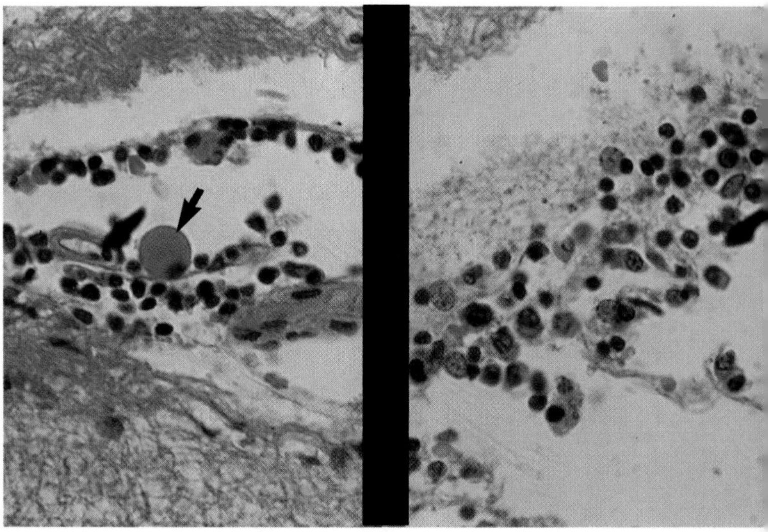

320 Plasma cells in subacute meningitis in multiple sclerosis.
Note Russell body (IgG storage) at left (arrow): Haematoxylin and eosin, × 250.

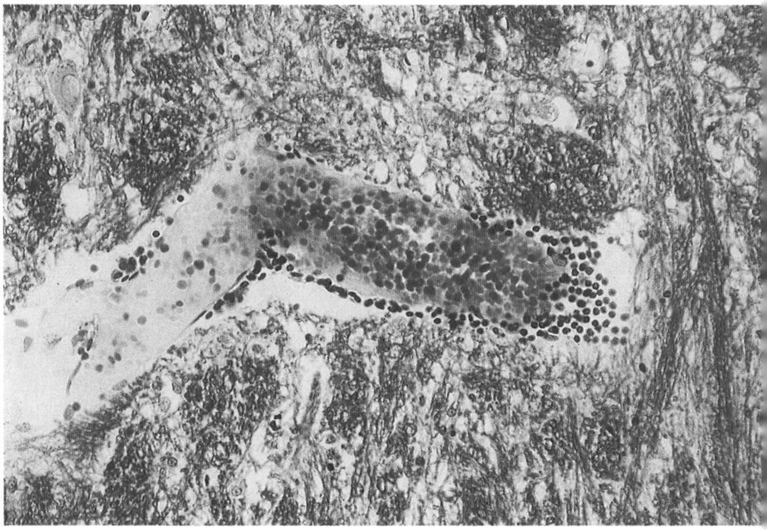

321 Dawson's finger at edge of active plaque: inflammatory infiltrate extending outwards from a plaque around a vein. Luxol fast blue, crystal violet, × 80.

322 Dawson's finger. As for **321**.
Haematoxylin-eosin, × 40.

323 Parallel rows of venules with perivascular infiltrate in central white matter near a plaque of multiple sclerosis. Haematoxylin-eosin, × 100.

Lymphocyte Cuffs · Venules · Dawson's Finger · Early Plaque

324 Centrifugal extension of multiple sclerosis along veins. The individual small lesions may then coalesce to form a large plaque, as in the periventricular region. *(Reproduced from Adams, 1977)*

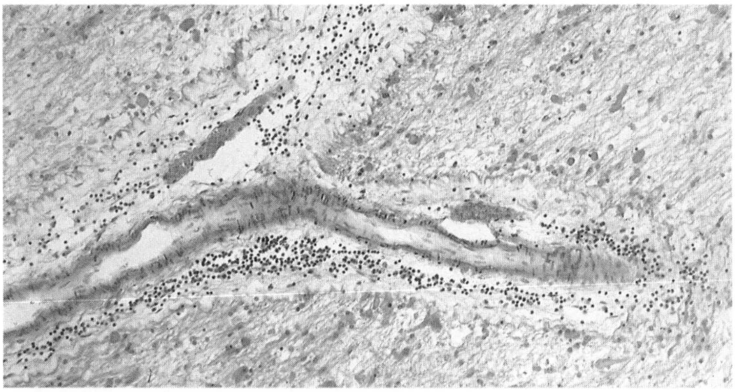

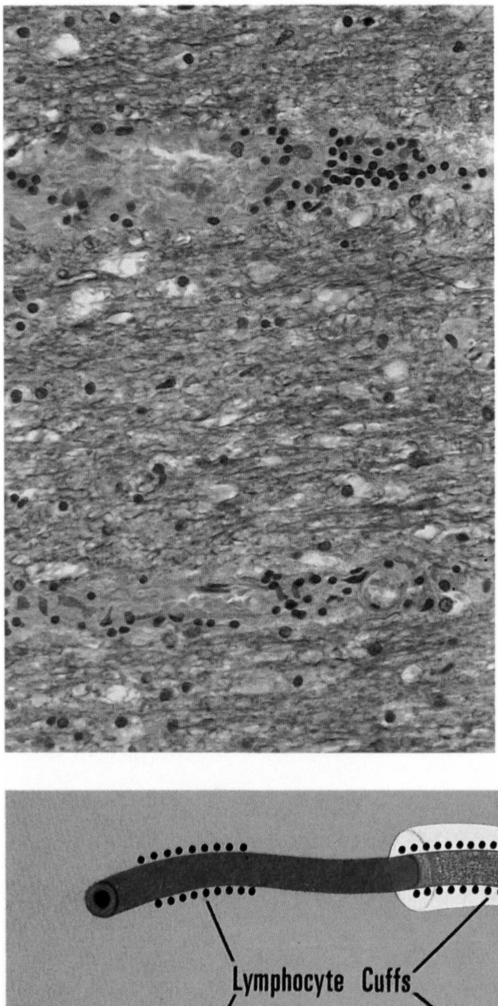

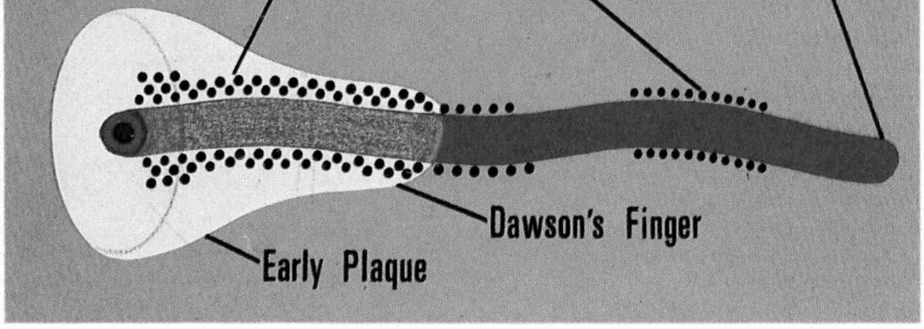

32

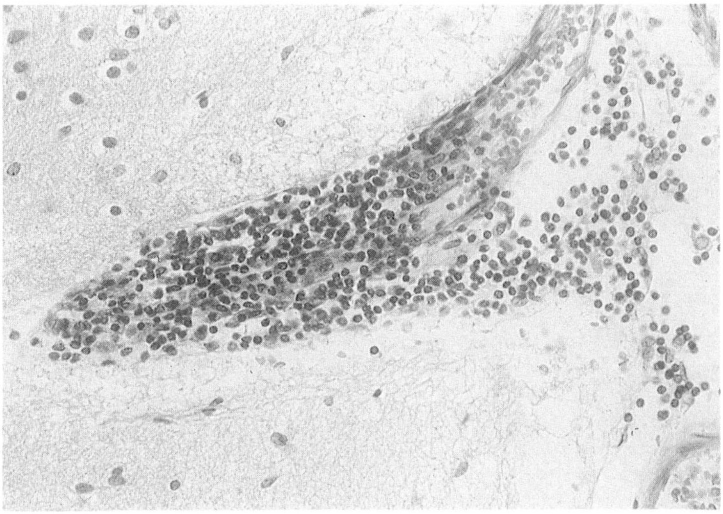

325 Lymphocytic meningitis in subarachroid space of cerebral sulcus in multiple sclerosis. Haematoxylin-eosin, × 80.

32

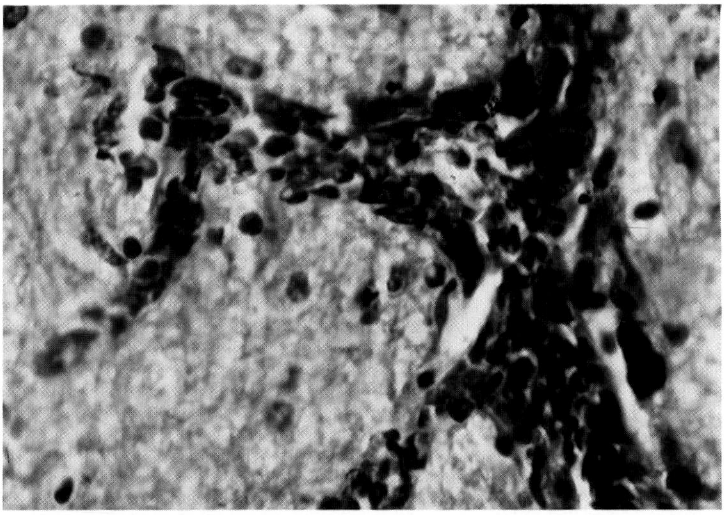

326 Lymphocytic emigration at venocapillary junction in white matter in multiple sclerosis. Heidenhain, × 350.

32

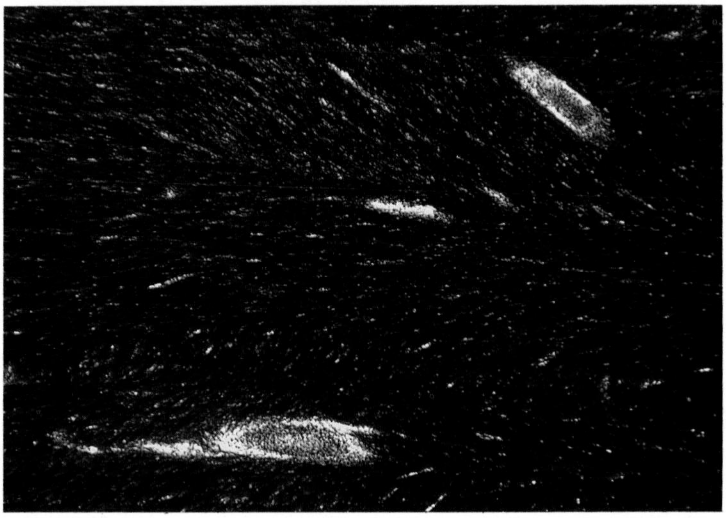

327 Oedema around venule in white matter in multiple sclerosis. Heidenhain, × 30.

328

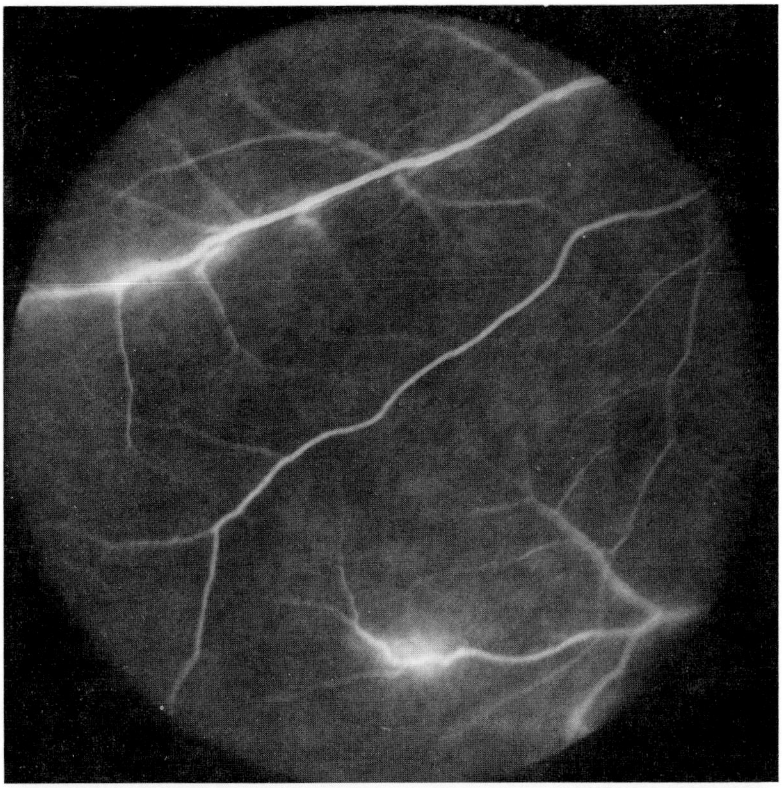

28 Perivenous sheaving in etina in MS. Fluorescence ngiography. *(Courtesy of Dr S. ightman and Profs. A.C. Bird nd W.I. McDonald)*

329

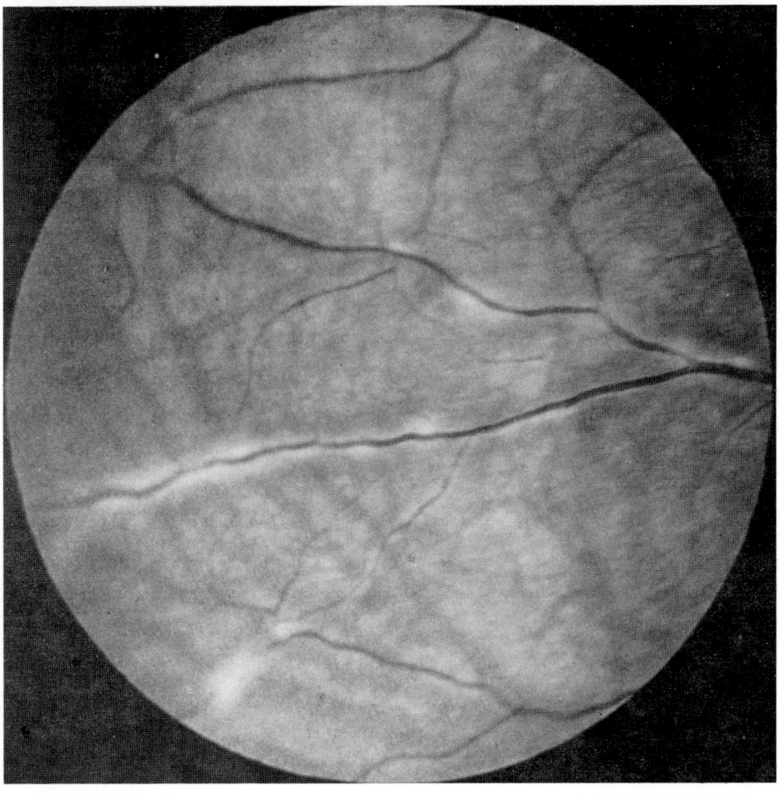

29 Perivenous sheaving in etina in MS. Low red hotography. *(Courtesy of Dr S. ightman and Profs A.C. Bird nd W.I. McDonald)*

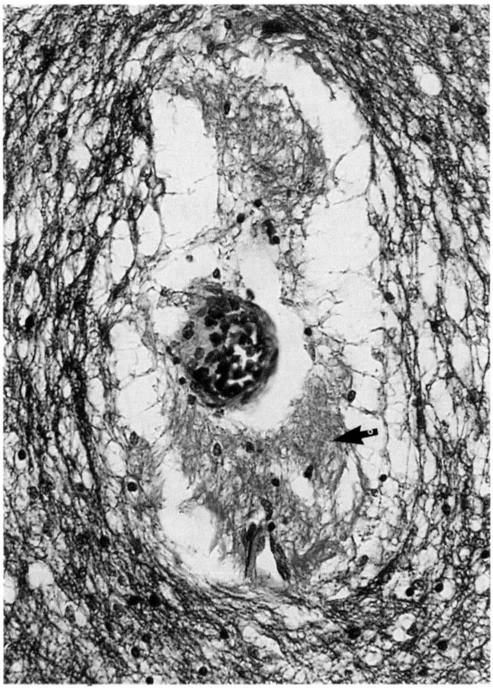

330

330 Fibrinous exudate (red-staining; arrow) around venule in active multiple sclerosis. Trichrome-MSB, × 80.

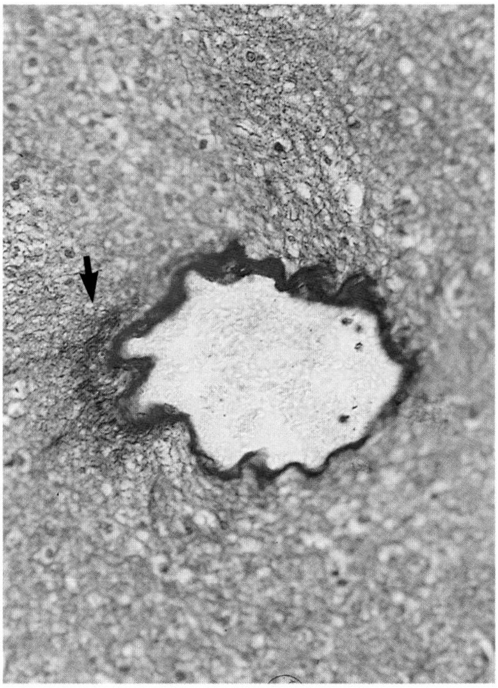

331

331 Fibrinous exudate as for 330, but blue staining (arrow). Phosphotungstic acid-haematoxylin, × 80.

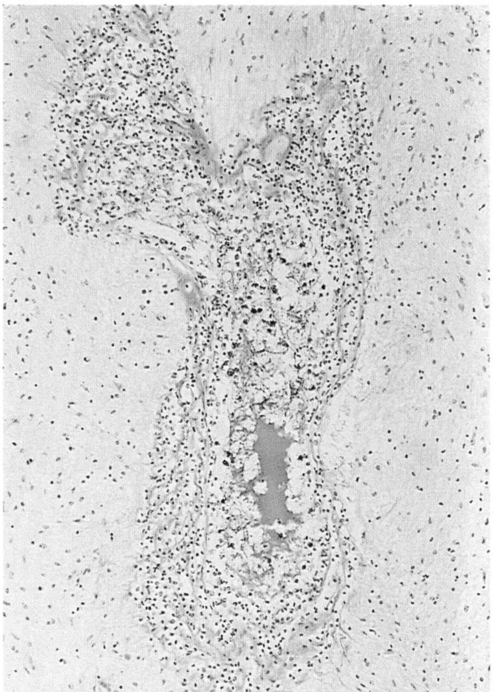

332

332 Fibrinous exudate around venule at centre of plaque of multiple sclerosis. Anti-fibrin-peroxidase, × 30.

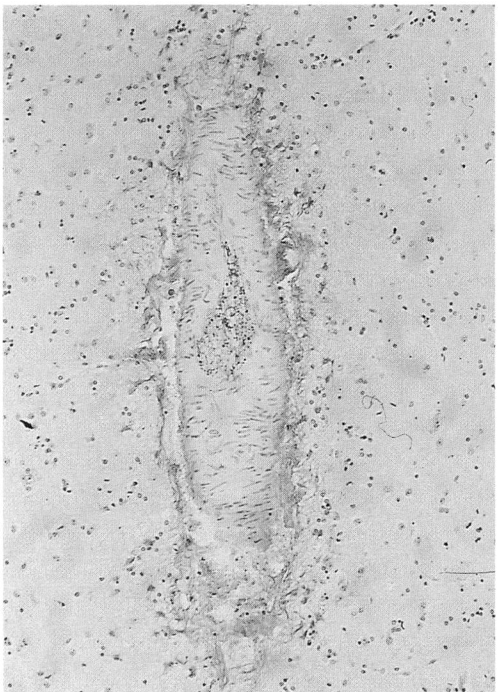

333

333 Fibrinous exudate around venule in white matter outside plaque of multiple sclerosis. Anti-fibrin-peroxidase, × 30.

334

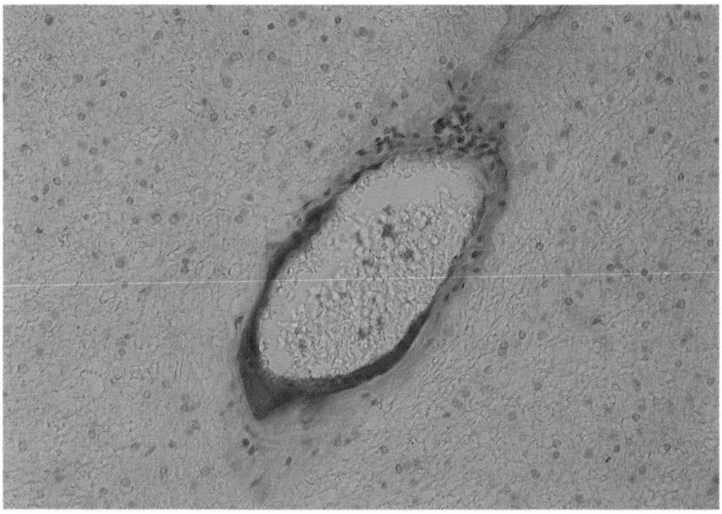

34 Permeability of vein in eriventricular plaque. Anti-IgG eroxidase, blue light × 30.

335

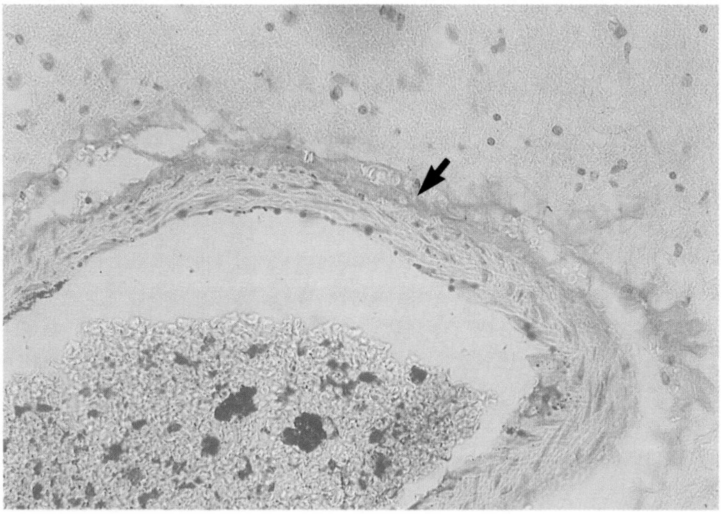

35 C_3-complement (arrow) around ein in periventricular plaque. Anti-$_3$-peroxidase, blue light, × 80.

336

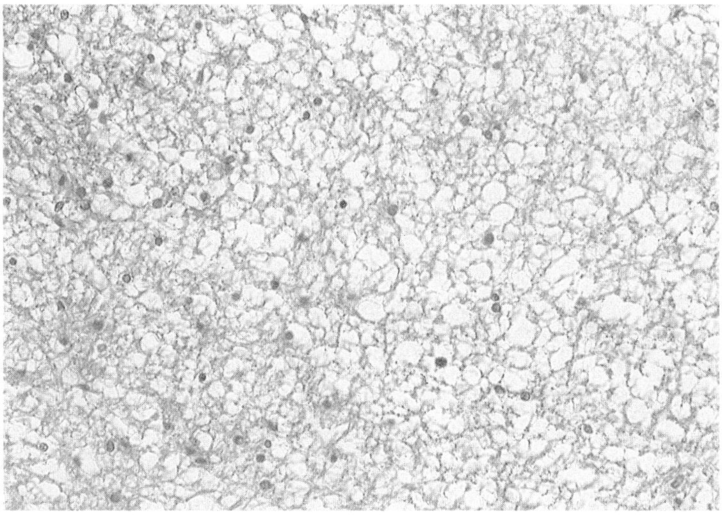

36 Vacuolar myelin in central white iatter in multiple sclerosis. laematoxylin-eosin, × 60.

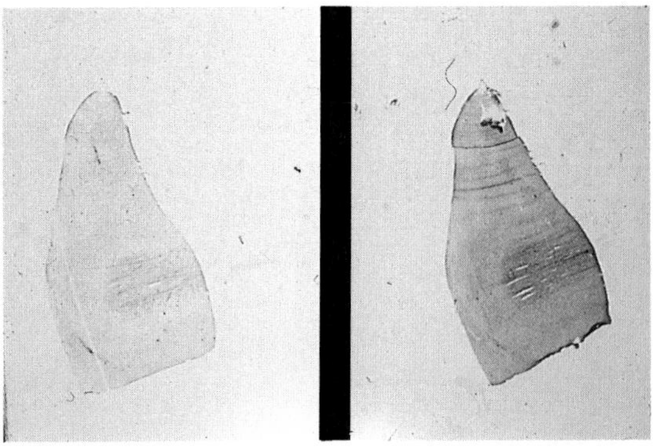

337 Early MS lesion in an acute case with 2-week clinical history. Note hypercellularity (increased enzyme activity) throughout lesion. Left: ATPase. Right; NADH-tetrazolium reductase, × 2.

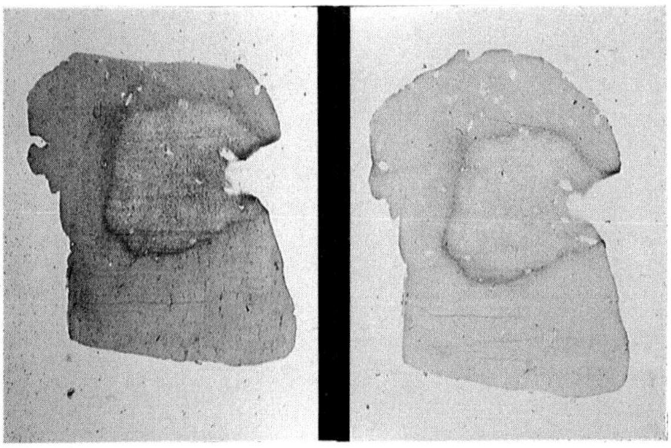

338 Active MS lesion with peripheral rim of hypercellularity (shown as increased enzyme activity). Left; ATPase. Right; NADH-tetrazolium reductase, × 2.

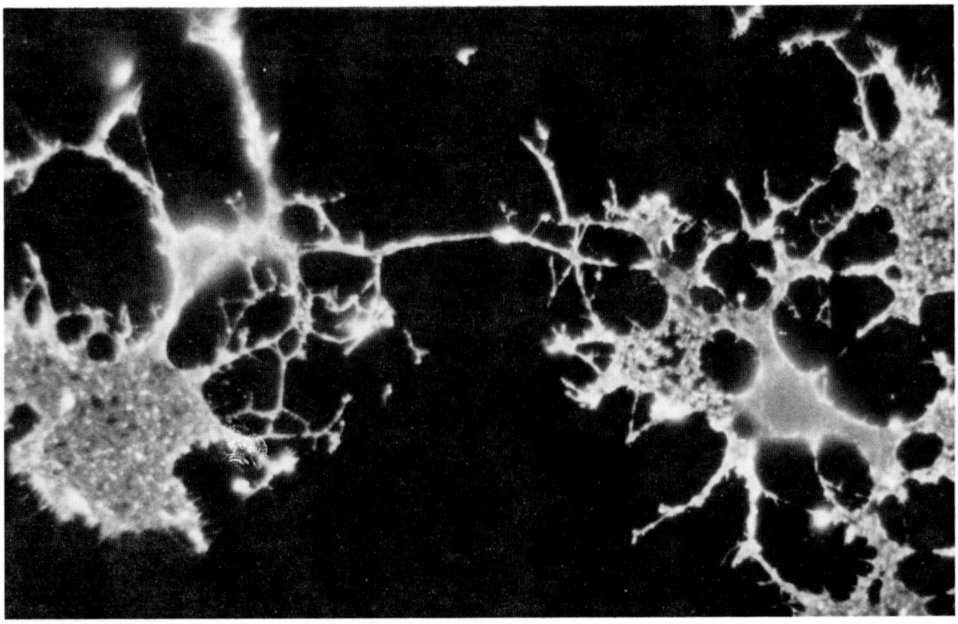

339 Oligodendroglia in culture stained by antigalactolipid-peroxidase, × 600. *(Courtesy of Professor M.C. Raff)*

340

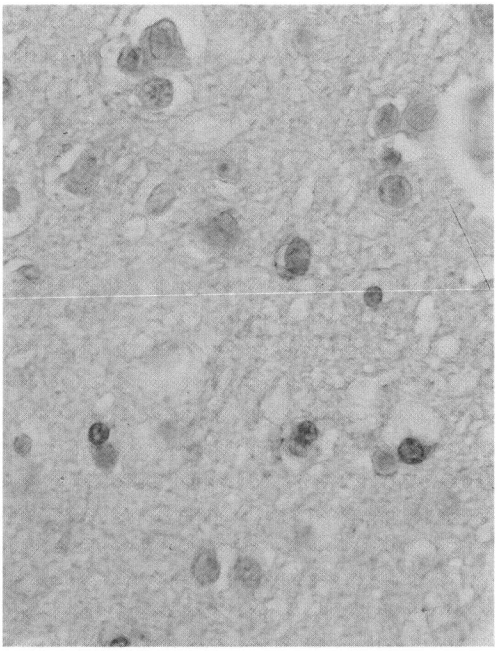

341

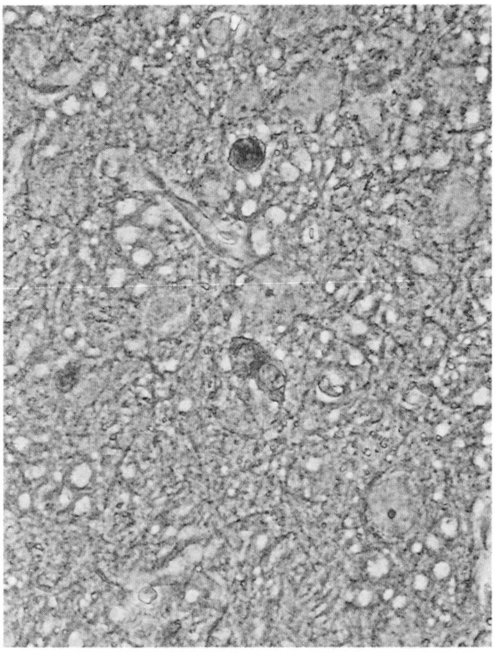

340 Human oligodendroglia stained by anti-carbonic anhydrase (II)-peroxidase, × 300. *(Courtesy of Dr N.A. Gregson)*

341 Human oligodendroglia stained by carbonic anhydrase-alkaline phosphatase, × 300. *(Courtesy of Dr N.A. Gregson)*

342

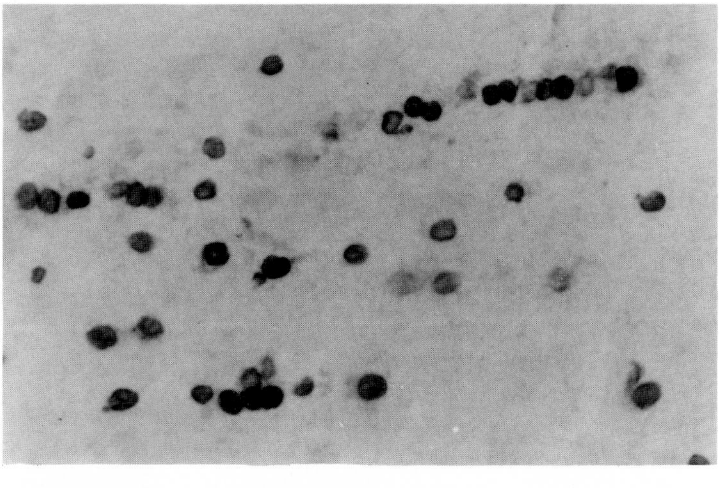

342 Human oligodendroglia stained by a mouse monoclonal antibody 14E – avidin/biotin peroxidase, × 300. *(Courtesy of Dr J. Newcombe)*

343

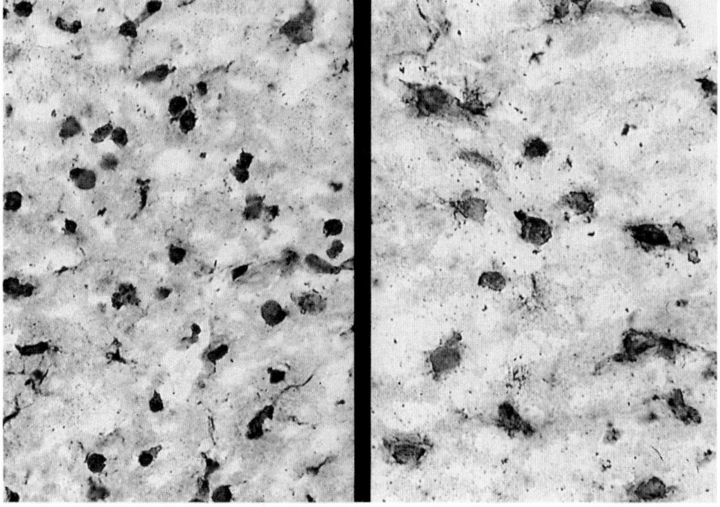

343 Left: Oligodendroglia (black) at edge of plaque of multiple sclerosis. Right: absence of oligodendroglia but abundant hypertrophic astrocytes (brown) in centre of plaque. Penfield silver carbonate, × 150.

344

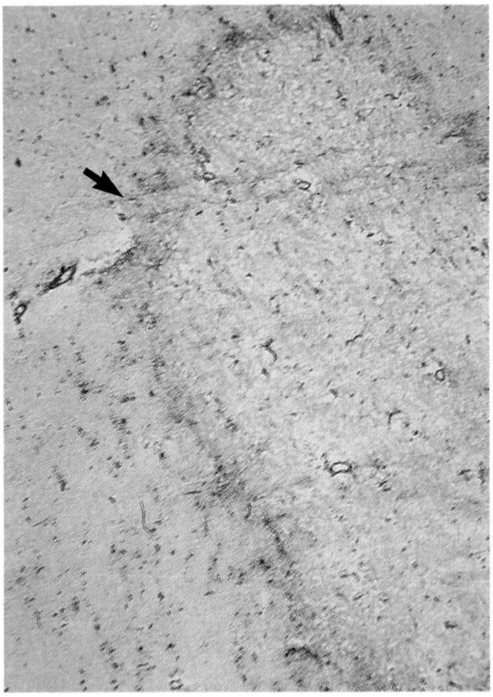

344 Proliferating rim of oligodendroglia at edge of active MS lesion. Haematoxylin-eosin, × 5.

345

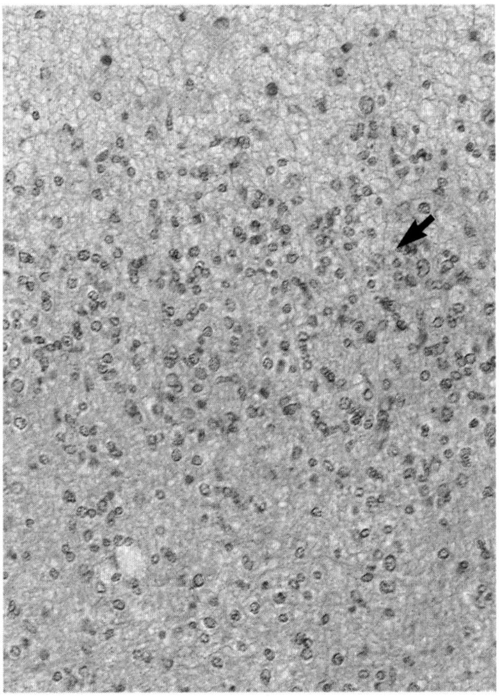

345 and **346 Higher power views of 344, to show cellular detail.** Most cells are oligodendroglia (round nuclei) but some astrocytic nuclei are also seen (larger, ovoid and more vesiculate nucleus). Occasional macroplage/microglial nuclei are elongated and sausage-shaped (see Hortega, 1930). Haematoxylin-eosin, × 100 and × 250.

346

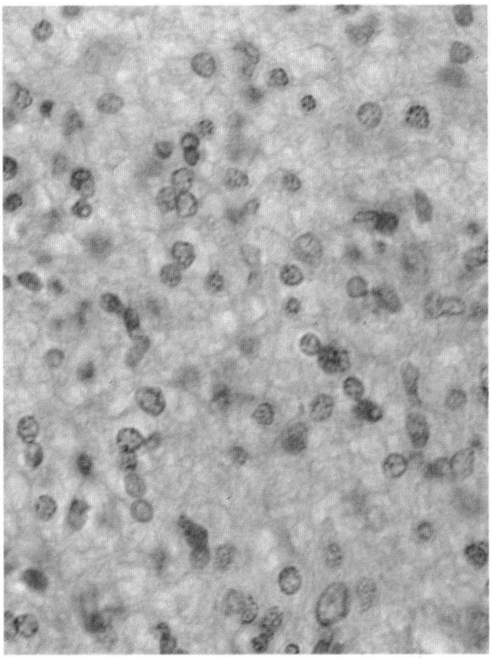

347

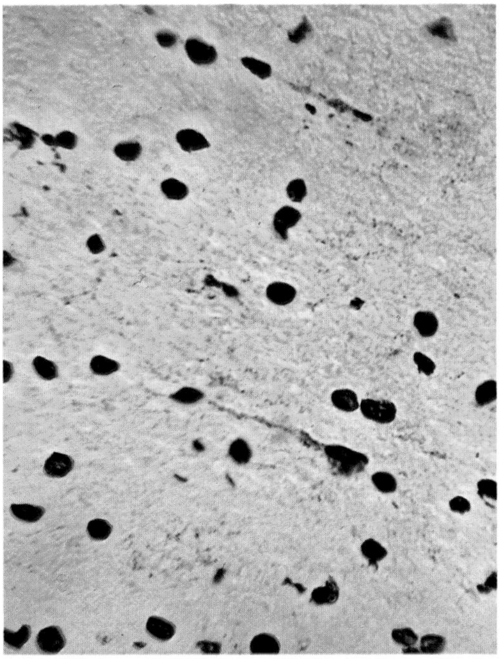

347 Oligodendroglia persisting at edge of MS plaque. Penfield silver carbonate, × 180.

348

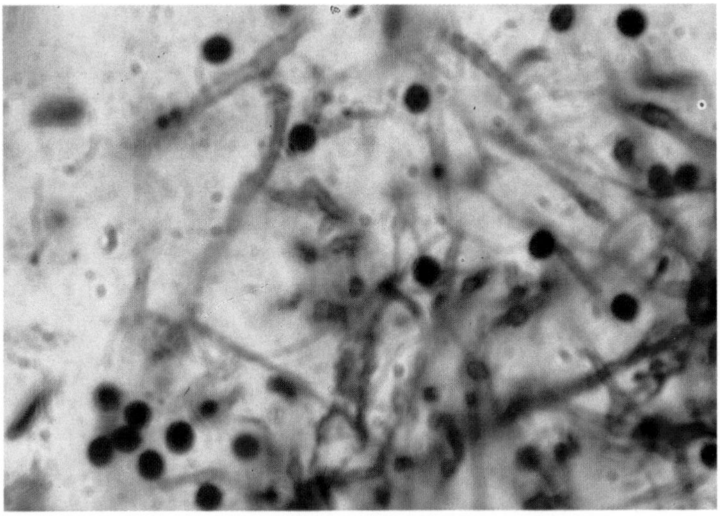

·48 Oligodendroglia persisting at ·lemyelinated edge of MS plaque. ·leidenhain, × 200.

349

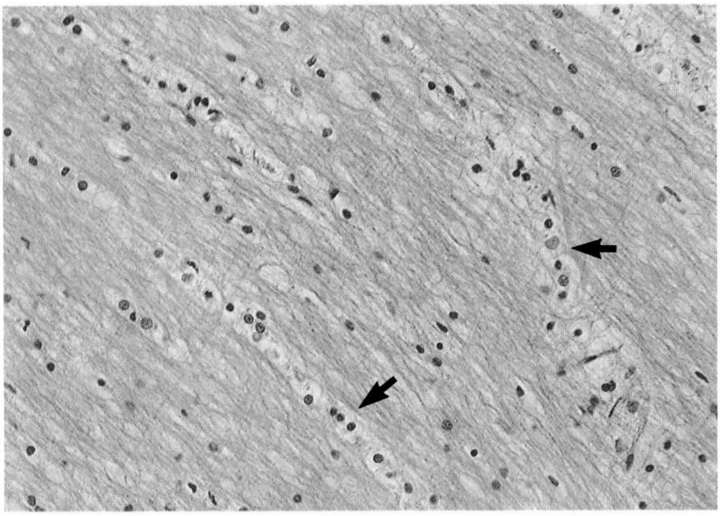

·49 Oligodendroglia near edge of ·IS plaque. Note perinuclear halo ·arrows) or cytoplasmic oedema ·'acute swelling'). Haematoxylin-eosin, ·< 100.

350

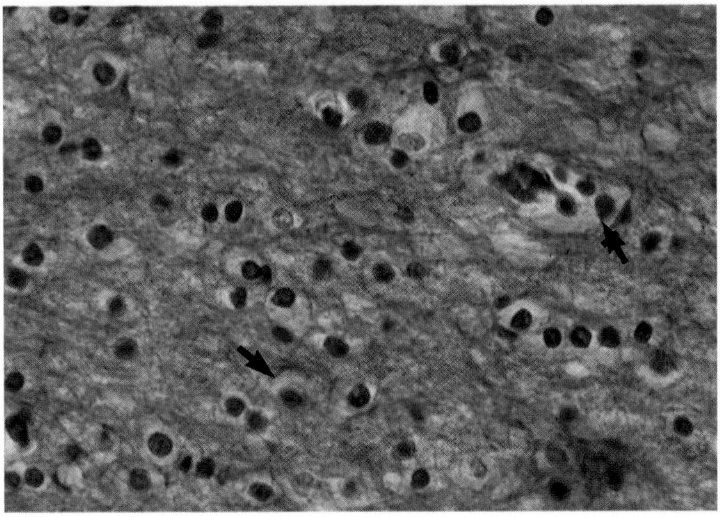

·50 Oligodendroglia in white matter ·n MS. Note acute swelling or ·ytoplasmic oedema. Phosphotungstic ·cid haematoxylin, × 300.

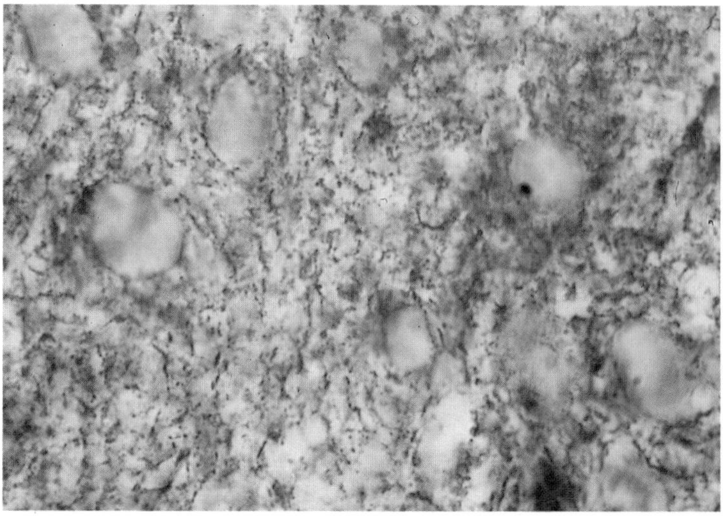

351 Increased oxidative activity in oligodendroglia in acute MS plaque. NADH-tetrazolium reductase, × 300.

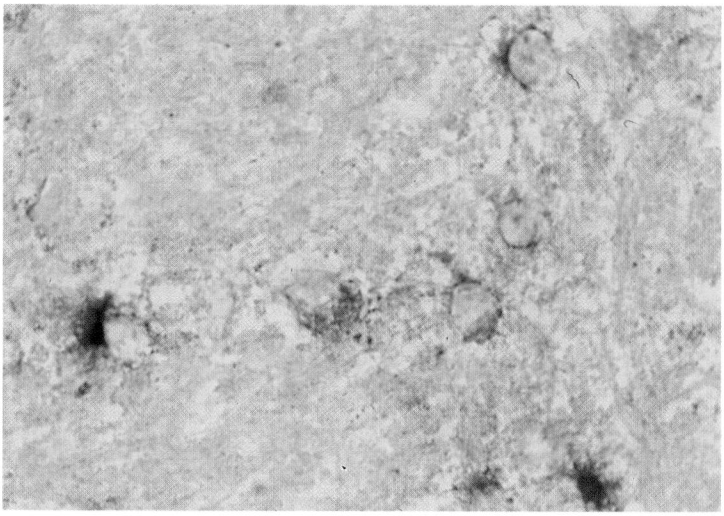

352 Normal oligodendroglia in human brain. NADH-tetrazolium reductase, × 250.

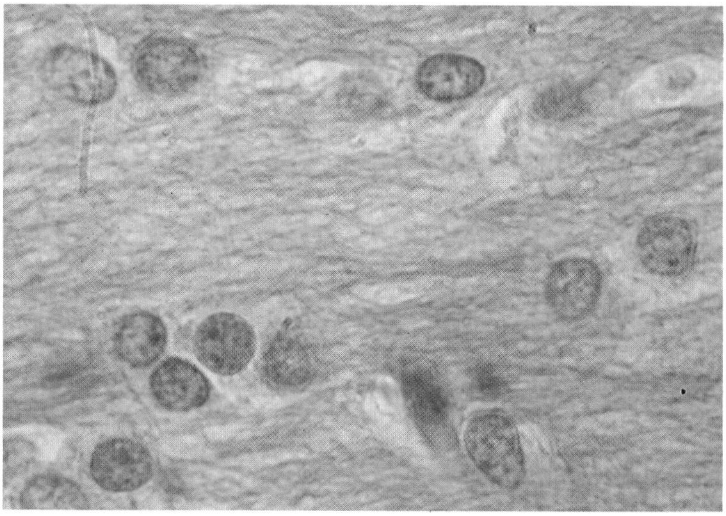

353 Hypertrophied oligodendroglia at edge of MS plaque. Haematoxylin-eosin, × 250.

354

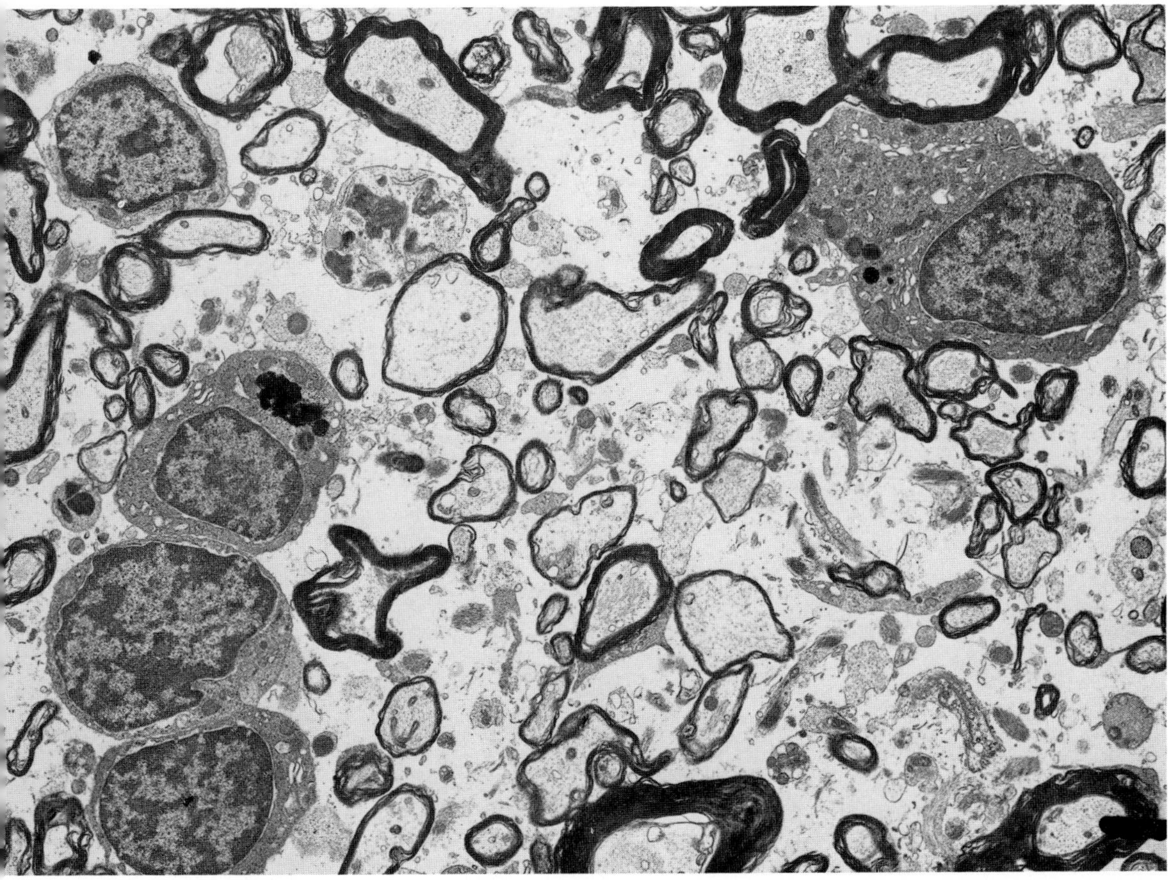

354 Chronic multiple sclerosis plaque. Note proliferation and hypertrophy of oligodendrocytes (dark cells). Note also inappropriately thin myelin which may represent demyelination, × 7,200. *(Courtesy of Professor C.S. Raine)*

355

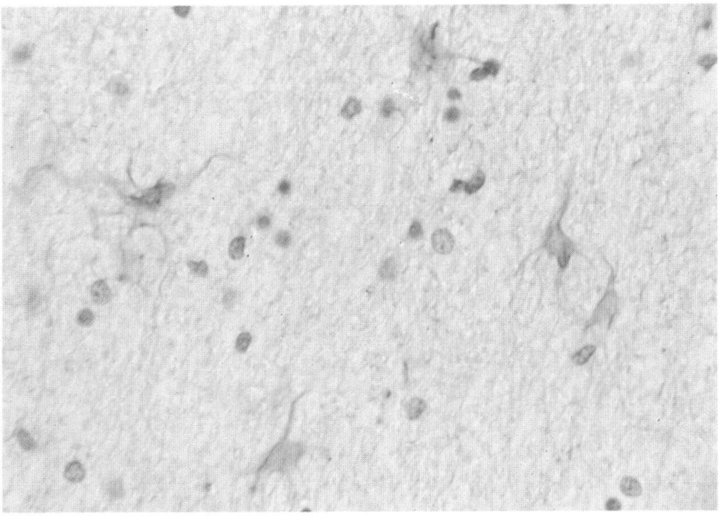

355 Normal fibrillary astrocytes. Glial fibrillary acidic protein (GFAP), × 150.

356

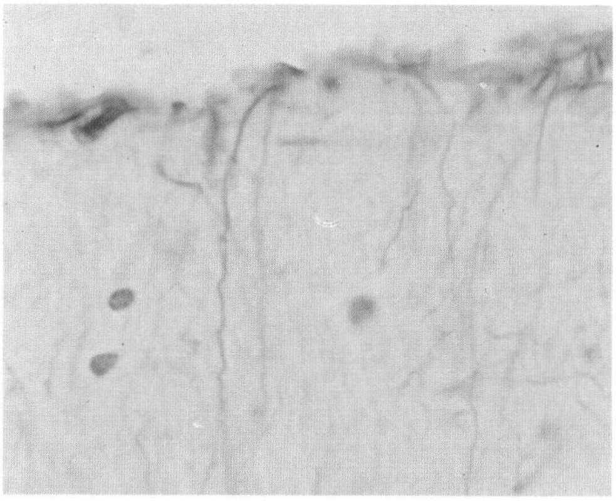

357

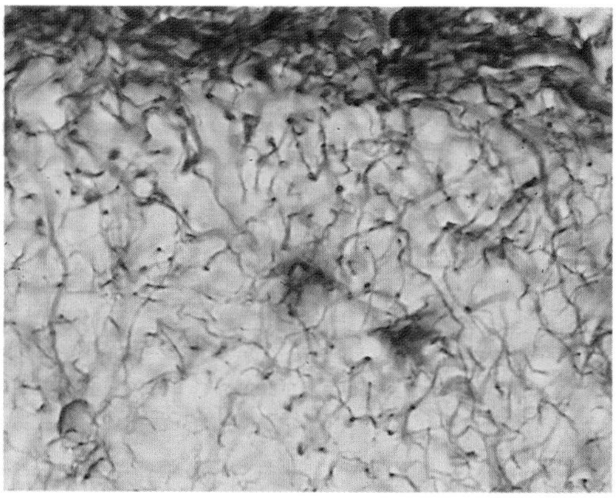

356 and **357 Subpial astrocytes.** Note long process passing deep into cortex (**356** top). Dense subpial condensation of astrocyte fibres (**357** top). GFAP, × 800.

358

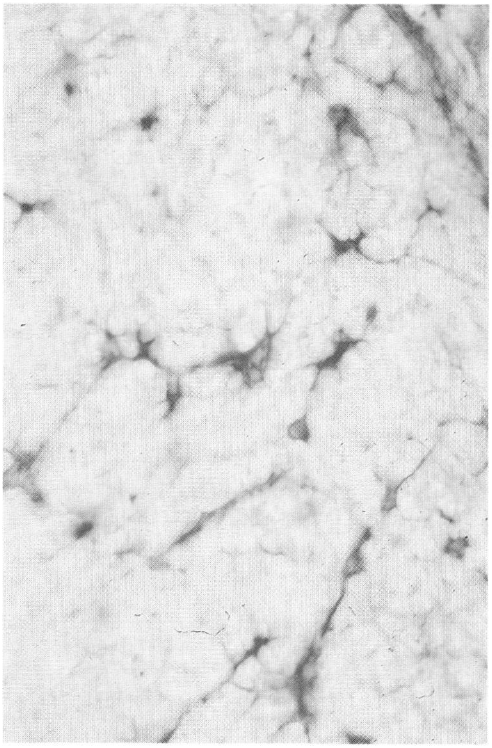

358 Normal astrocytes. They are seen here performing their conduit function. Channels are formed from blood vessels (top right), interconnecting with other astrocytes and passing into the parenchyma of the brain to nourish neurones. Lactic dehydrogenase, (nitroblue tetrazolium), × 200.

359

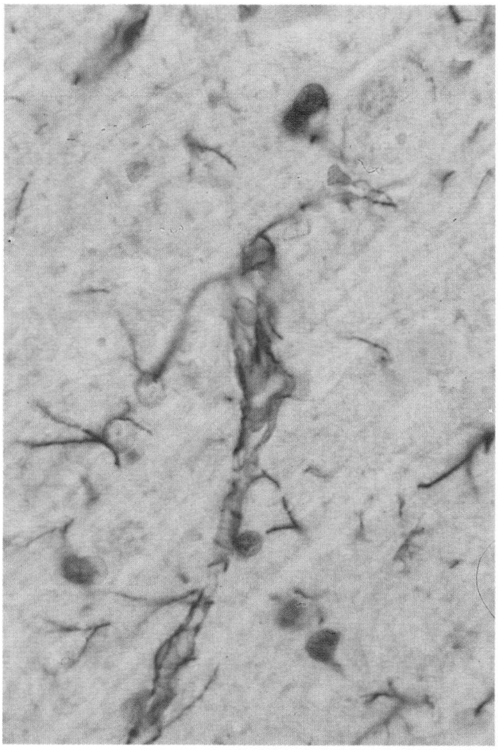

359 Interrelationships between glial fibres (blue), oligodendroglia (brown) and a blood vessel (centre right). Double staining with GFAP-alkaline phosphatase (blue) and carbonic anhydrase II – peroxidase, × 200. *(Courtesy of Dr N.A. Gregson)*

360

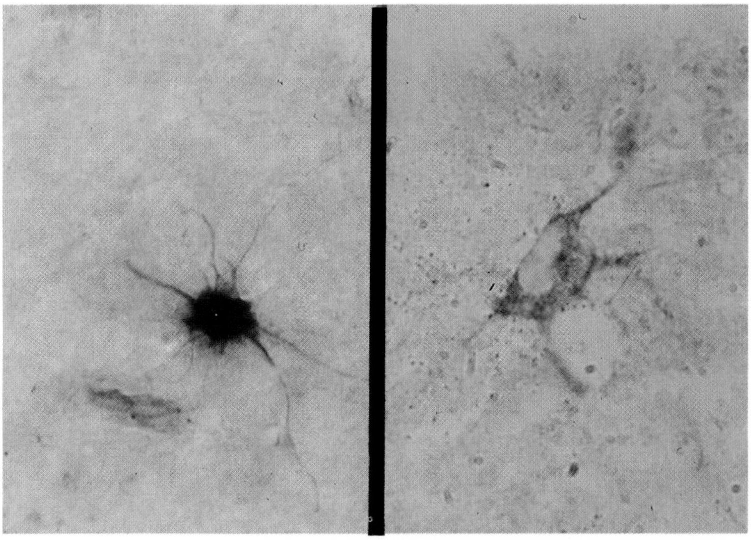

60 **Astrocytes near MS plaques.** eft: showing fibrillary astrocyte with nlarged cell body and creased lactic dehydrogenase ctivity. Right: protoplasmic strocyte in MS with enlarged cell-ody, glucose-6-phosphate ehydrogenase (NBT), both × 250.

361

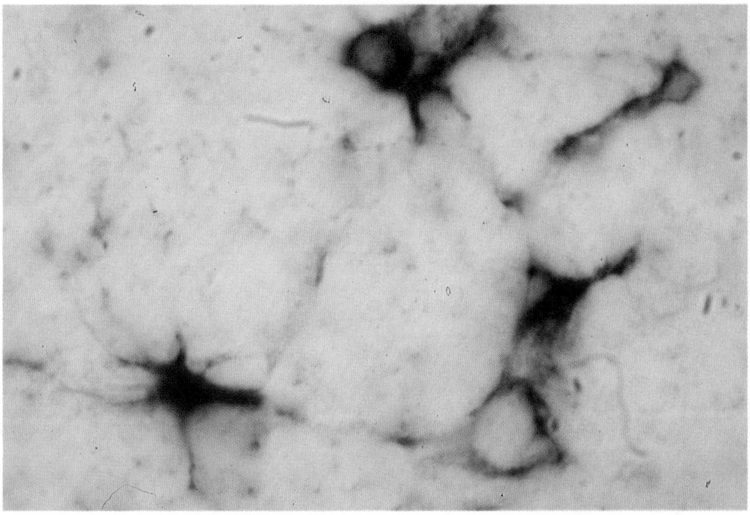

1 **Reactive astrocytes near laque in MS.** Increased NADH-trazolium reductase activity, 350.

362

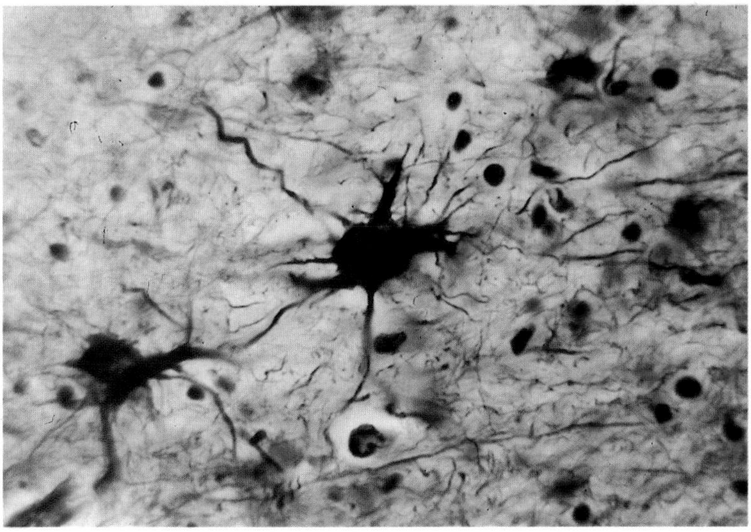

2 **Fibrillary astrocytes at edge f chronic MS plaque.** Note nlarged cell-body. The term 'spider ell' can be seen to be appropriate r these reparative gliotic cells. ajal gold sublimate, × 250.

363 Proliferation of reactive astrocytes in a plaque in acute multiple sclerosis. Anti-vimentin peroxidase, × 160.

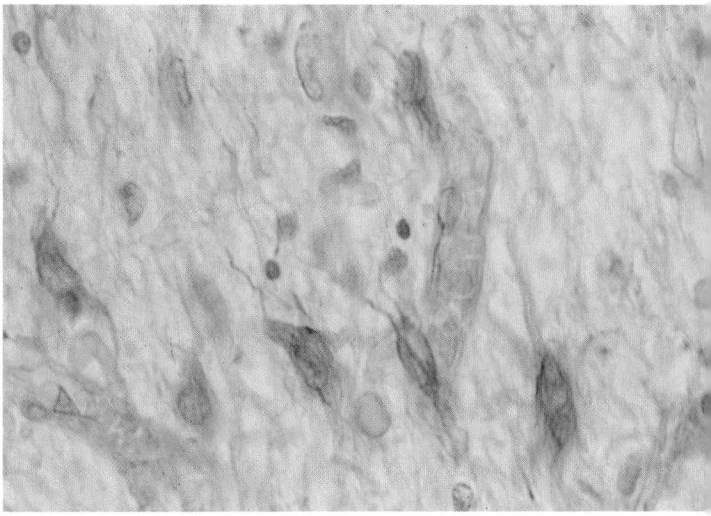

364 Astrocytes at edge of chronic plaque of multiple sclerosis (associated with formation of Rosenthal fibres). Anti-vimentin, × 160.

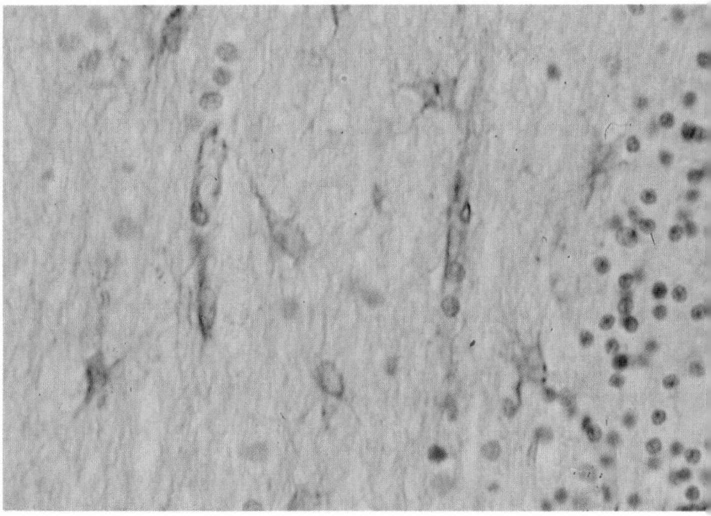

365 Fibrillary astrocytes (spider cells) at edge of MS plaque. GFAP (blue filter), × 160.

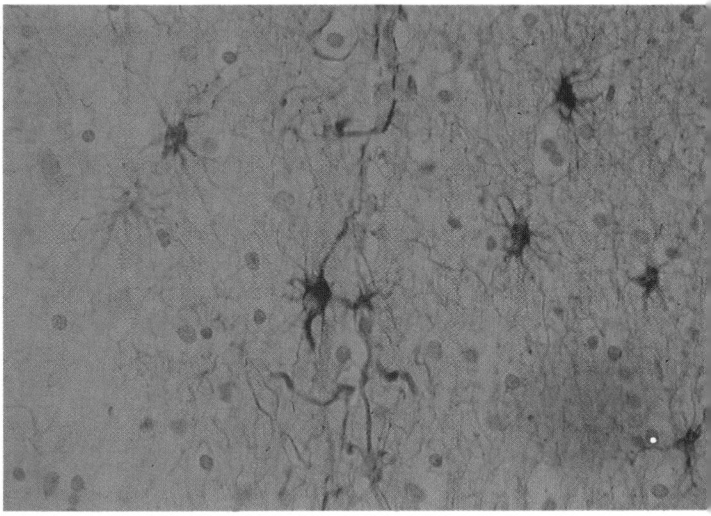

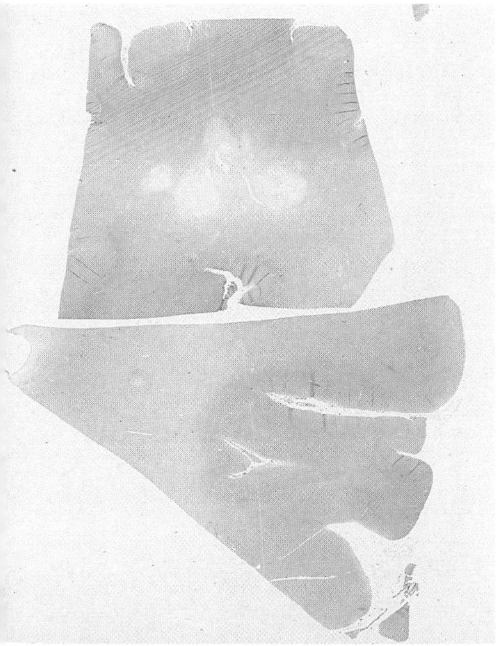

366

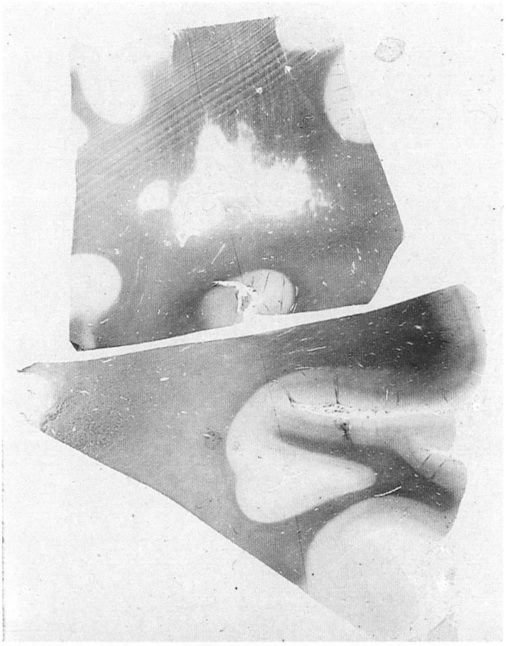

367

66 to **368**: **366** (H & E), **367** (Luxol), and **368**
ɬolzer). Chronic MS plaque repaired by
strocytic fibrillary gliosis (**368**), × 2.

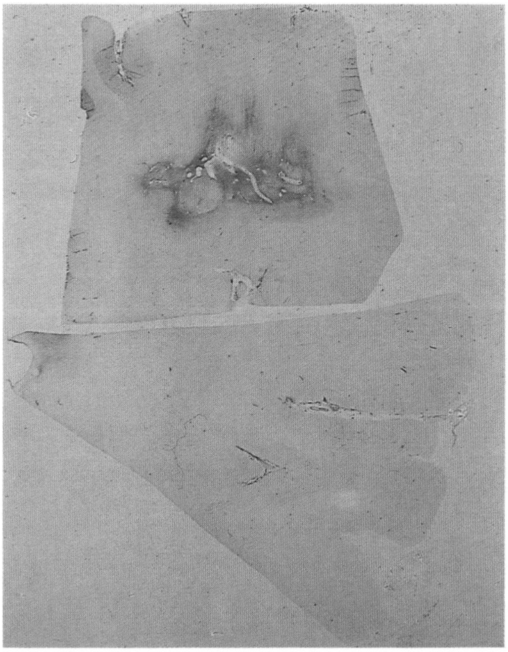

368

369

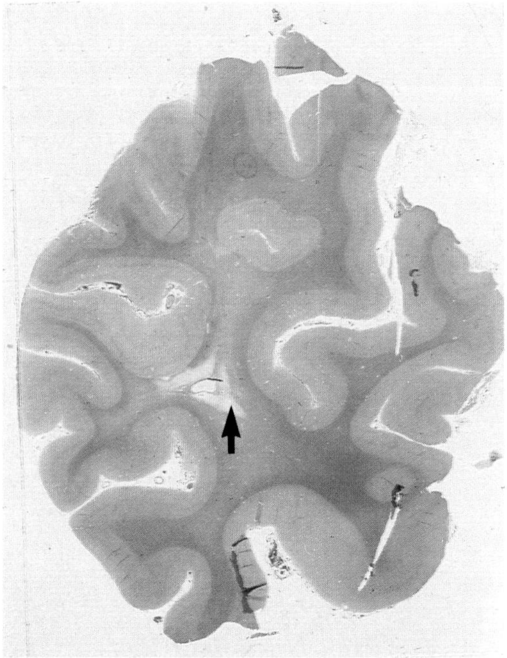

370

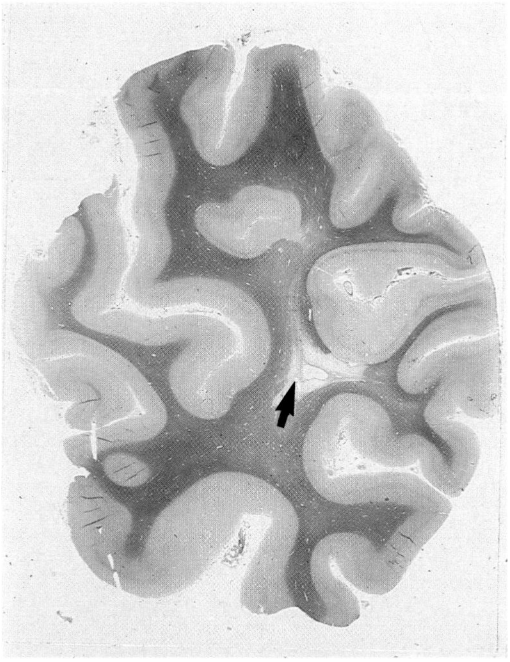

369 to **371**: **369** (H & E) **370** (Luxol), and **371** (Holzer). Chronic periventricular plaque, with extension into central white matter repaired by fibrillary gliosis (**371**), × 1.

371

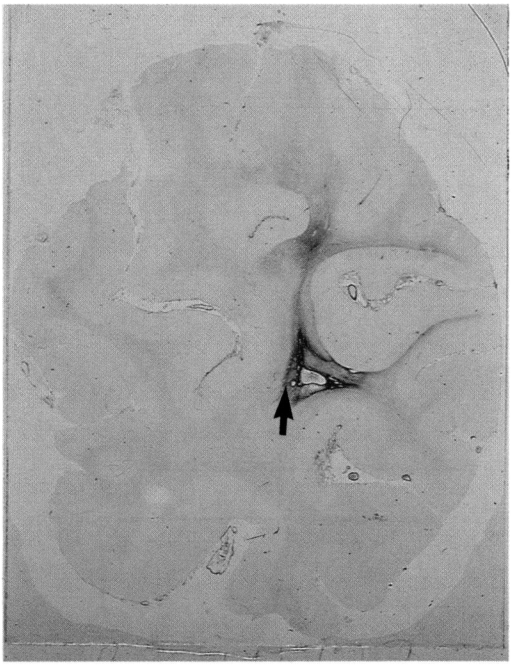

372

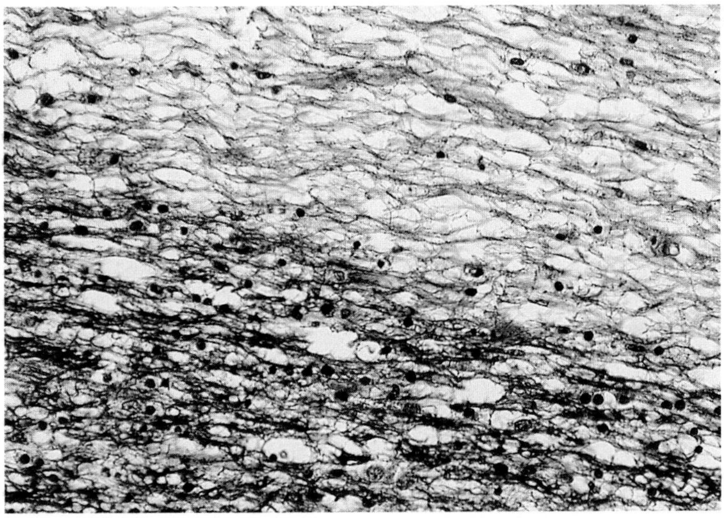

·72 Isomorphic gliosis (parallel ows of astrocyte fibres at top) in epair of chronic burnt-out MS laque. Phosphotungstic acid aematoxylin, × 100.

373

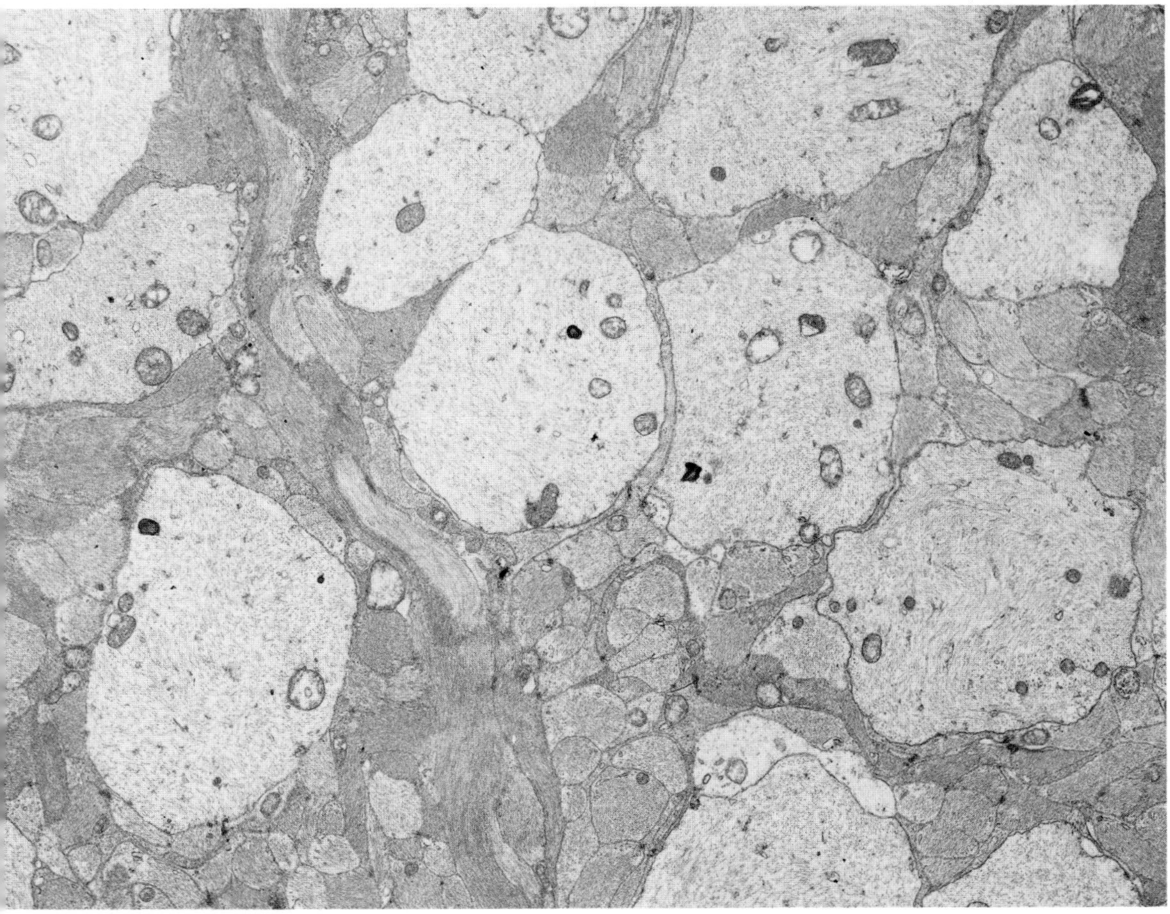

73 Chronic MS in spinal cord with gliotic demyelination'. Note umerous astrocyte processes and lemyelinated axons, × 10,000. *Courtesy of Professor Cedric Raine).*

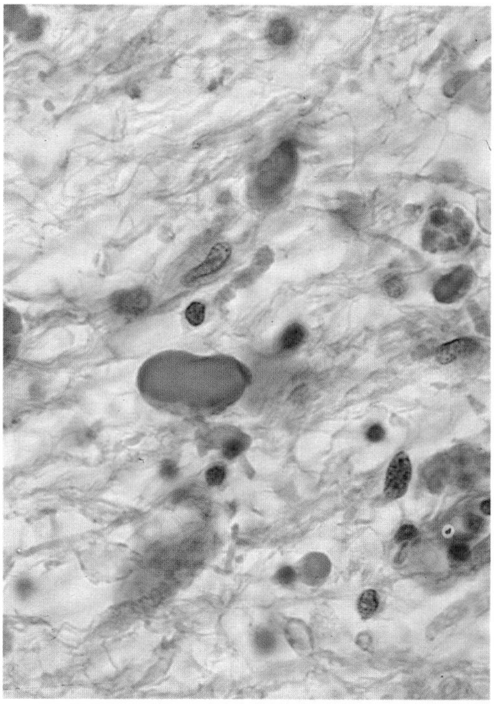

374

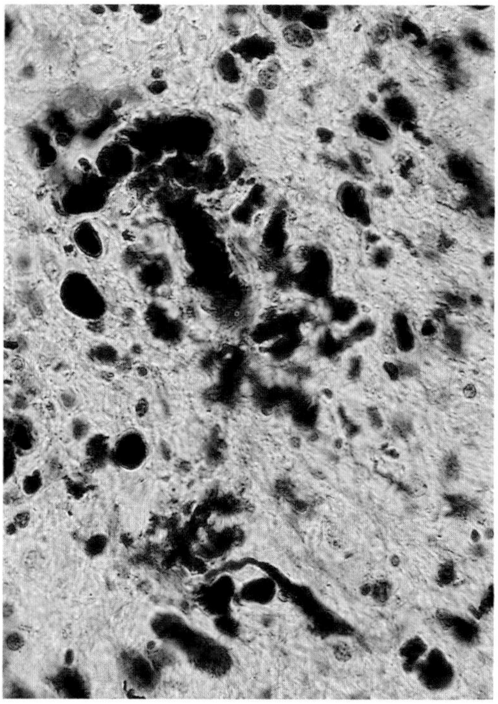

375

374 to **380** **Rosenthal fibres** (RF) in an area of astrocytic gliosis in subacute MS, stained by various methods (all × 200): haematoxylin and eosin (**374**), phosphotungstic acid haematoxylin (**375**), Holzer (**376**), Gros-Bielchowsky (**377**), Heidenhain (**378**), GFAP (**379**) and vimentin (**380**). RF may appear round, elongated, ovoid, sausage- or tadpole-shaped, in part depending on the plane of section.

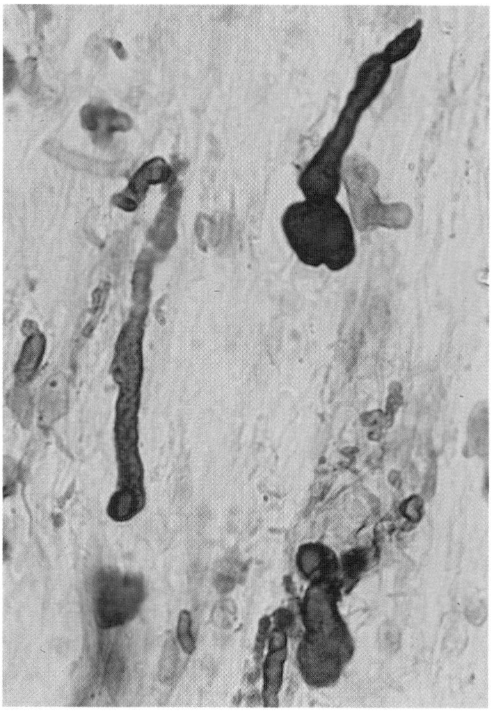

376

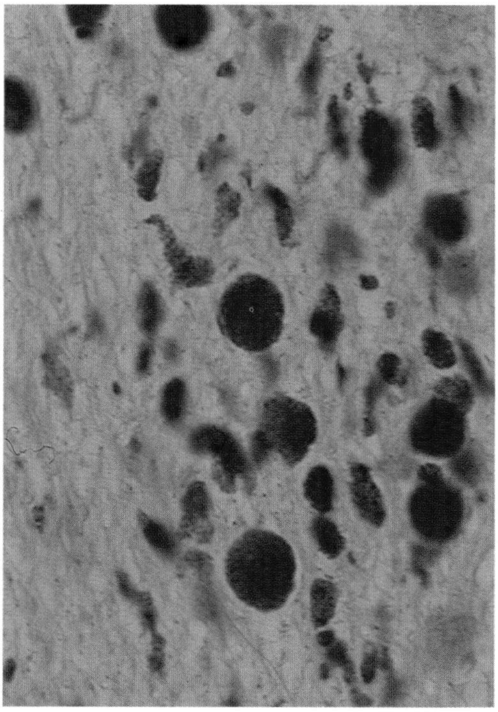

377

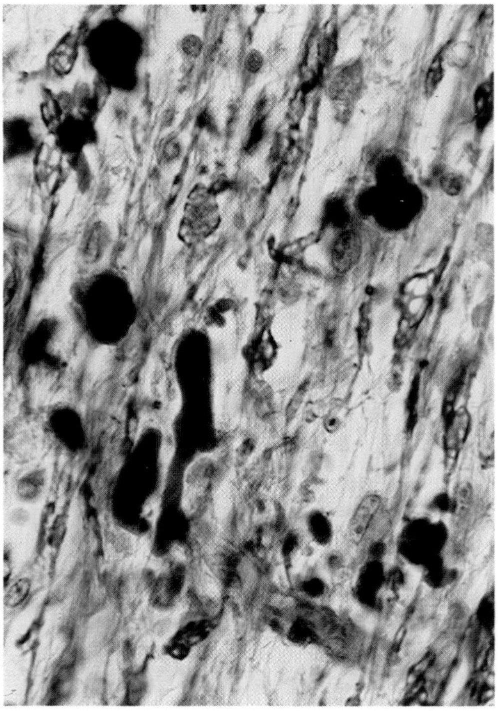

378

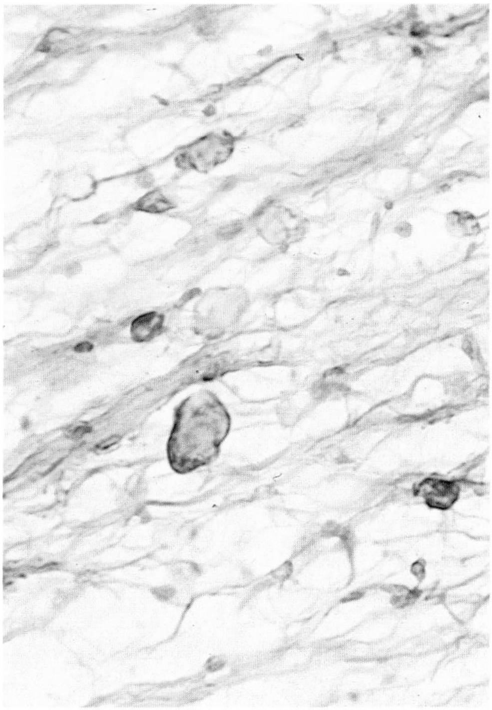

379

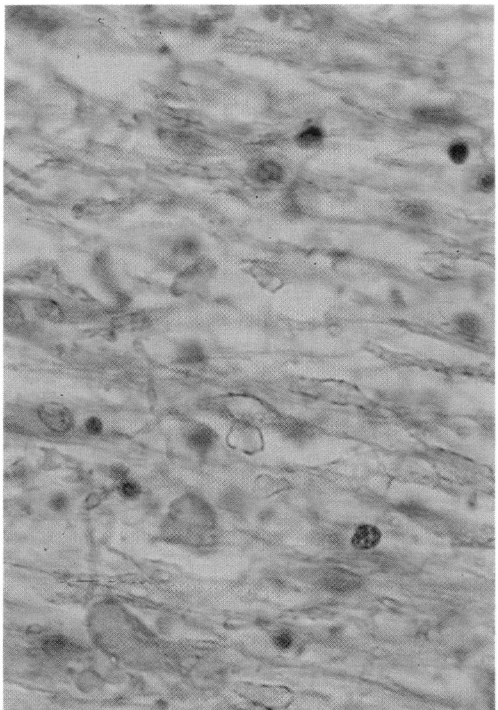

380

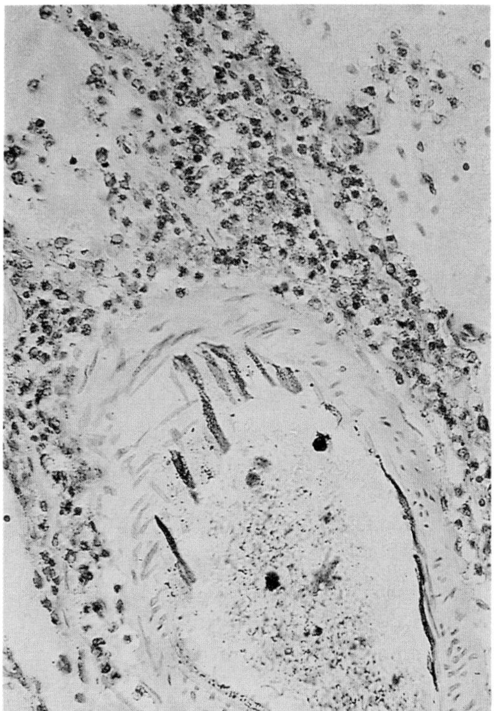

381

379 and **380** Note surface staining only of some RF for GFAP **379** and negative reaction for vimentin **380**.

381 Haematogenous macrophages emigrating through vein wall in an acute MS plaque. Muramidase (anti-lysozyme), peroxidase-anti peroxidase, × 60.

382

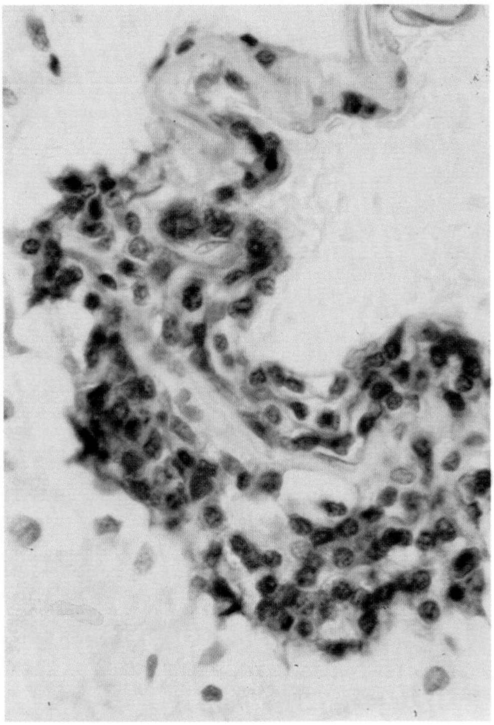

382 Haematogenous macrophages in vein wall and perivascular space in active MS. Muramidase, × 150.

383

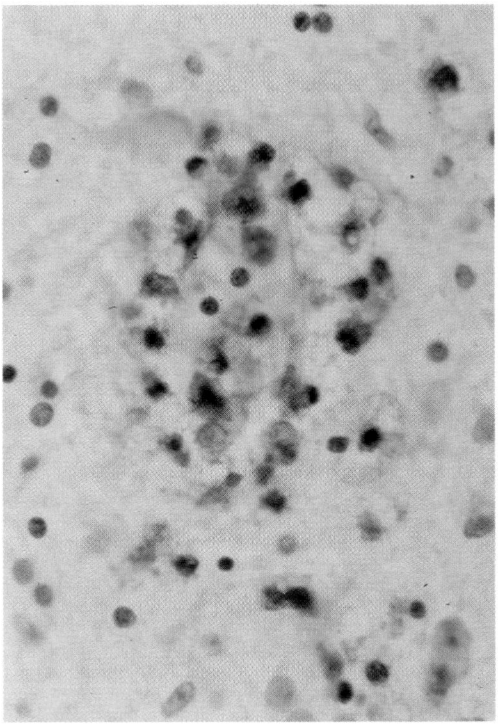

383 Focal haematogenous macrophages within an acute MS plaque, Muramidase, × 150.

384

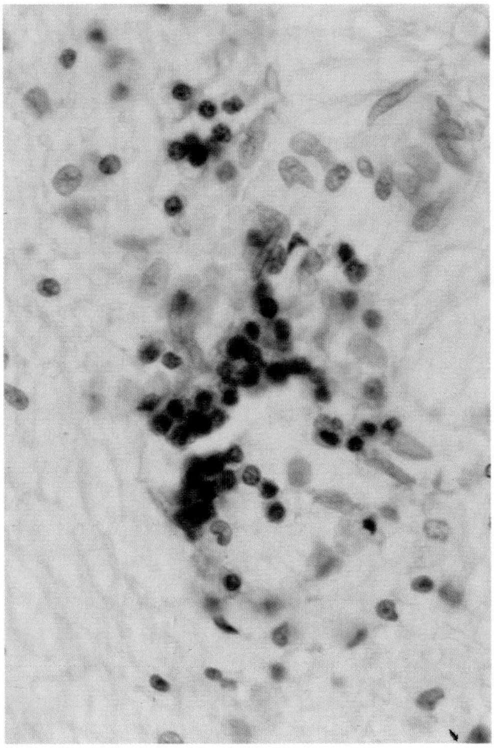

384 As for 383, MAC monoclonal antibody for macrophages, × 160.

385

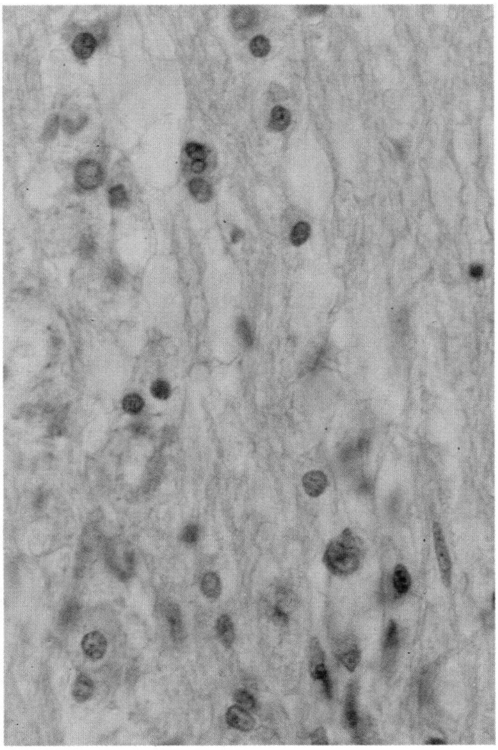

385 Vimentin in haematogenous macrophages in acute MS (also see **364**). Anti-vimentin, PAP, × 150.

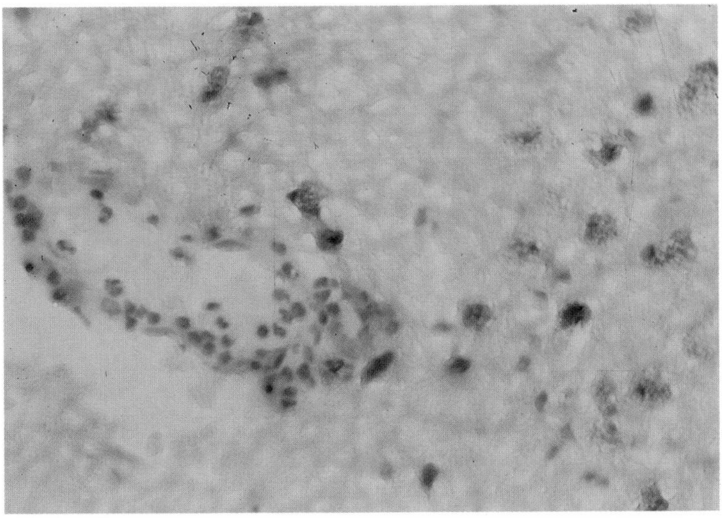

386

386 Acid esterase in macrophages in active plaque of MS. α-Naphthyl acetate esterase, × 100.

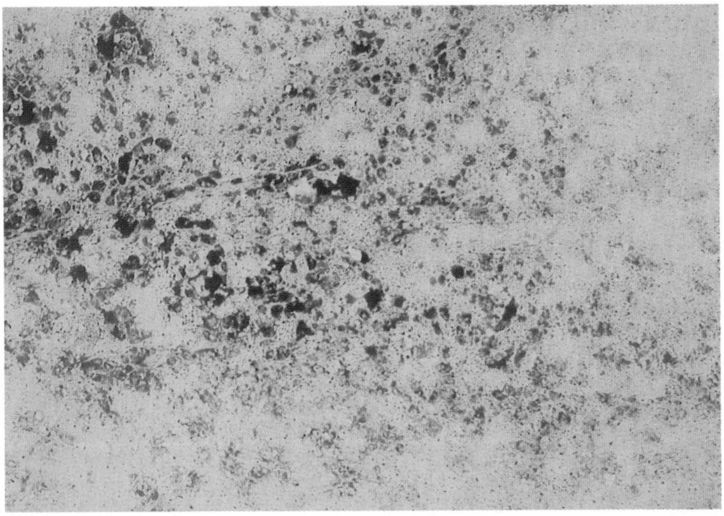

387

387 Active plaque of MS with infiltration of esterase-positive-macrophages. Endogenous microglia are not stained. Indoxyl-acetate esterase, × 50.

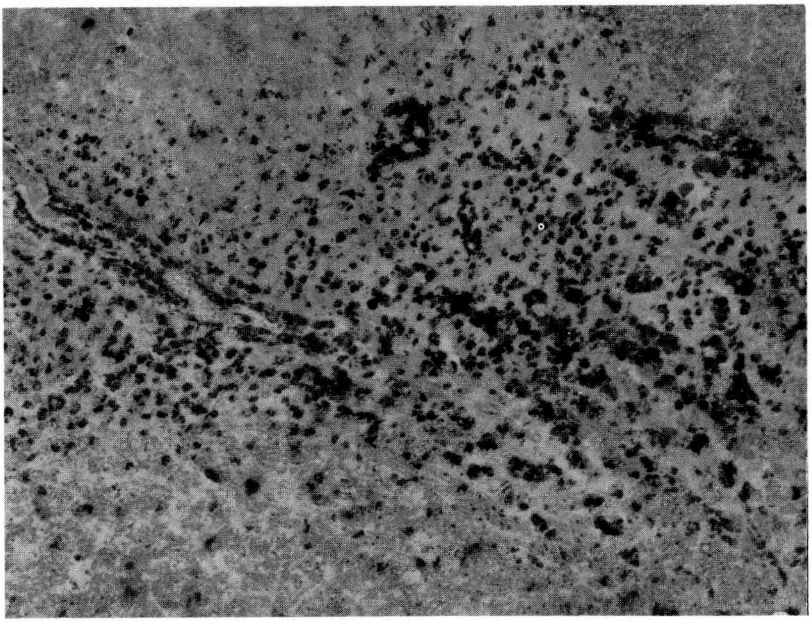

388

388 Acid phosphatase in macrophages (and possibly astrocytes) at edge of early plaque of MS. α Naphthyl phosphate – hexazotised pararosanilene, × 94.

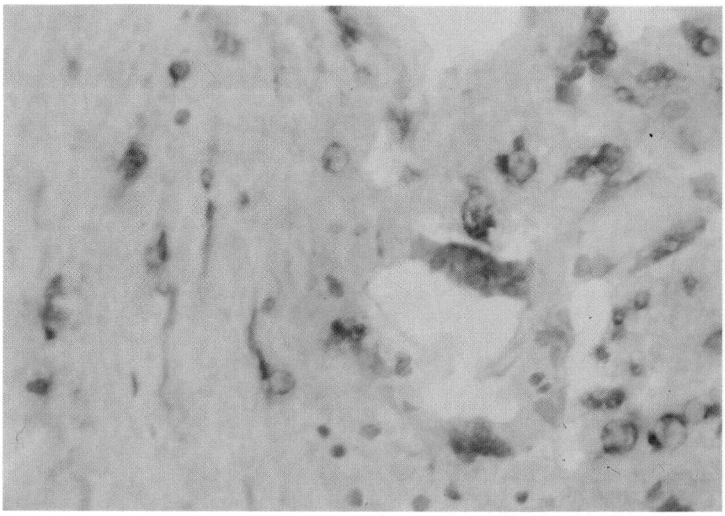

389 Macrophages in active MS plaque stained by the pan-macrophage marker EBM-11. A much wider range of macrophages is stained than with markers for recently recruited haematogenous macrophages (**381** to **385**). EBM-11 indirect peroxidase, × 160. *(Specimen by courtesy of Dr M. Esiri)*

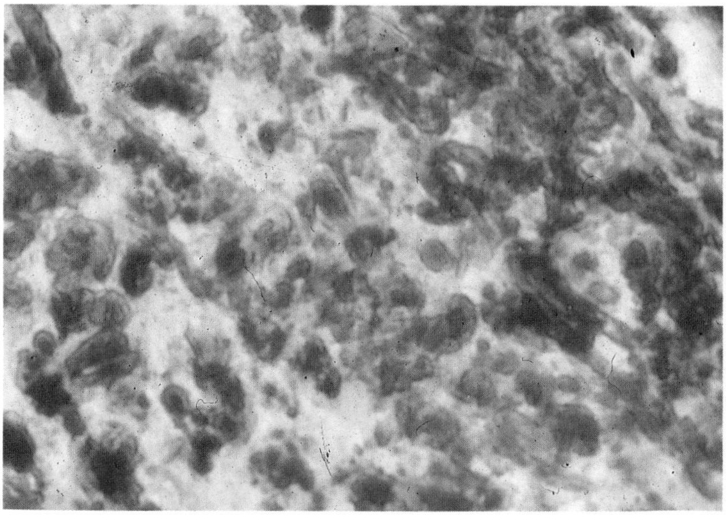

390 Macrophages at edge of active MS lesion showing blue staining 'myelinic' material and pink esterified cholesterol. Nile blue sulphate, × 200. *(After Adams, 1958)*

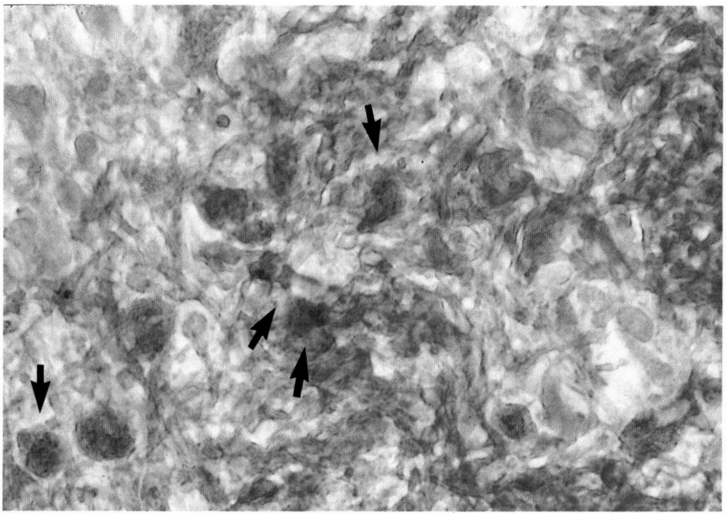

391 Macrophages at edge of acute lesion of MS. Some cells show mixed blue and red staining indicating partial myelin breakdown. Solochrome cyanin – oil red O, × 150.

392

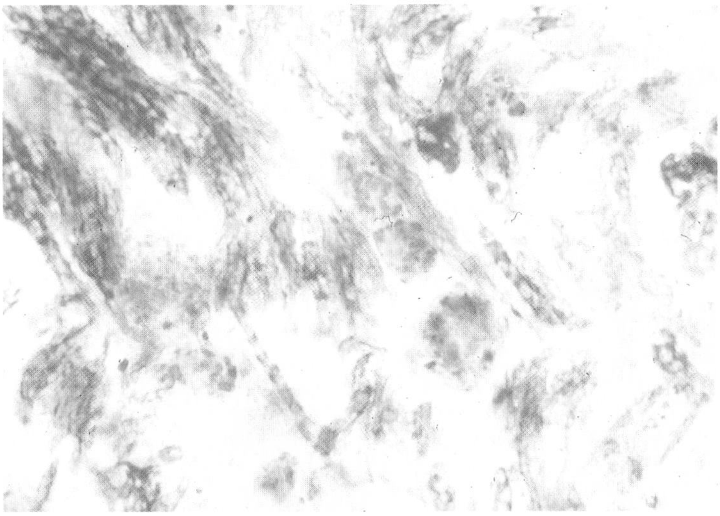

392 Perivascular macrophages in an acute plaque of MS showing blue staining 'myelinic' material. Solochrome cyanin – oil red O, × 100.

393

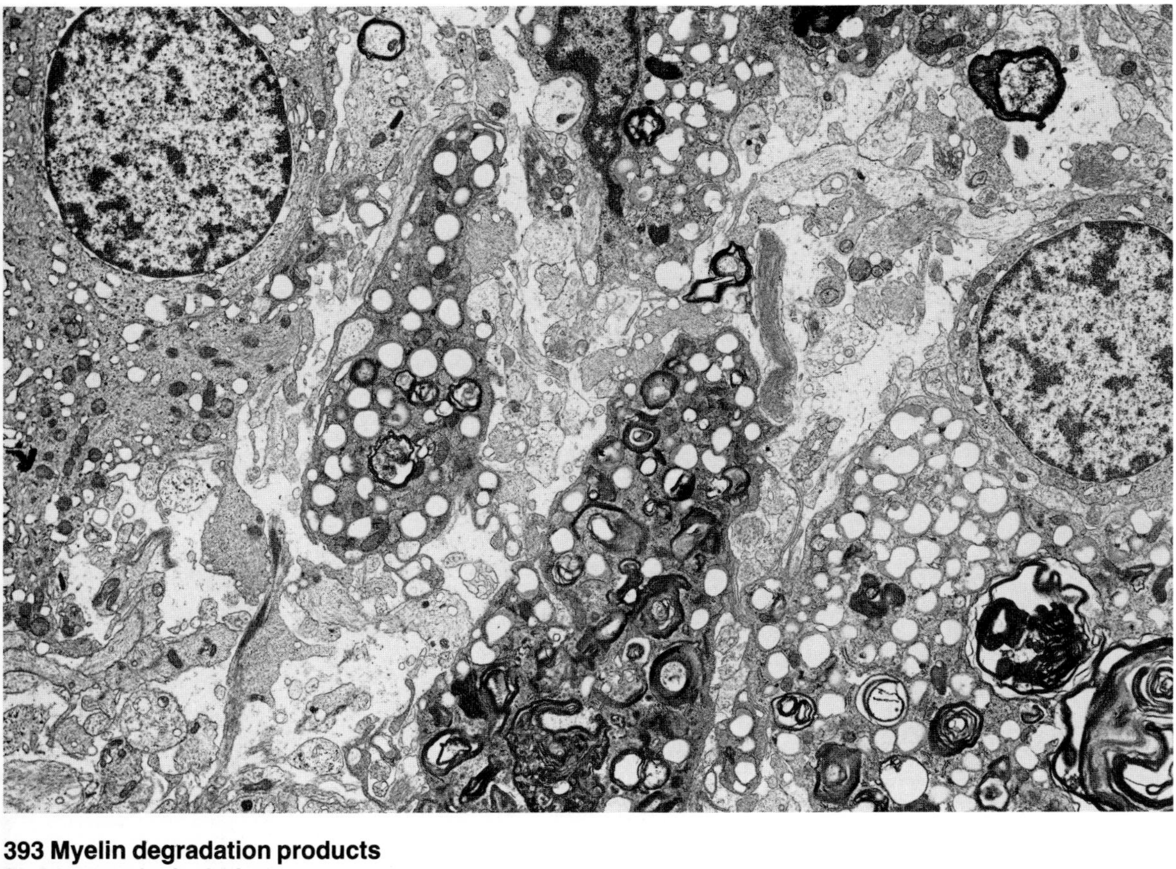

393 Myelin degradation products (lipid vacuoles) within four macrophages and two surviving oligodendrocytes (left and right) in active MS plaque, × 7,200. *(Courtesy of Professor C.S. Raine)*

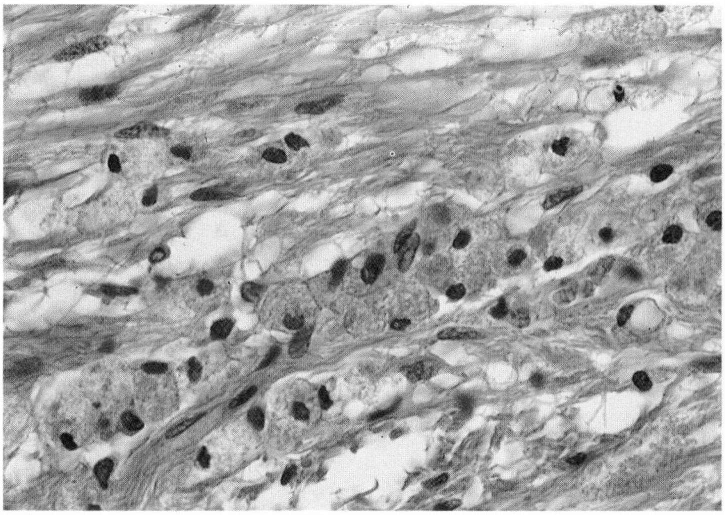

394 An acute case of multiple sclerosis with usually massive, sometimes confluent infiltration of foam cells (macrophages) throughout the plaque. Haematoxylin and eosin, × 250.

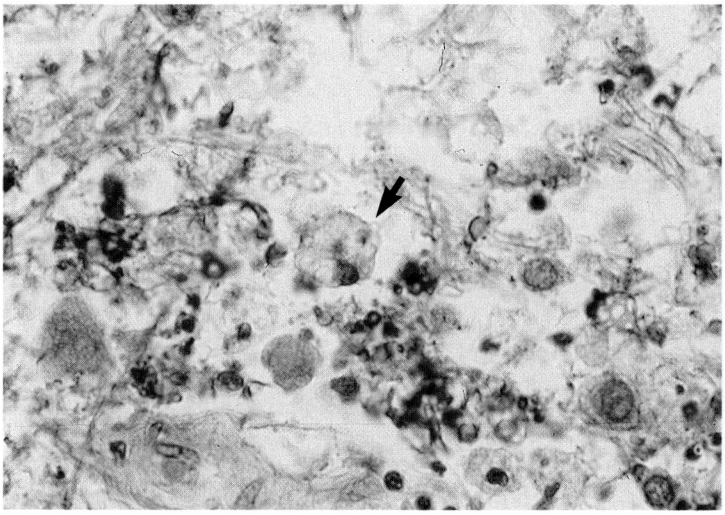

395 Foamy macrophage (centre) in close apposition to partly demyelinated axons at edge of active MS plaque. Phosphotungstic acid-haematoxylin, × 250.

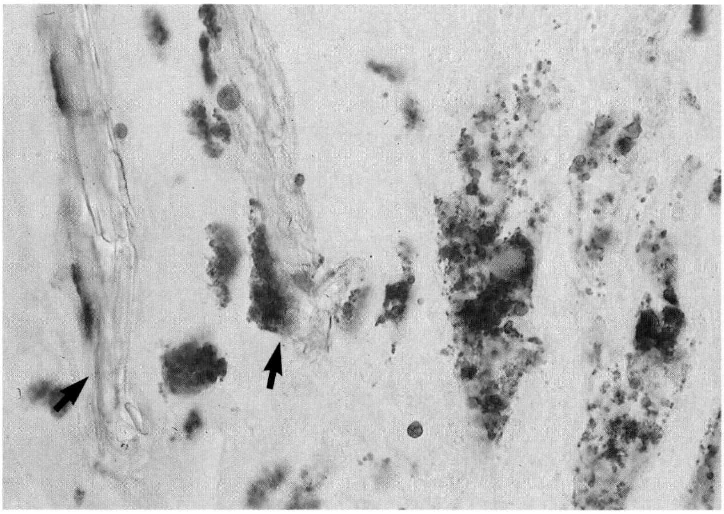

396 Macrophages in atherosclerosis digesting a cholesterol crystal (arrows). Fatty acids are blue (Nile blue oxazine) while esterified cholesterol is pink (Nile blue oxazone), × 350.

397

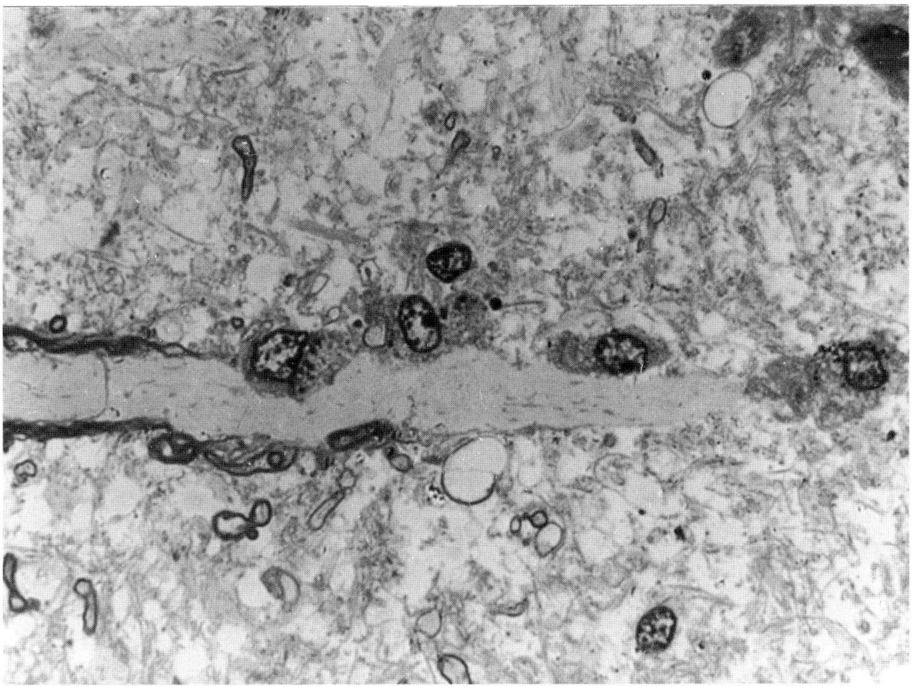

397 Edge of chronic active plaque of MS. Macrophages can be clearly seen to be digesting myelin along the course of an axon (centre and right). Myelin sheath surrounding axon at left. The important question is whether this is secondary digestion of an already damaged sheath or a primary macrophage assault on the myelin. Plastic section, toluidine blue, × 1250. *(Courtesy of Professor C.S. Raine)*

398

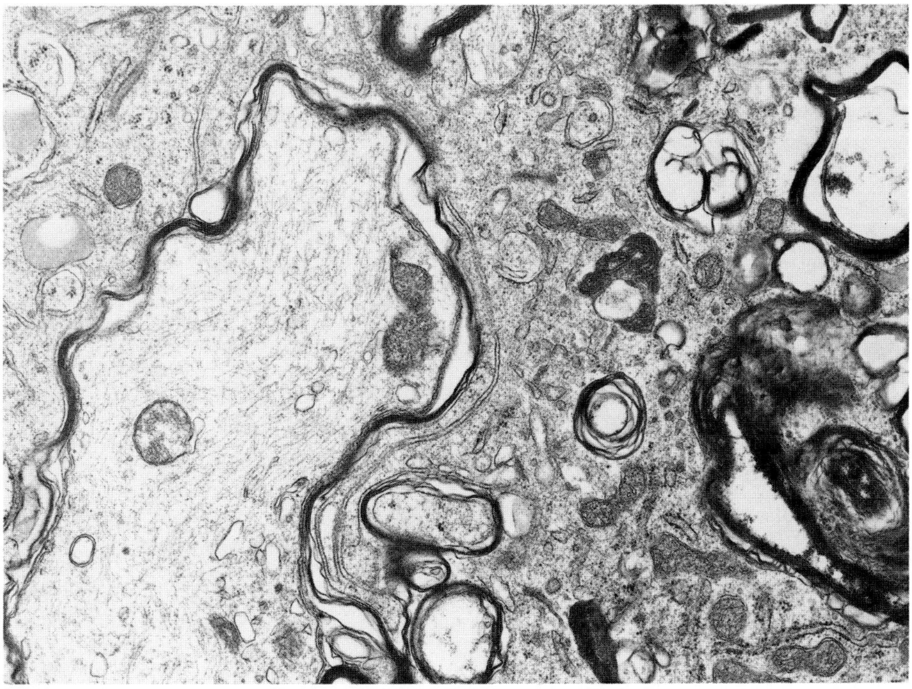

398 Macrophage (at right) in close opposition to axon (at left). The macrophage is full of lamellated debris (myelin breakdown products), while the axon is surrounded on all sides by thin incomplete disorganised myelin, × 24,000. *(Courtesy of Professor C.S. Raine)*

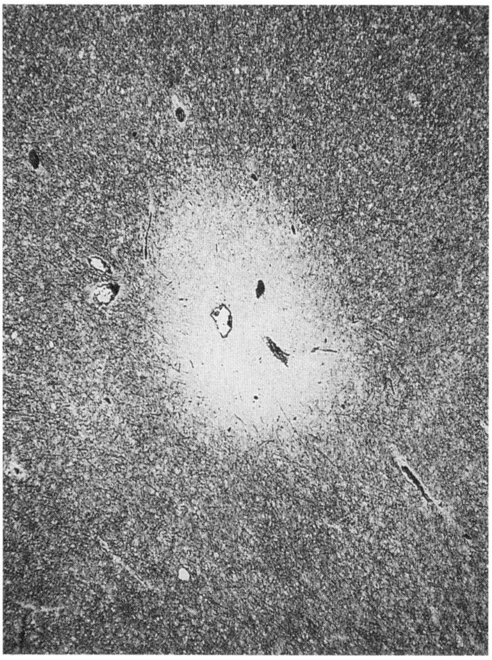

399

399 A small inactive chronic plaque of MS, which probably is an aborted lesion. Note prominent central vein. Trypan blue, × 15.

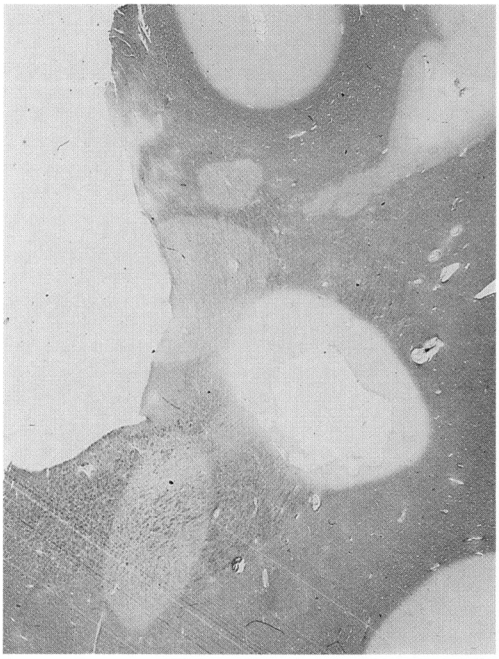

400

400 Three shadow plaques and other smaller lesions surrounding a confluent demyelinated periventricular plaque. The plaques are uniformly partly demyelinated and may not proceed further. Luxol fast blue, × 1.

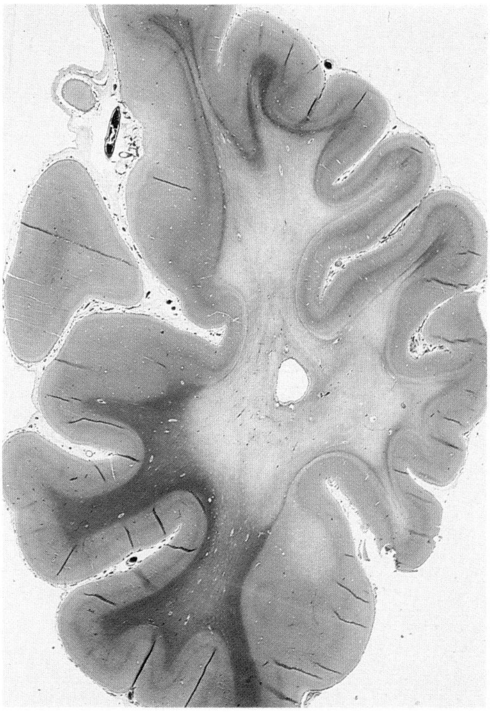

401

401 Chronic active plaque with sclerosis of most of the central white matter, but activity continues in an area of residual white matter at the left bottom. Loyez, × 3.

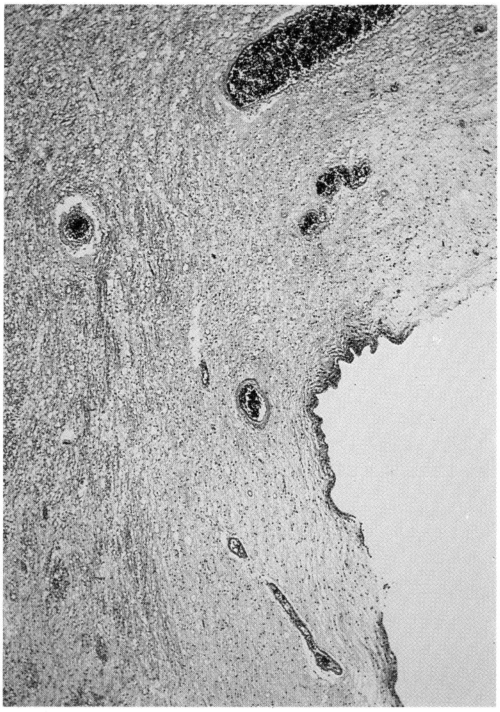

402

402 Chronic periventricular plaque of MS in a man of 92 years of age. There is slight mononuclear infiltration around the veins at centre, but no other signs of progression. Trichrome-MSB, × 10.

403

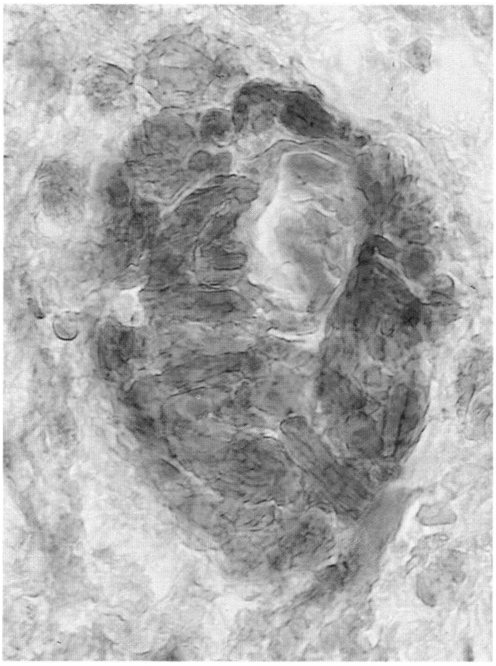

404

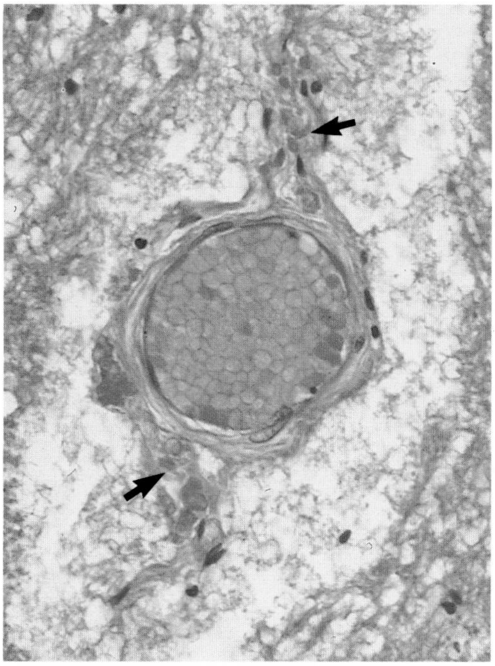

403 Perivascular accumulation of lipid-filled macrophages in active plaque, Oil red O, × 150.

404 Perivascular accumulation of pigmented lipid (lipofuscin) in a chronic plaque of MS. Haematoxylin and eosin, × 100.

405

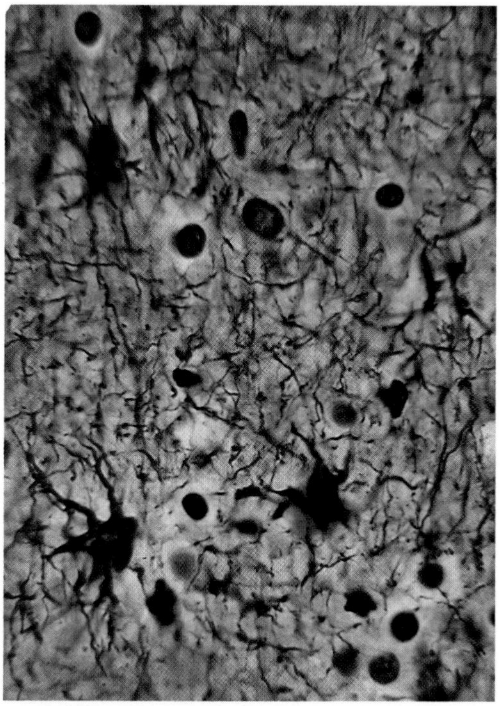

406

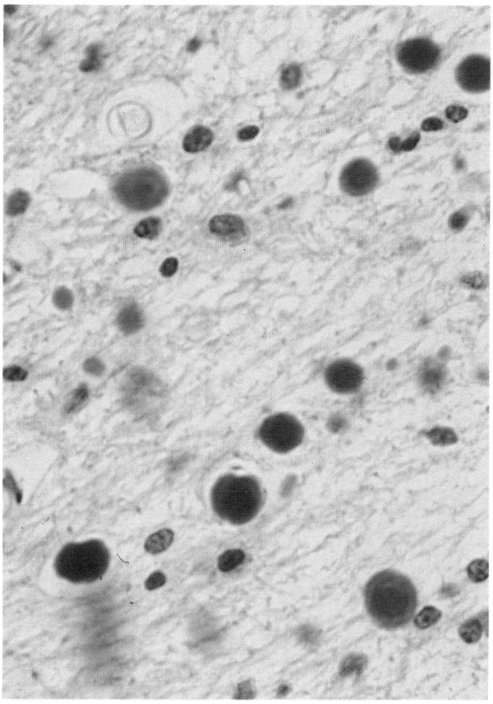

405 Fibrillary astrocytosis ('spider' cells) in chronic MS. Cajal gold sublimate, × 150.

406 Corpora amylacea. These degenerative bodies are common in MS and in the ageing brain. Phosphotungstic acid-haematoxylin, × 120.

407

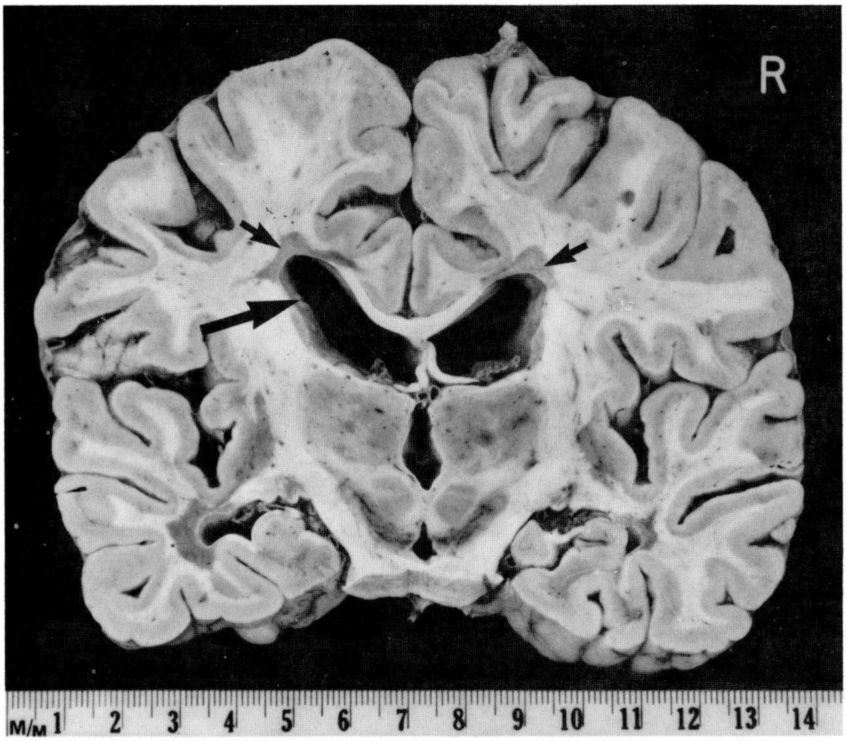

407 Granular ependymitis on lateral surfaces of lateral ventricles (large arrow) in presence of periventricular plaques of multiple sclerosis (small arrows), × ⅔.

408

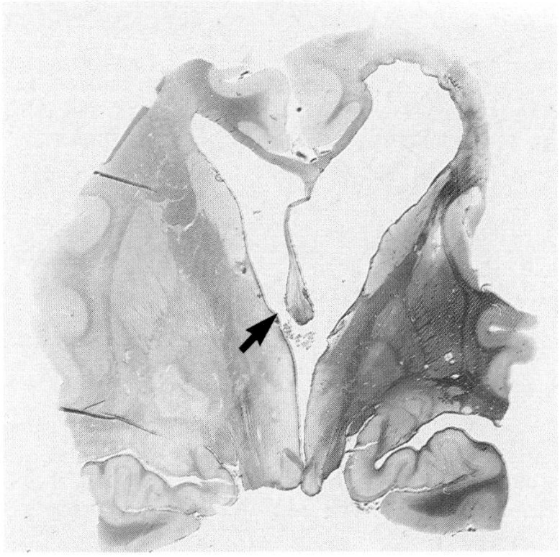

409

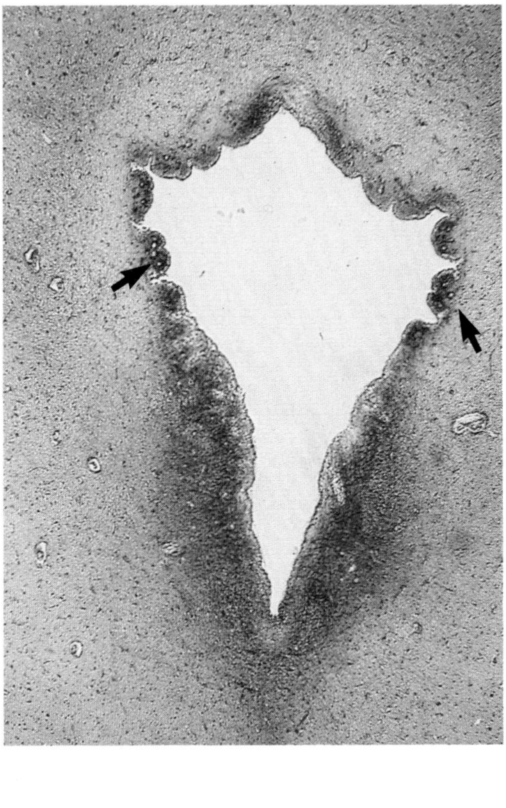

408 Granular ependymitis in wall of the IIIrd/lateral ventricles in multiple sclerosis at level of anterior pillars of fornix/mamillary bodies, × 1.

409 Granular ependymitis in aqueduct in multiple sclerosis. Phosphotungstic acid haematoxylin, × 10.

410 Granular ependymitis in lateral ventricle in multiple sclerosis. Note focal areas of deficient ependyma and replacement by a glial nodule (arrows). Van Gieson, × 5.

411 Two exuberant ependymal granulations near a sub-ependymal vein in multiple sclerosis. IIIrd ventricle, phosphotungstic acid-haematoxylin, × 30.

412 Normal ependymal lining to ventricular system. Haematoxylin-eosin, × 250.

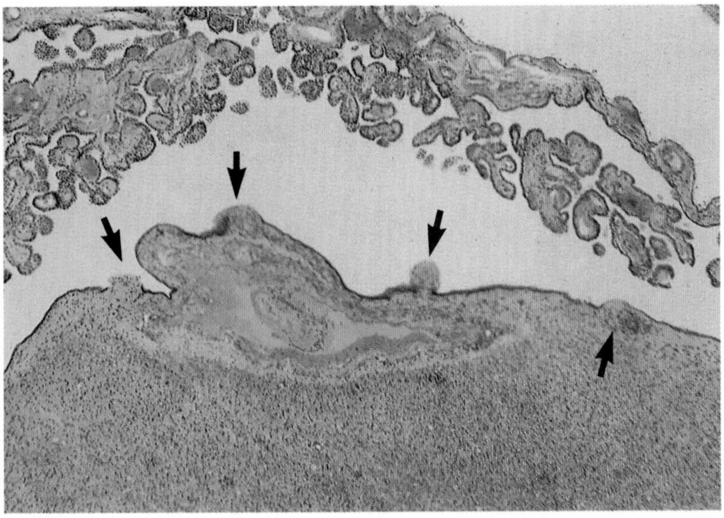

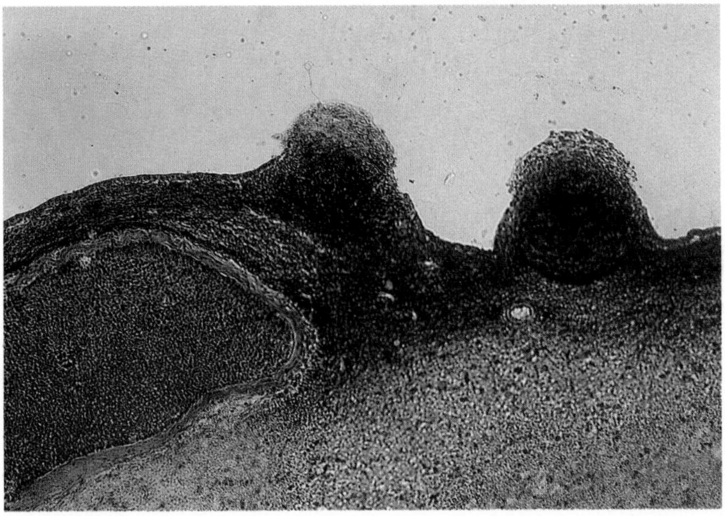

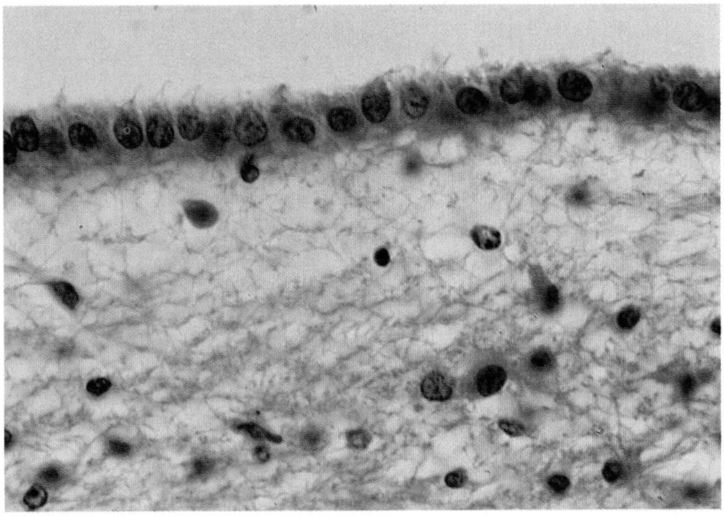

41

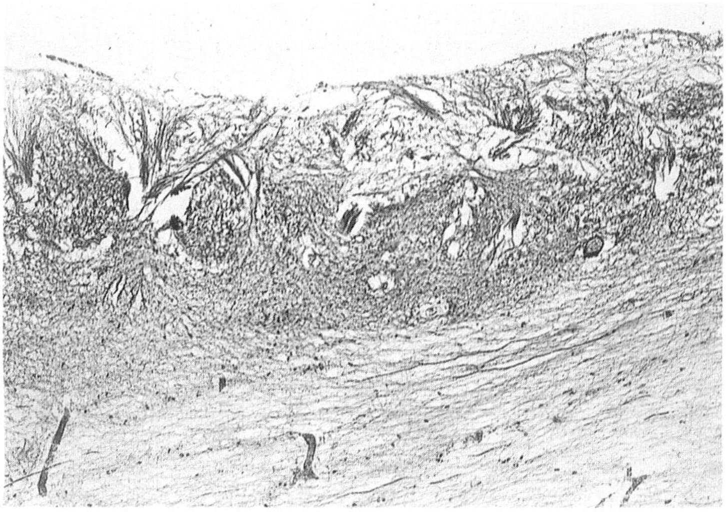

413 Glial fibres in ependymal granulation. Holzer, × 100.

41

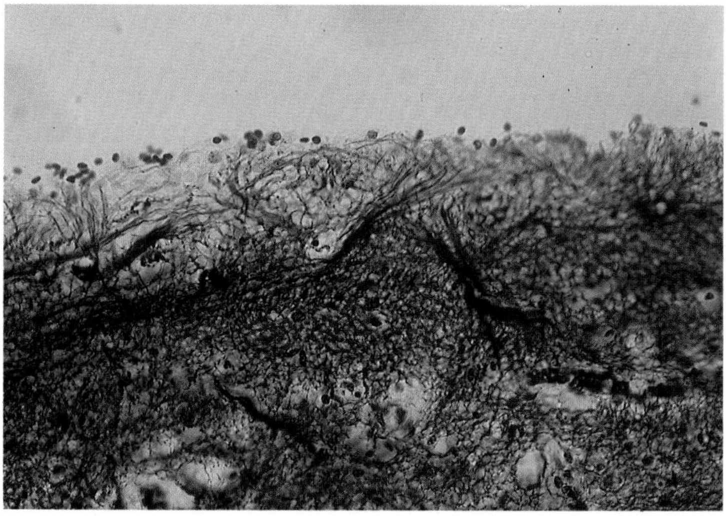

414 Glial fibres in ependymal granulation. Phosphotungstic acid haematoxylin, × 100.

41

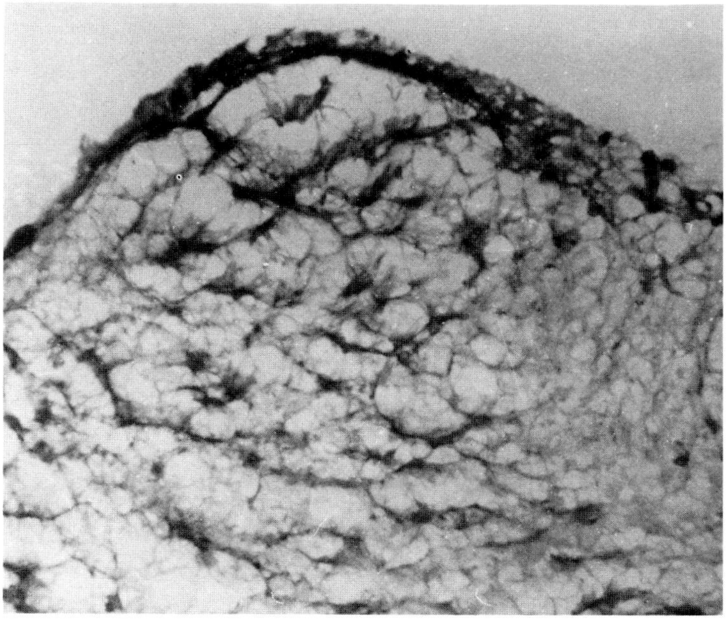

415 Granular ependymitis in aqueduct. Astrocytic proliferation within nodule shown by GFAP, × 200.

416

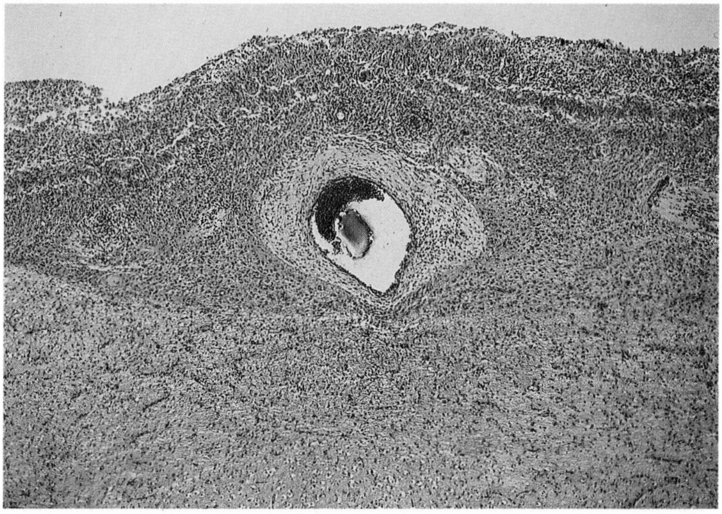

16 Acute ependymitis associated vith severe purulent meningitis, aematoxylin and eosin, × 40.

417

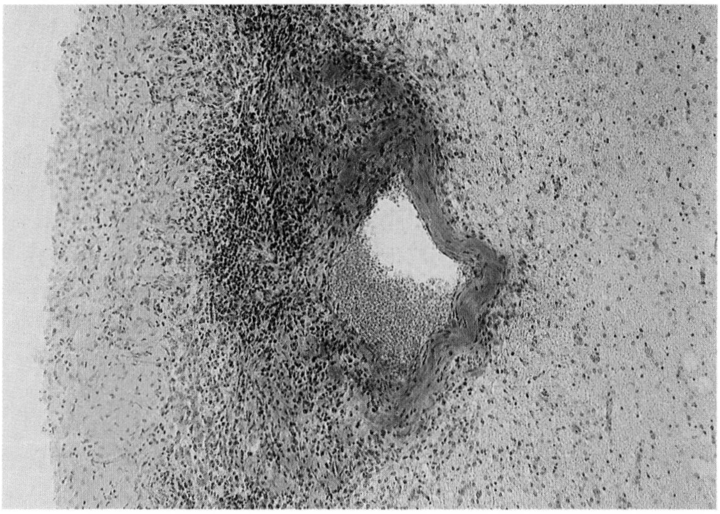

17 Acute ependymitis, in purulent ıeningitis. Van Gieson, × 80.

8 Vascular aspects of multiple sclerosis

It has been realised for over 100 years that the lesions of multiple sclerosis are centred on veins, although it is obviously not easy to establish this relationship in very large confluent lesions (Rindfleisch, 1873; Dawson, 1916 a, b, c; Putnam and Adler, 1937; Schienker, 1949; Fog, 1965). Small lesions almost invariably show a vein at their centre, while one or more inflamed veins or venules are often seen coursing through areas of diffuse myelin damage (**323**) characterised by myelin pallor and oedema.

This 'dependence' of the plaque upon a vein has led to the oft repeated conclusion that the causative agent has spread from the blood to the CNS (*see* Dawson, 1916a, b, c and many authors since). The high frequency and early appearance of periventricular plaques (*see* Chapter 6) presumably led Dawson to consider that the causative agent might spread into the brain from the CSF. However, Fog's (1965) studies showed that lesions spread out from the ventricles along small veins and venules as Dawson's fingers (*see* Chapter 6; **321** and **322**). Histomorphometry has shown that periventricular plaques have a more definite geometric relationship to periventricular veins (**418**) than to the ventricular lining or ependyma (Adams *et al.*, 1987).

Simple observation of early lesions, stained in the gross (**419**) or conventionally sectioned, shows that periventricular lesions – before they become confluent – are circular in outline as though encircling a vein rather than arising from the ependyma (**420**), and a vein can often be seen in the centre of the smaller early periventricular lesion (**421**). Histomorphometry shows that the 'centroid' of the plaque is based on the periventricular (subependymal) vein rather than on the centroid of the ventricle (Adams *et al.*, 1987). Hence, it seemed reasonable to infer that the early periventricular lesion is caused by something originating in the blood rather than the CSF. Although soluble material can diffuse from the subarachnoid space to the cerebral perivascular space (Wagner *et al.*, 1974), inflammatory cells and particulate matter are stopped by the pial membrane which separates the true perivascular space from the true subarachnoid space in the meninges (Hutchings and Weller, 1986; Alcolado *et al.*, 1988). Thus, the inflammatory infiltrate around cerebral veins in MS is more likely to be derived from the blood in the lumen of the vessel than from the subarachnoid CSF.

Inflammatory lesions in and around veins

Perivascular cuffing with lymphocytes has been recorded on numerous occasions in and around the MS plaque (*see* Chapter 7). However, the vein wall is also involved in this inflammatory process in that the inflammatory infiltrate is sometimes confined to the vein wall only (**422** and **423**; Adams *et al.*, 1985; Tables 6 and 8 in Chapter 7). It could be argued that this picture only reflects passage of inflammatory cells across the vein wall, but against this is evidence that the vein wall may itself be damaged. In the brains of 70 cases of MS examined, we have observed the following evidence of vascular (vein wall) damage in 21 of these patients (Adams, 1988):

Intramural fibrinoid deposition	5
Recent haemorrhages round veins	10
Mixed recent and old haemorrhages with siderocytes	2
Perivenular iron deposition (old haemorrhages)	21
Venular thrombosis or encrustations	4

The fibrinoid deposition within the vein wall in some cases of MS is evidence of leakage of plasma (**424** to **428**) and is evidence of a local vasculitis (plasmatic vasculosis), but without the intensity of that seen in an arteritis (**123**).

The recent perivenular haemorrhages are of more debatable significance (**429**), as these could be held to occur as an agonal event. However, the resemblance between the haemorrhage in MS depicted in **430** and the ring haemorrhages seen in acute haemorrhagic leukoencephalopathy (**431** and **432**; *see* Chapter 2) is noteworthy. Indeed, this relationship has been commented upon elsewhere (Chou, 1982). Similar perivenular ring haemorrhages may be seen in the leucoencephalitis accompanying Bechcet's disease (Chapter 3), Binswanger's disease (Feigin and Budzilovich, 1980) and in the vasculomyelinopathy of cerebral malaria (Toro and Roman, 1978). MS plaques occasionally develop large haemorrhages, which have required surgical evacuation (Jankovic *et al.*, 1980).

Iron (haemosiderin) deposition as an indication of previous haemorrhage is frequently seen around the veins (**433** to **435**) of MS plaques or at the edge of the lesion (**436**). A similar deposition of haemosiderin is seen in some 75 per cent cases of vasculitis causing peripheral neuropathy (**138** and **139**). As noted above, 30 per cent of our 70 MS cases show iron deposition (haemosiderin) around blood vessels: a higher frequency of iron was recorded by Craelius *et al.*, (1982) in a small series of 5 cases. Occasional cases show old haemosiderin in the vein wall with a later episode of recent haemorrhage (**437** and **438**). This is strong evidence that at least some of the venous haemorrhages in MS represent progressive damage to the vein wall.

Perivascular iron deposition in the brain occurs in association with vascular disease in about 9 to 11 per cent of non-MS subjects over 70 years of age. For these reasons the deposition of iron in the brain in MS could be regarded as non-specific (Walton and Kaufman, 1984). However, detailed consideration of the distribution of iron deposition in MS reveals that the iron was related to veins in or at the edge of plaques in all but one case. In occasional cases the iron pigment accumulated as an incomplete pallisade at the edge of the plaque (**436**). The conclusion is that the plaque-related perivenular haemosiderin is a specific feature of the disease. Lumsden (1970) reviewed the evidence that there may be a disorder of iron metabolism and splenic haemosiderosis in MS but, in view of the above evidence, it seems more likely that the haemosiderin reflects damage to the vein wall, which in severe cases (see above) can be regarded as a mild vasculitis. Allen *et al.*, (1978) found no evidence of splenic haemosiderosis in the records of 71 autopsied cases of MS.

Thrombosis has been previously described in the veins of MS plaques and was linked with the pathogenesis of the disease (Putnam, 1937), but later it was realised that such thrombi were the result rather than the cause of the plaque (Dow and Bergland, 1942; Zimmerman and Netsky, 1950; Macchi, 1954). Although the increased platelet stickiness in MS (Caspary *et al.*, 1965; Wright *et al.*, 1965) has been linked with thrombosis as a pathogenic factor, such thrombi and encrustations are features of older lesions (**439**) and have little to do with the active stage of the disease. It is hardly surprising that a chronic mild vasculitis or vasculosis should result in occasional thrombotic occlusions: thrombosis is a common event in all grade of vasculitis, ranging from inflamed varicose veins to polyarteritis nodosa. Indeed, it seems that stimulated or activated macrophages are a potent source of thromboplastin (Spillert *et al.*, 1986).

Platelet adhesiveness is increased by saturated fatty acids and by animal (saturated) fat (Coma Report, 1984). However, the borderline therapeutic value of adding polyunsaturated fatty acids (PUFA) to the diet in MS is unlikely to be related to platelets, but rather to the mild immunosuppressive action of PUFA (Chapter 5). Lysolecithin also increases platelet stickiness (Andreoli *et al.*, 1973), presumably by altering the surface properties of the platelet.

The prolonged effect of inflammatory or traumatic damage to the vein wall in the MS brain leads to eventual marked scarring and collagenisation of the vein, as shown in **440** to **444**. Such collagenisation of cerebral veins is also seen in hypertensive subjects and in senile normotensive patients (Cervos-Navarro and Roggendorf, 1983). Some veins in MS appear to have undergone collagenous degeneration or hyalinisation (Rindfleisch, 1873; Allen, 1981). The veins in MS, hypertensive and senile subjects also become tortuous and sometimes appear to have proliferated (**443**). Petrescu and Marcovici (1971) have pointed out that there is an excess of reticulin fibres in and around vessels associated with plaques: this again indicates reparative venular thickening in the MS lesions.

The collective evidence above does suggest that the vein wall is specifically damaged in MS, but this damage is confined to the CNS and does not occur in other tissues. Clearly, the intensity of the reaction is much less than that in vasculitides such as polyarteritis nodosa, and is consistent with Lumsden's (1970) concept of MS as a 'slow tempo' disease and with Lendrum's (1963) concept of plasmatic vasculosis in mild form.

In passing, it should be mentioned that a number of artefacts may be seen in and around blood vessels in autopsied tissue. Figures **445** and **446** shows postmortem bacterial colonies and calcinosis in vessel walls that resemble iron deposition, while **447** shows postmortem fungal hyphae or bacillary filaments superficially resembling a network of fibrin strands.

Venous drainage and the localisation of MS plaques

An interesting hypothesis has been proposed by Schelling (1986), who points to the proximity of periventricular plaques of the third and lateral ventricles to the collecting (subependymal) veins which drain into the great vein of Galen and, thence, into the sigmoid sinus and internal jugular vein. Schelling has suggested that reflux back-pressure within these cerebral veins would damage their walls and could explain some of the findings described above. Even if not directly related to the initial pathogenesis of MS, reflux pressure on a cerebral vein wall, previously damaged by inflammatory disease, could well exacerbate tissue reactions or promote a local relapse.

The primary lesions of multiple sclerosis seem to arise, as mentioned above, around periventricular veins, and around the aqueduct. The veins draining these areas (septal, subependymal, posterior ventricular and inferior ventricular) drain into the internal cerebral veins and from thence into the great vein of Galen (Johanson, 1954; Padget, 1956; **448**). The superior cerebellar vein drains into the great vein of Galen; the anterior cerebellar vein drains much of the cerebellum, pons and medulla and drains into the superficial petrosal sinus and thence into the transverse sinus. Hence, those areas of the brain where plaques most commonly begin (apart from the optic pathway) mainly drain into the Galenic or petrosal systems. In fact, forceful injection of the jugular veins at postmortem leads to extravasated area around the ventricles resembling human MS plaques (Schlesinger, 1939).

There are no valves in these veins or sinuses but some control is exerted over blood flow by sleeves or pads of cavernous (erectile) tissue around these vessels (Le Gros Clark, 1940; Balo, 1950). Obstruction to venous blood flow in the Galenic system is known to cause a mild hydrocephalus, as there is only a poor anastomosis between the internal and external cerebral veins (Bailey, 1934). Venous blood flow from the brain may also be controlled by sympathetic extracranial venoconstriction, presumably located partly in the jugular vein (Pearce and Bevan, 1983). Failure to regulate arterial pressure changes leads to the linear transmission of arterial pulse waves to cerebral veins and the CSF (Portnoy *et al.*, 1983; Lazorthes, 1961). Such pulsatile pressure in the CSF or subependymal veins could well influence the course of MS lesions, particularly by causing focal changes in permeability. Myogenic autoregulation fails when arterial transmural pressure exceeds arterial vasomotor tone, and this can be caused by arterial vasodilation, systemic hypotension, hypercapnea, increased intracranial pressure, or failure of arterial smooth muscle to contract (Portnoy *et al.*, 1983). All these factors, together with sudden changes in the standing head of hydrostatic pressure within the jugular system, could well exert stresses on the subependymal regions of the brain.

On a different tack the periventricular lesions of MS have been related to infection of the cavernous sinus, which has a close anatomical relationship to the third ventricle and optic chiasm (Gay and Dick, 1986). The infection of the cavernous sinus was attributed to penetration of organisms into it from the nasal sinuses via thin bone lining the sinuses or the cribriform plate in the base of the skull. This idea is strengthened by the observation of a high frequency of chronic sinusitis in MS patients (Gay *et al.*, 1986).

Centrifugal spread of MS

Whatever the merits of the above two hypotheses, the lesions of MS do commonly arise around the ventricular system (third, lateral and fourth ventricles, and the aqueduct). Dawson (1916 a, b, c) and Fog (1964, 1965) both pointed out how lesions extend outwards as Dawson's fingers, along the course of veins from the third and lateral ventricles into the central white matter of the hemispheres (Chapter 6). The disease would seem to start near the ventricular surface, around the draining subependymal veins (Adams *et al.*, 1987), and spread centrifugally into the brain. Further examination of our material shows that lesions more frequently occur in the cerebellar peduncles, pons and medulla than in the cerebellar white matter (**251** to **265**). The former sites are closer to the aqueduct and fourth ventricle and, in the early stages, bear a close relationship to them. Dawson's fingers can be seen extending out from plaques around the fourth ventricle into the reticular formation, olives and middle cerebrallar peduncle, or from the aqueduct into the substantia nigra and basis pedunculi (**248** to **250**). Furthermore, the optic chiasm abuts on the anterior termination of the third ventricle (**246**) and, as mentioned in Chapter 6, optic neuritis (including the whole optic pathway) is seen in 90 per cent or more of patients with MS. This further evidence of centrifugal spread from the periventricular or periaqueductal regions again supports the view that MS is an outward progressing disease, commencing around the collecting veins in the subependymal region of the ventricular system.

Venous permeability in MS

As discussed in Chapter 7, venous permeability eems to be increased in and around active MS plaques, as shown by the oedema, fibrin and complement seen in such lesions (**327**, **330** to **335**), by postmortem permeability studies (Broman, 1947; 1964), by magnetic resonance imaging (**240**, **241** and **243**), by scintigraphy (Engell *et al.*, 1984) and, in periphlebitis retinae, by vitreous fluorophotometry (**328** and **329**; Engell *et al.*, 1986; Lightman *et al.*, 1987). We have been unable to detect any gross change in the vessel wall in small veins and at the venocapillary junction. The characteristic enzyme of the endothelium of such vessels, alkaline phosphatase, remains normal (C.W.M. Adams and J.F. Hallpike, unpublished observations; **449**), but anti-factor VIII peroxidase has not yet been tested in MS tissue. Although cerebral permeability may be determined by astrocytes or by microfilaments controlling tight junctional opposition (Janzer and Raff, 1987; Bottaro *et al.*, 1986), electron microscopy has not, from the limited material examined to date, apparently revealed any increase in endothelial vesicular transport or opening of intercellular gap-junctions in the MS plaque. The integrity of the basement membrane and occasionally reported occurrence of fenestrations in cerebral vascular endothelium are further factors to be considered.

Vasculitis and MS

Apart from the mild form of vasculitis (plasmatic vasculosis) seen in small veins and venules in or around MS plaques described above (Table 6 in Chapter 7) (Adams *et al.*, 1985; Adams, 1988), there have been a number of reports of vasculitides (particularly systemic lupus erythematosus) accompanying or resembling MS (Allen *et al.*, 1979b; Meloff, 1980; Tanphaichitr, 1980). In addition, a family has been described with multiple cases of SLE in one generation and multiple cases of MS in the next. However, there were no shared HLA haplotypes between the two disease groups (Sloan *et al.*, 1987). It is perhaps to be expected that supposedly autoimmune diseases, partly or wholly expressed as disorders of (or involving) blood vessels, should share certain clinical and pathological features.

Conclusions

In this chapter, it has been suggested that vascular (venous) damage is an important factor in the pathogenesis of multiple sclerosis; such damage comprises recent and past haemorrhage, fibrin deposition and collagenous thickening or repair of the vein wall. This damage appears to result from inflammatory agents entering the vein wall from the lumen, rather than from the perivascular space. In MS the main localisation of lymphocytes (both T and B cells) is in the perivenular region while lymphocytes (T cells) are sparse at the demyelinating edge (usually not more than 1 per × 40 field) and even more sparse in the parenchyma. This view of the primacy of the vascular lesion in MS is supported by the role of vascular endothelium in presenting MHC Class II antigens (*see* Chapter 9), the antigenic and immunogenic properties of endothelial cells (Tsukada *et al.*, 1987; Tanaka *et al.*, 1987), the presence of both T and B lymphocytes (concerned with both cellular and humoral immunity) and of Tac cells (with interleukin-2 receptors) in the perivascular infiltrate (Woodroofe *et al.*, 1986) and the presence of perivenous lymphocytic infiltrates in all 20 cases in a study on acute MS (Adams *et al.*, 1989). It is difficult to avoid the conclusion that the perivenous process sets up an initial 'bystander' or other autoimmune reaction, which then damages the myelin sheath at the periphery and activates macrophages to consume the altered myelin.

418

418 Subependymal periventricular vein. These veins drain into the Galenic system.

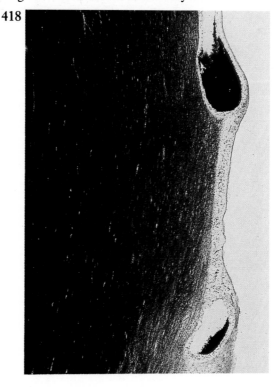

419

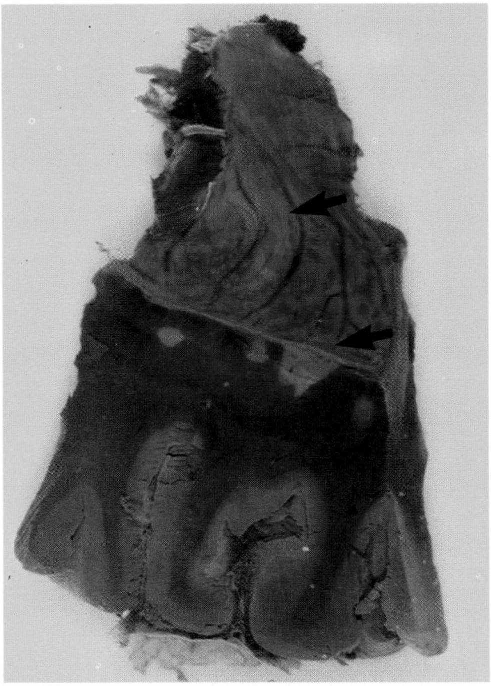

419 Block of brain in multiple sclerosis. At the right is the outer ependymal surface of the lateral ventricle, under which are subependymal veins surrounded by sleeves of demyelination. These sleeves are seen in cross section in **421**. Nile blue sulphate, × 1/3.

420

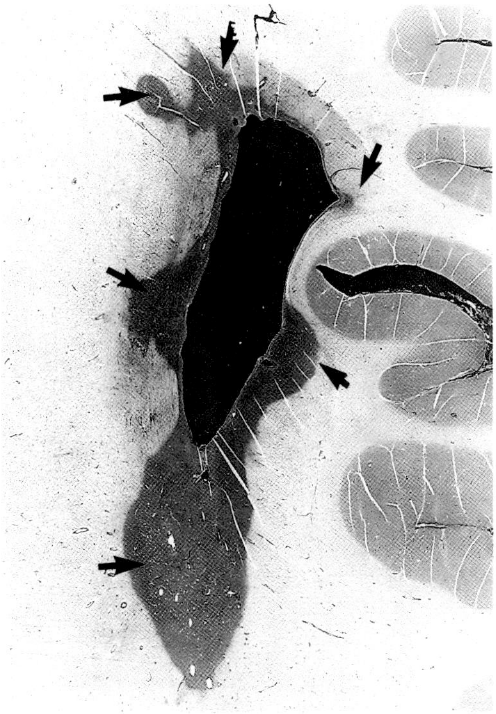

420 Negative image of periventricular plaques (used for histomorphometry) to show relationship of plaques to the lateral ventricle and subependymal veins, × 1.

421

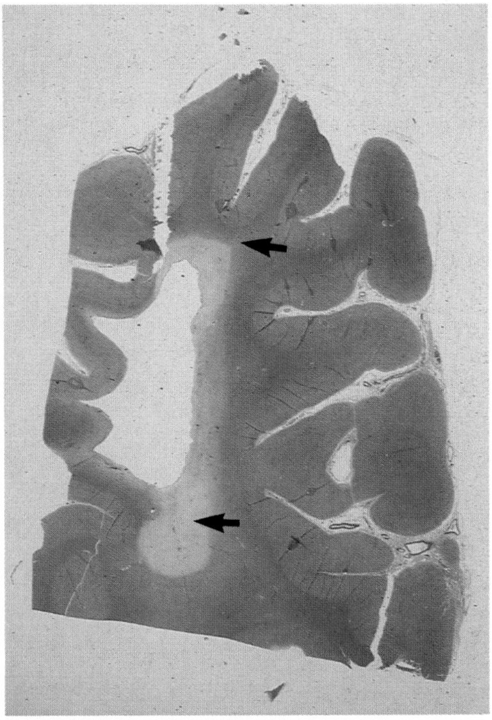

421 Periventricular plaque (lateral ventricle) to show relationship of constituent lesions to blood vessels (arrows). Haematoxylin-eosin, × 1.

422

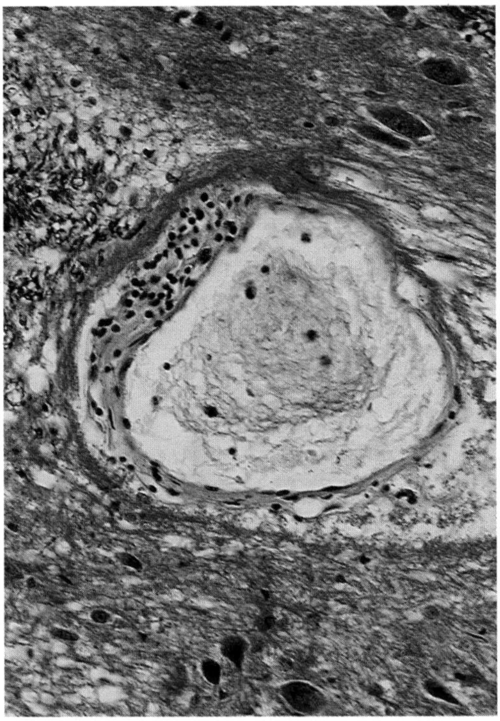

422 Infiltration of vein wall near plaque with predominant lymphocytes. Trichrome, × 100.

423

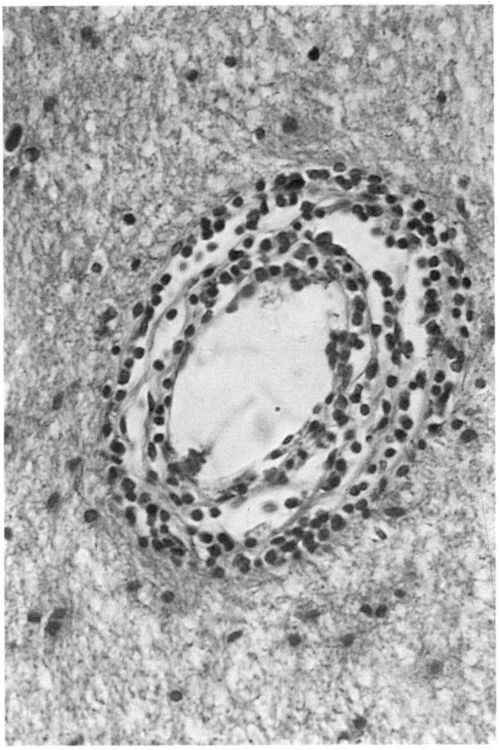

423 As for 422. Trichrome-MSB, × 200.

424

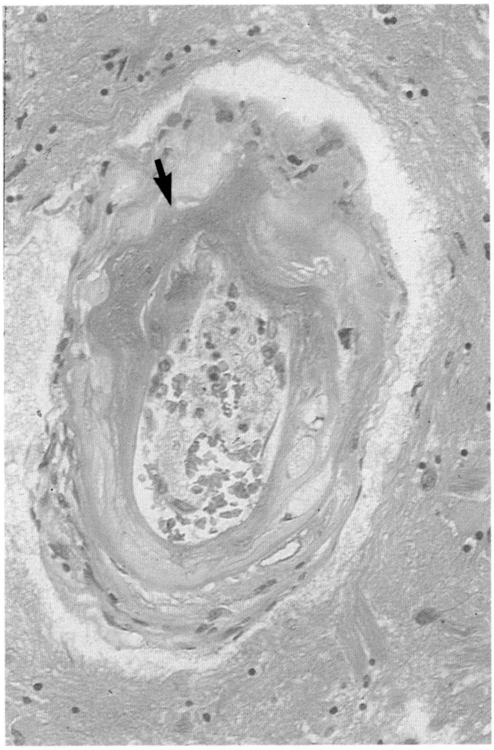

424 Fibrin (arrow) in vein wall in plaque of multiple sclerosis. Haematoxylin-eosin, × 150.

425

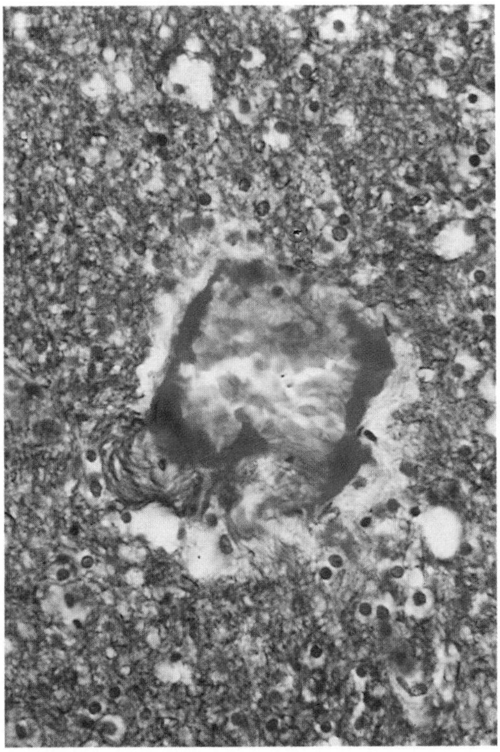

425 Fibrin (stained red) in vein wall outside plaque. Trichrome-MSB, × 100.

426

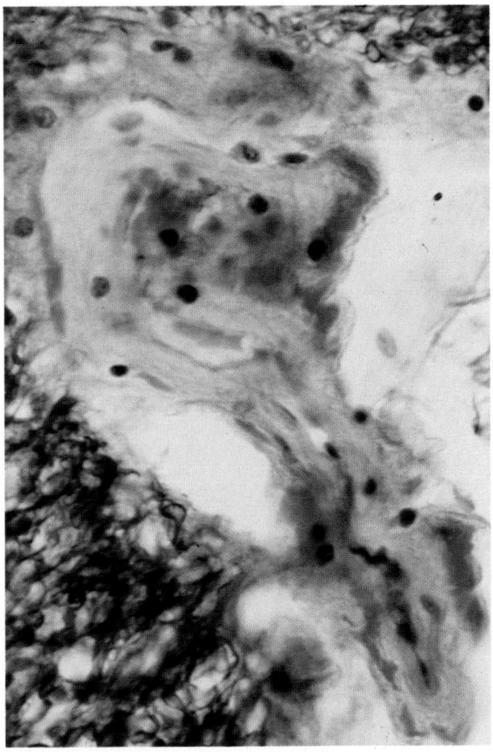

426 Fibrin in vein wall near multiple sclerosis plaque. Trichrome-MSB, × 200.

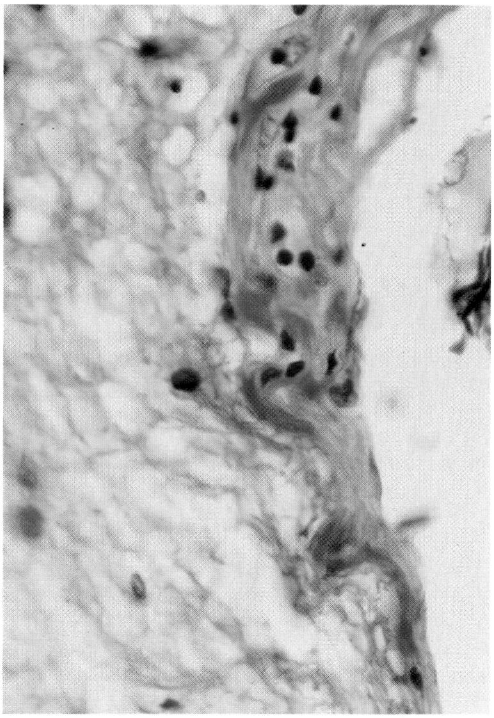 427

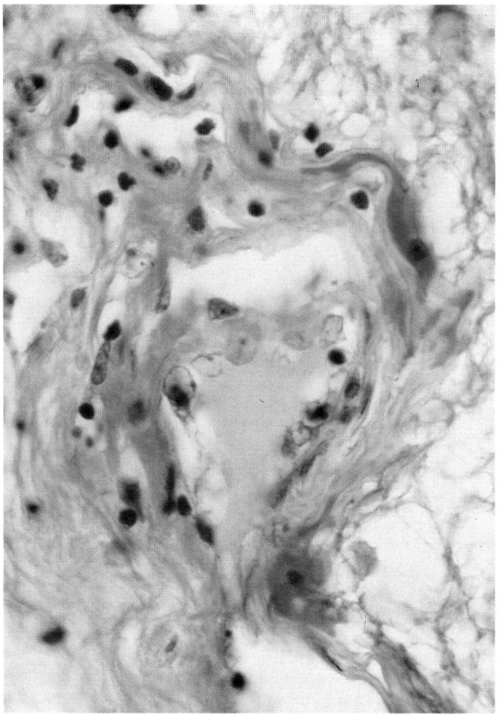 428

427 and **428 Fibrin (stained red) in vein wall in multiple sclerosis.**.Note lymphocytic infiltration in **428**. Trichrome-MSB, × 200.

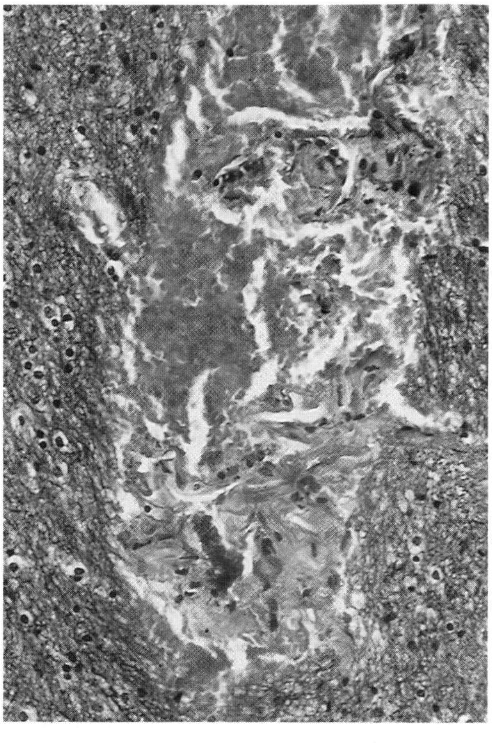 429

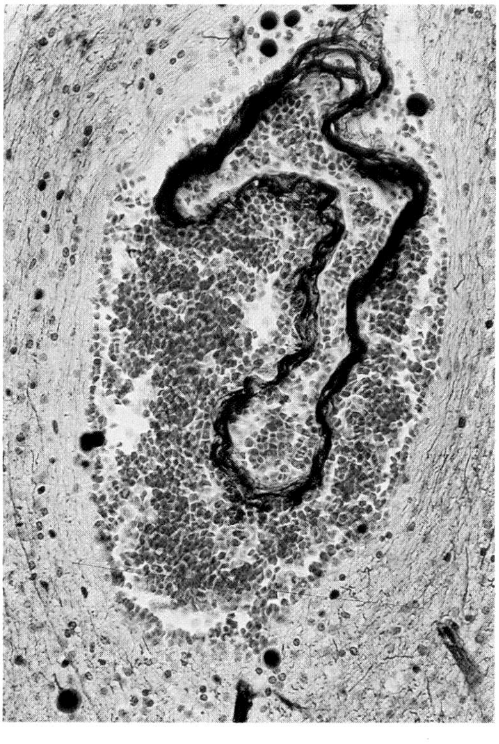 430

429 Another venous haemorrhage in multiple sclerosis. Trichrome-MSB, × 100.

430 Haemorrhage from vein in plaque. Gros-Bielschowsky, × 25.

431

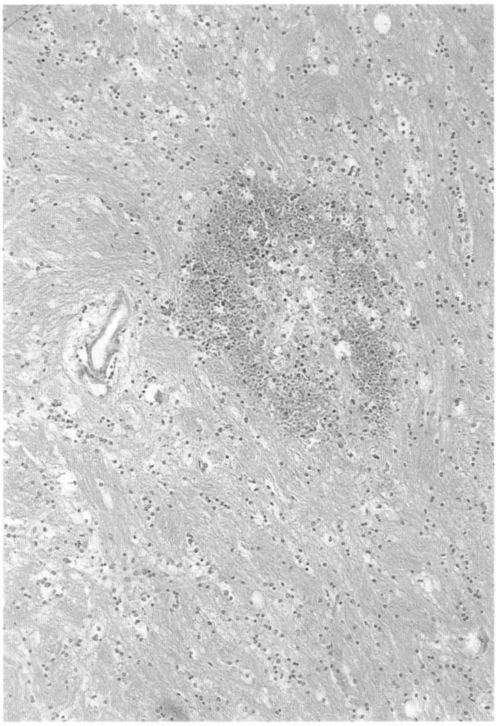

431 Ring haemorrhage in acute haemorrhagic leucoencephalopathy. Haematoxylin and eosin, × 25.

432

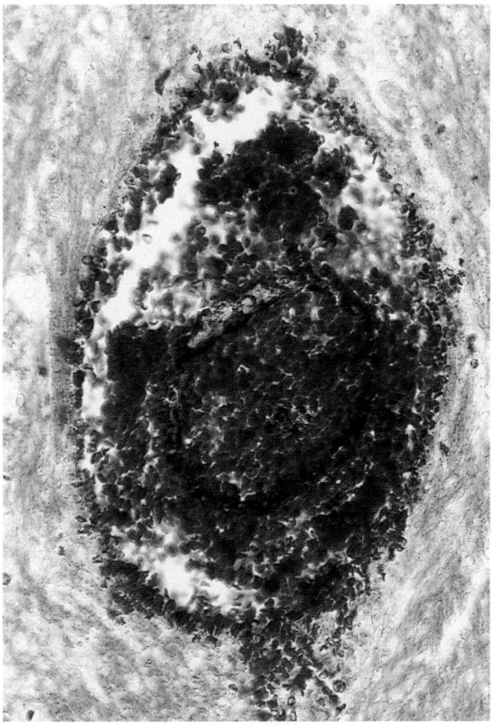

432 Haemorrhage into vein wall and perivascular space in acute haemorrhagic leucoencephalopathy. Phosphotungstic acid haematoxylin, × 40.

433

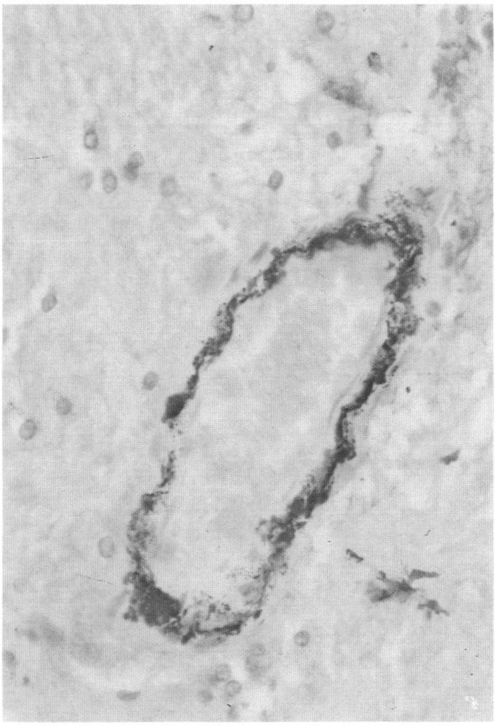

433 Old haemorrhage into vein wall and perivascular space in multiple sclerosis. Perl's ferrocyanide for haemosiderin (iron), × 50.

434

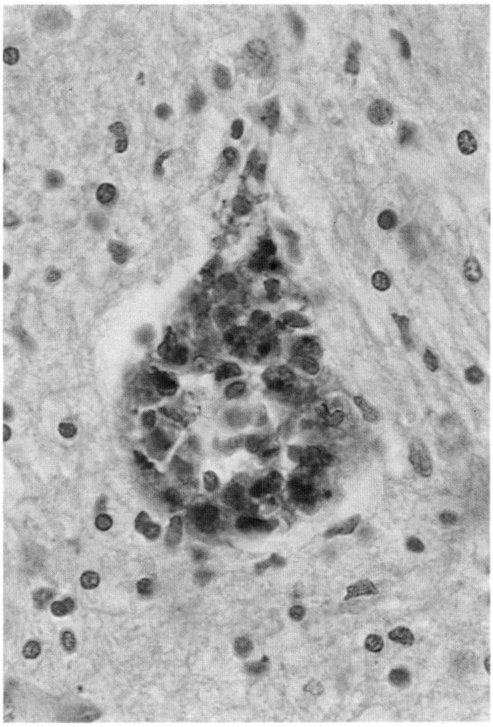

434 Other old perivenular haemorrhage to show haemosiderin. Perls' method, × 200.

435

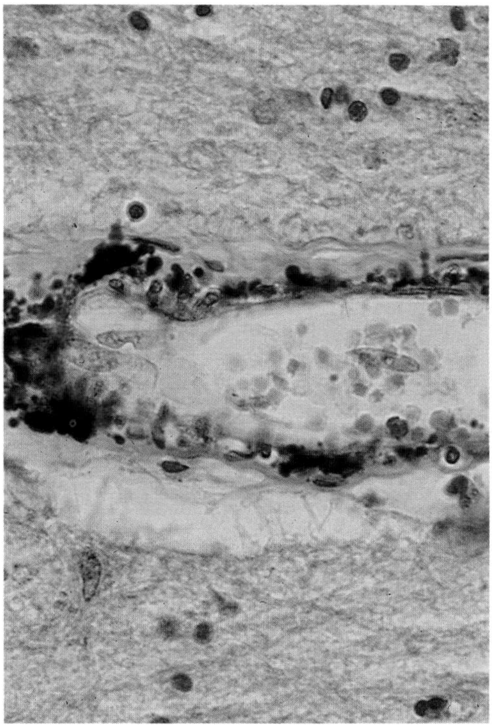

435 Old perivenular haemorrhage in MS plaque. Perls' method × 150.

436

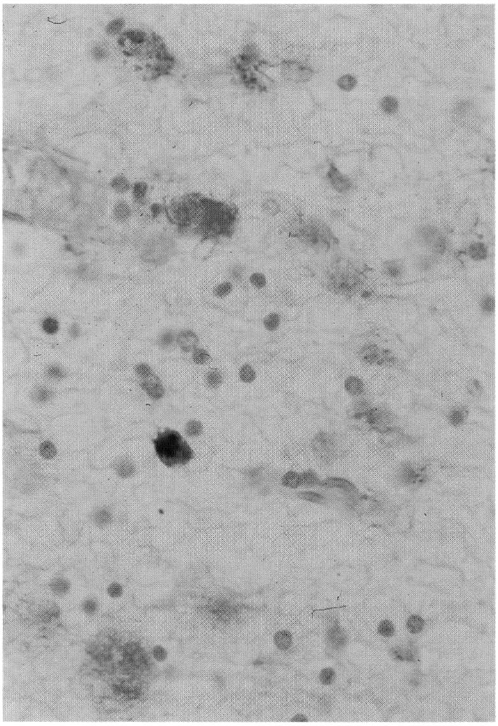

436 Old haemorrhage with haemosiderin forming a pallisade at the edge of a plaque of multiple sclerosis. Perls' method, × 200.

437

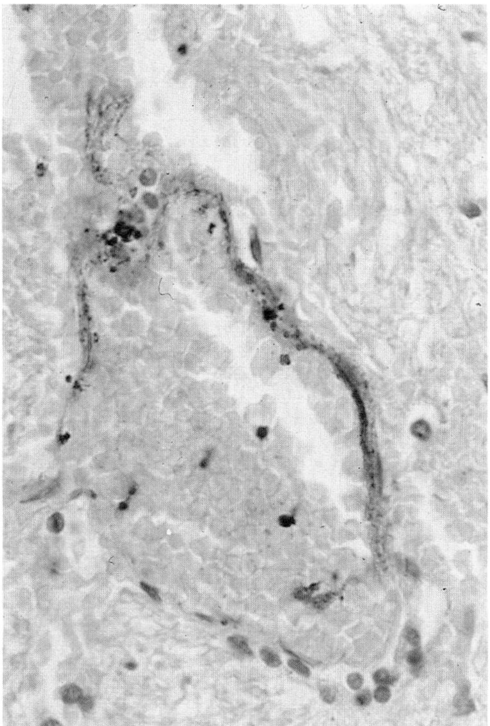

438

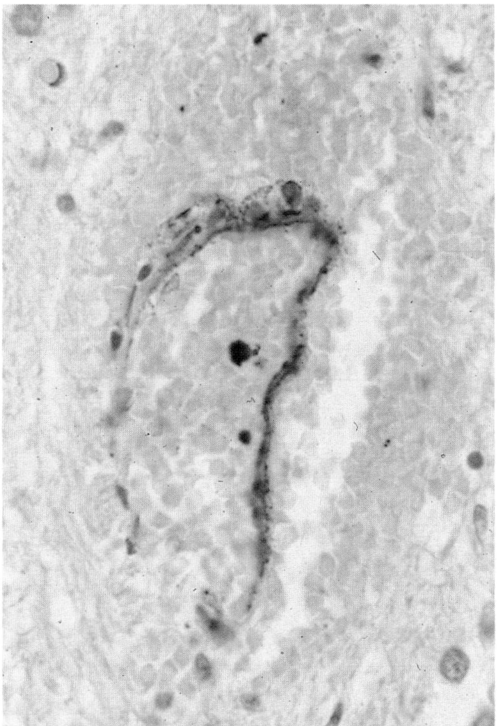

437 and **438 Recent haemorrhages around vein wall in plaques of multiple sclerosis.** The presence of haemosiderin (brown) in the wall of the vein indicates that haemorrhage had occurred on a previous occasion. Haematoxylin-eosin, × 50.

439

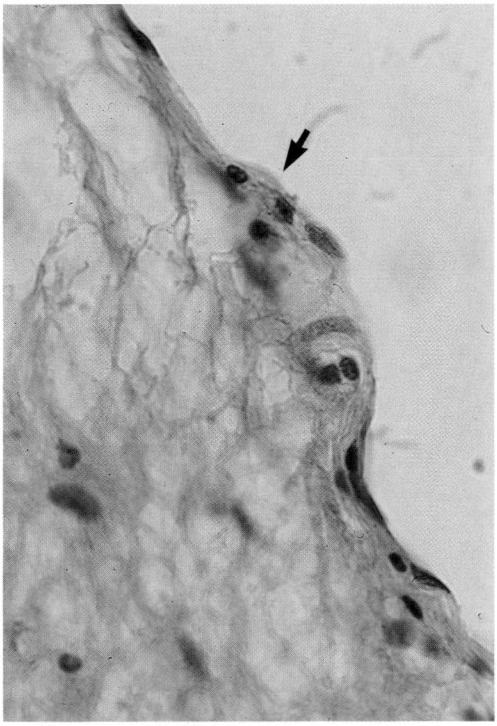

439 Encrustation of old organised thrombosis on vein wall in multiple sclerosis. Haematoxylin-eosin, × 300.

440

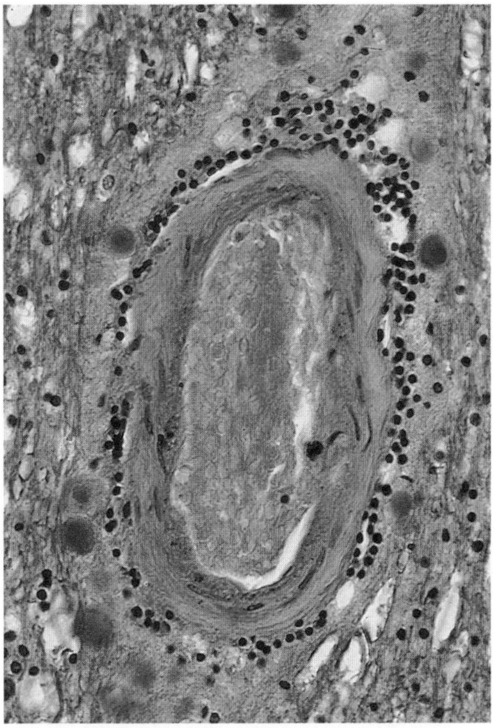

440 Hyalinised vein wall (resembling an artery) with perivascular lymphocytes in multiple sclerosis. Note fairly recent thrombosis. Haematoxylin-eosin, × 50.

441

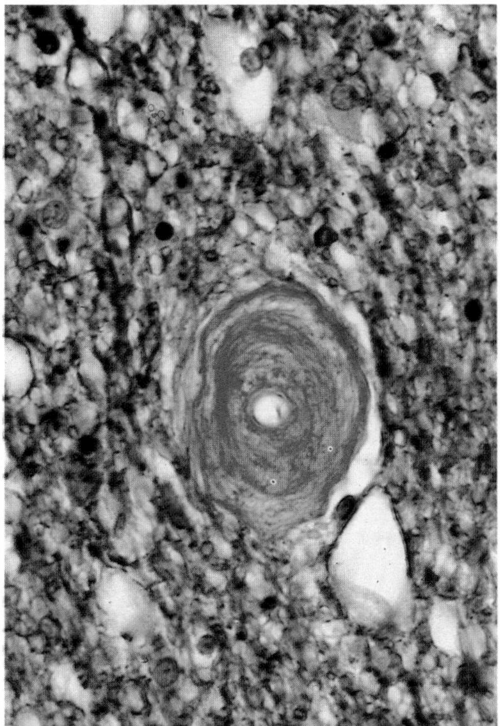

441 Hyalinised collagenised vein in plaque of patient with multiple sclerosis and severe hypertension. Van Gieson-elastic, × 50.

442

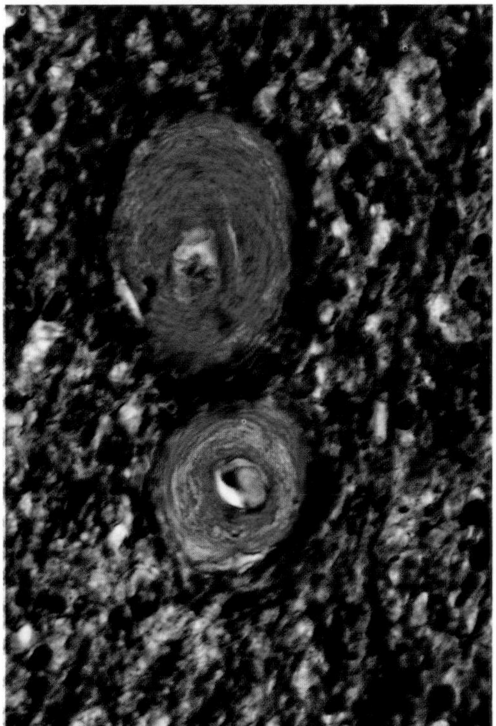

442 Hyalinised collagenised vein near plaque in normotensive patient with multiple sclerosis. Van Gieson-elastic, × 50.

443

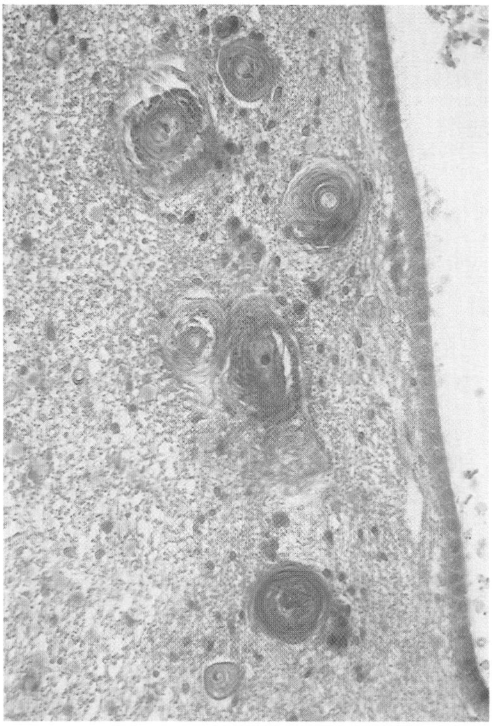

443 Proliferation of thick-walled hyalinised veins in a periventricular plaque of multiple sclerosis. Van Gieson-elastic, × 30.

444

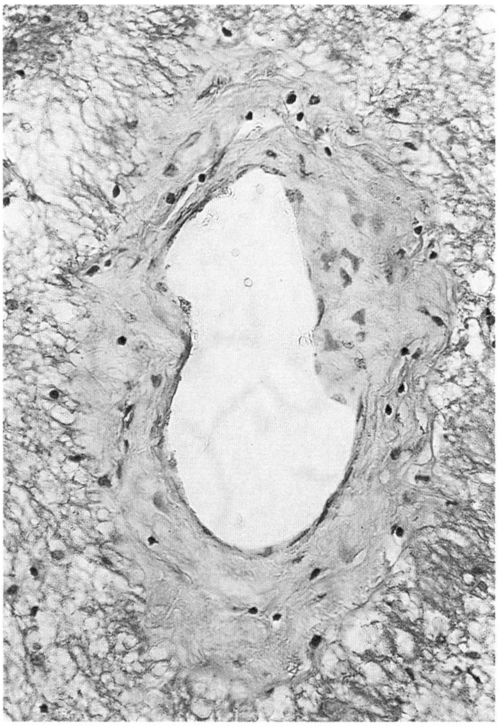

444 Thickened collagenised vein wall in periventricular plaque in multiple sclerosis. Note organising encrustation on wall. Trichrome-MSB, × 60.

445

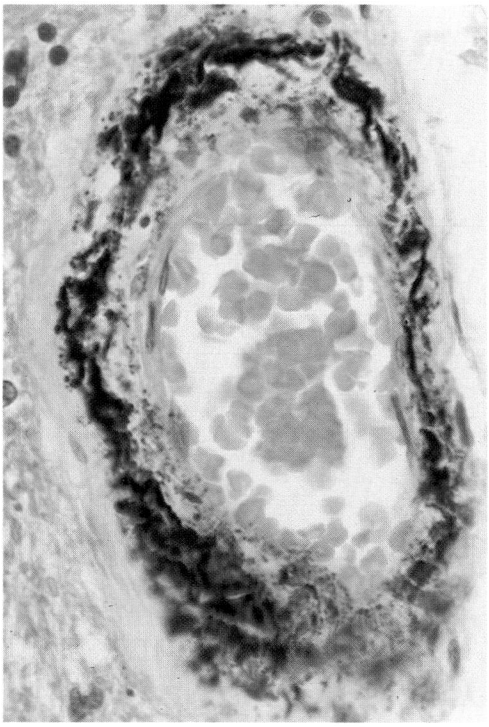

446

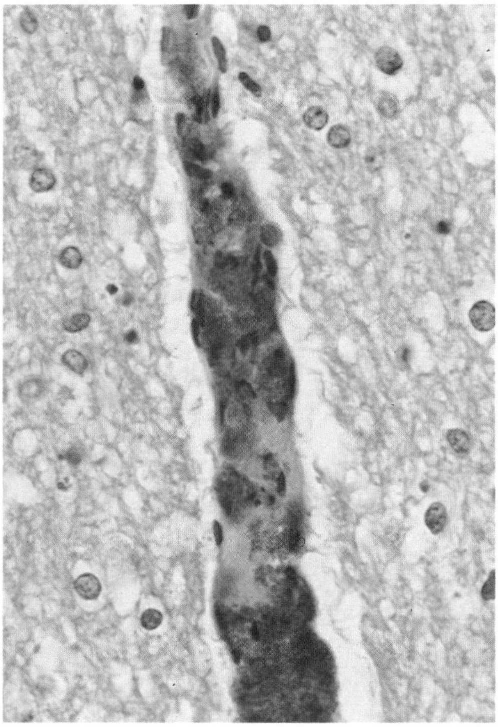

445 and **446 Artefacts. Calcinosis and possibly bacterial growths in vessel walls resembling iron.** Haematoxylin-eosin, × 150.

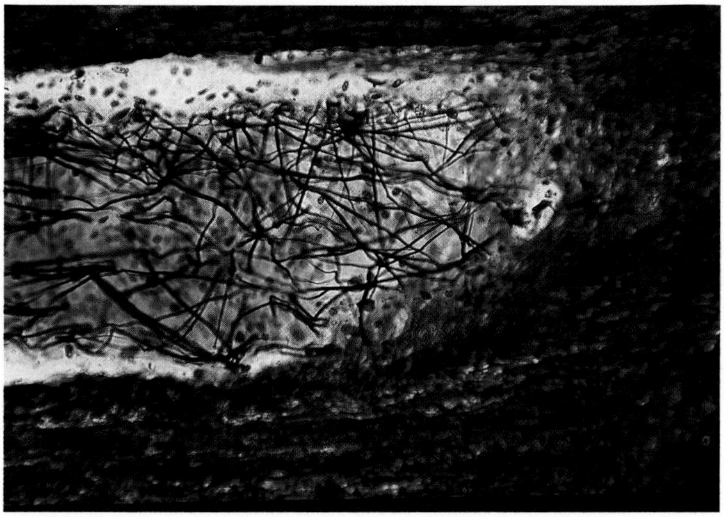

447

447 Artefact. Fungal intervascular growth resembling fibrin. Heidenhain, × 100.

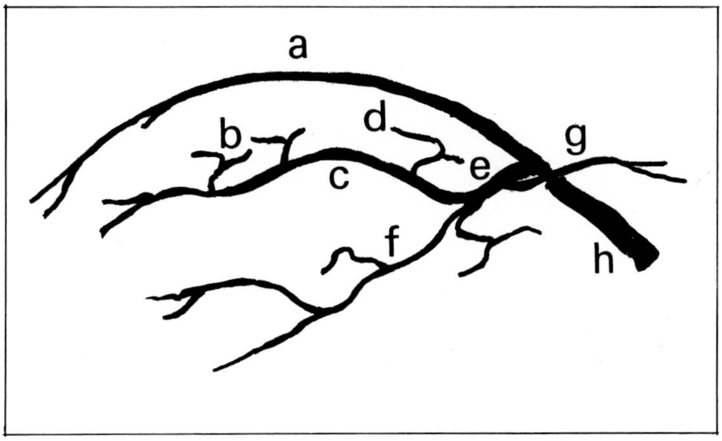

448

448 Internal cerebral (Galenic) venous system (*redrawn after Johanson, 1954*).
a Inferior longitudinal sinus
b Thalamostriate vein
c Internal cerebral vein
d Vein of posterior horn
e Great cerebral vein of Galen
f Basal vein
g Superior cerebellar vein
h Straight sinus

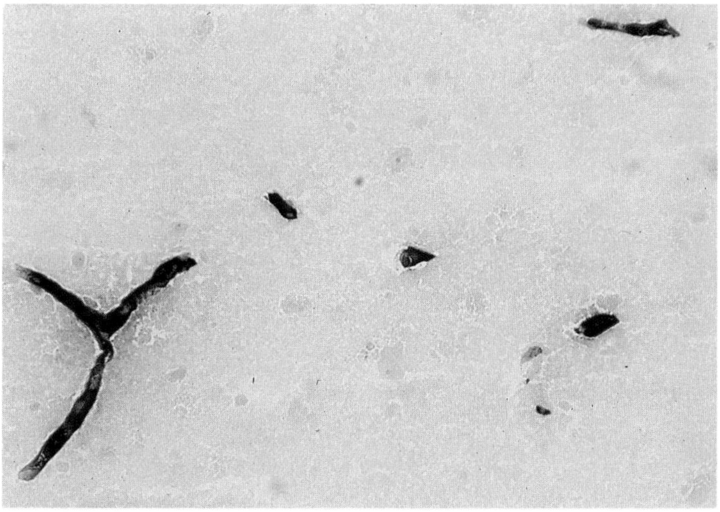

449

449 Normal alkaline phosphatase activity in wall of vessels in plaque of multiple sclerosis. Lead-cobalt method, × 20. *(C.W.M. Adams and ?.F. Hallpike, unpublished)*

9 The immunology of multiple sclerosis

The immunology of MS can be regarded from several aspects:

1 Circulating antibodies and their relationship to viral diseases
2 The cellular immunology of MS
3 Autoimmunity & EAE

Circulating antibodies

Although a search for a specific virus or antibody in MS has been at best inconclusive, it is tacitly assumed that a viral infection is the underlying pathogenic mechanism of MS. The many viruses and other micro-organisms that have been isolated or identified may represent either a spectrum of microbes that can cause the disease or are passenger or contaminant viruses. It could further be argued that the disease is caused by an unknown virus, or is an abnormal reaction to an identified virus.

The raised serum antiviral antibodies which have been detected in MS patients (measles, varicella, mumps, etc.; Adams and Imagawa, 1962; Ter Meulen and Stephenson, 1983) could represent humoral (B cell) immune overactivity in MS (anamnestic reaction: *see* Chapter 5). However, such humoral immune hyperactivity might only be a feature of active or relapsing MS and might not be evident in the burnt-out case. There is no direct evidence that any particular virus or incomplete virus is the specific cause of MS but, for example, a minor episode of measles encephalitis might be one of a number of damaging events to the brain in childhood, leading to the subsequent development of MS (*see* Chapter 5).

The serum in MS shows little change in the total level of immunoglobulins, but circulating immune complexes are present in most cases (Goust *et al.*, 1978). However, there is no direct evidence that these can cause demyelination, and demyelination is not a feature of circulating immune complex diseases (Leibowitz, 1983).

The role of glycolipid haptens (Arnon *et al.*, 1980), serum demyelinating factors and antimyelin and antioligodendroglial antibodies (Abramsky *et al.*, 1977) in MS is quite uncertain and not enough evidence is yet available for a firm conclusion to be made, but it is not unreasonable to suppose that any disease resulting in the primary or secondary destruction of myelin may result in the production of an antibody to a myelin constituent. Hence, such antibodies have relevance to myelin breakdown in a wide range of diseases but are not specific to MS (Traugott *et al.*, 1979; Brostoff, 1984).

Cellular immunology of MS

CSF and blood

The CSF in MS shows an increase in total immunoglobulins, a k/λ pattern different from that in plasma, and a number of oligoclonal bands. Oligoclonal bands are not specific to MS and are found in other CNS infections stimulating antibody production within the CNS (Thompson *et al.*, 1979; Salmi *et al.*, 1983). They probably represent the restricted clones that can be produced from the relatively small number of CSF lymphocytes in MS (see Walsh and Tourtellotte, 1983), and may well be specific for each plaque (review by McKhann, 1982). Oligoclonal bands are not known to play any part in MS, and might be said to be searching for a pathogenic role. Immune complexes are also found in the CSF in MS (Coyle, 1987), but they are present in some other neurological diseases and are, therefore, non-specific.

The proportion of T cells increases in the CSF, doubtless a reflection of the increased content of lymphocytes in brain, cord and CSF in the active disease. These changes imply that the active phase of MS is characterised by increased cellular (T cell) immunity, even though the level of the general humoral or antibody (B cell) response may remain static.

T cell subset methods, using peripheral blood and CSF lymphoctyes, in general show a reduced proportion of T suppressor to T helper cells (Th/Ts increases) in relapses or in the chronic progressive form of the disease (Bach *et al.*, 1980; Arnason, 1983; Antel *et al.*, 1986; Kuroda and Shibasaki, 1987). The suppressor-inducer T cell subset was found to be decreased in most cases of progressive MS but not in acute MS (Morimoto *et al.*, 1987). This accords with De Graaf *et al.*, (1987) who found raised T helper cells in progressive disease, but not in the episodic relapsing form of MS. Indeed Rose *et al.*, (1987) found a fall in T helper cells 1-2 months before a relapse. By contrast, Bellamy *et al.*, (1985) found an increase of activated lymphocytes (Tac cells) with interleukin-2 receptors in active but not chronic MS.

Immunocytochemistry

Immunocytochemical methods confirm that humoral immunity plays a part in plaques, but the amount of immunoglobulin deposited is only modest. As with the cellular inflammatory features of the lesion, the process seems often to proceed in 'slow tempo' (Lumsden, 1970).

Immunoglobulin G (IgG) and complement have been demonstrated in neuroglia, around blood vessels, at the edge of active plaques and in the subependymal region in MS brains (**450** and **451**; Simpson *et al.*, 1969; Esiri, 1977, 1980; Adams *et al.*, 1987). Earlier studies with fluorescence labelling have now been largely superseded by the peroxidase method, which allows much more precise histological interpretation. These newer techniques show that IgG is more abundant in hypercellular plaques and in those that are active (Esiri, 1980). IgG has also been found capping macrophages in active MS plaques (Prineas and Graham, 1981).

Macrophages are discussed in detail in Chapter 7, but it should again be mentioned that activated macrophages (as evident from their immunoglobulin capping) could play a role in the demyelinating process (Prineas, 1985). However, there remains the uncertainty whether such macrophages are the initial mediators of the disease, or simply a secondary or scavenger response to previously damaged myelin (**452** to **454**; *see* Chapter 7).

Lymphocytes are readily recognised in formalin fixed tissue by using the anti-common leucocyte antigen (PD7/26; CD45; 455). However, separate identification of T cells and B cells requires the use of unfixed tissue, either using immuno-staining methods or non-specific esterase to show the paranuclear body of the T cell. Results on MS plaques show that there is a greater proportion of T cells than B cells therein; B cells are mainly located in the perivascular space as is further shown by the frequent occurrence of plasma cells. However, there is no final concensus as to changes in suppressor T cells (Booss *et al.*, 1983; Traugott and Raine, 1982; Traugott *et al.*, 1983; Hauser *et al.*, 1986; McCallum *et al.*, 1987).

Immunocytochemical studies on fresh MS plaques reveal that most of the lymphocytes in the perivascular cuff are T cells, particularly suppressor T cells (T_s; CD8). Raine (1984) recorded that a few T_h cells (CD4) may be found scattered in the parenchyma, whereas Booss, Esiri *et al.*, (1983) observed T_h cells (CD4) in the perivascular cuff but not in the parenchyma. T_s cells were located both in the perivascular space and in the parenchyma. The latter group (McCallum, Esiri *et al.*, 1987) subsequently found that T_s cells in the white matter around the plaque are decreased in numbers in active disease but increase in controlled static disease, while the T helper (Th) cells sited at the demyelinating edge remain constant in numbers. This implies that the rather scanty peripheral suppressor T cells (T_s) at the active edge may locally control and limit the established disease.

Although the results in plaques have not been consistent, the general tenor is that the active phase is accompanied by a local hypersensitivity reaction, with increased or normal amounts of helper cells and reduced suppressor cells. The illustrations presented here of plaques of active MS show considerable perivascular infiltrates of both T_s and T_h cells (**456** to **459**), but T cells at the periphery of these active lesions were usually scanty, and outnumbered by those in the perivascular space.

For T cells to recognise antigens, it is necessary for the 'presenting cell' to provide the Major Histocompatibility Complex Class II antigen (Ia). Not all cells in the nervous system can present Class II antigens, but it seems that macrophages, endothelial cells and perhaps astrocytes can all express this 'Ia restricted T cell receptor' (Fontana *et al.*, 1984; Traugott and Raine, 1985; Hayes *et al.*, 1987). Hence, such cells are required to initiate the early stages of an immune reaction in the nervous system, as the T cell is incomplete on its own. Macrophages expressing Ia are found in large numbers in the acute MS plaque (Traugott *et al.*, 1983).

T lymphocytes from MS subjects, exposed to encephalitogenic peptide, are cytotoxic for neonatal rat glial cells (Frick, 1982). This seems to be a reasonably specific in vitro feature of MS and reflects altered cell-mediated immunity in the disease.

A local hypersensitivity reaction in the vicinity of myelin has been held to cause demyelination as a result of the so-called 'bystander reaction' (Wisnewski, 1977; Wisnewski and Bloom, 1975; Wisnewski *et al.*, 1980). This idea would suppose that the lysosomal products of the inflammation accompanying a hypersensitivity reaction would cause myelin breakdown in the same way as shown for lysosomal cathepsins (*see* Chapter 4). In fact any inflammatory reaction resulting in the release of myelinolytic lysosomal enzymes would constitute a bystander reaction. The role of the inflammatory process in demyelination is further discussed in Chapter 7. The abundance of lymphocytes in the perivascular compartment contrasts with the sparsity of such cells at the periphery of the lesion. This reinforces the view that the vascular lesion is the initiating factor or at least plays a very important early role in the pathogenesis of MS.

Autoimmunity and relationship to EAE

Immunity serves a useful function when directed against an invading or endogenous harmful antigen. However, a response which comes to be directed against the hosts' own tissues is autoimmune and harmful. In MS autoimmunity is widely held to be a result of a previous infection by an unspecified neurotropic virus.

Experimental allergic encephalomyelitis (EAE) is the archetype of an autoimmune disorder in the nervous system, even though it was first produced by the cannibalistic mechanism of injecting brain or cord suspensions between individuals of the same species. The experimental aspects of the disease concerning the antigens and use of Freund's adjuvant are set out briefly in Chapter 4.

The idea that MS may have an autoimmune component largely originated by analogy with EAE, where there is a perivascular locally demyelinating inflammatory lesion and where T cells are again much more prominent than B cells. EAE does not itself much resemble MS. Although the perivenular infiltrate in EAE (*see* Chapter 4) has some resemblance to that in MS, the extent of demyelination is nowhere nearly as extensive as in MS. Furthermore, EAE is a monophasic disease unlike MS. However, chronic relapsing EAE (CREAE; *see* Chapter 4) does bear closer resemblance to MS, particularly as regards its relapsing course (Raine, 1983) and immunochemical changes, including local increase in T helper cells (Traugott *et al.*, 1986). Nevertheless, the pathogenesis of EAE or CREAE is artificial, does not show the same anatomical preference, depends on a non-specific antigen and cannot be taken to have a direct bearing on the pathogenesis of MS.

Conclusions

In Chapter 8, it was suggested that vascular (venous) damage is an important factor in the pathogenesis of multiple sclerosis; such damage comprises recent and past haemorrhage, fibrin deposition and collagenous thickening or repair of the vein wall. This damage appears to result from inflammatory (including immune) agents entering the vein wall from the lumen, rather than from the perivascular space.

In MS the main localisation of lymphocytes (both T and B cells) is in the perivenular region while lymphocytes (T cells) are generally sparse at the demyelinating edge (usually not more than 1 per × 40 field) and even more sparse in the parenchyma. This general view of the primacy of the vascular lesion in MS is supported by the role of vascular endothelium in presenting MHC Class II antigens, the antigenic and immunogenic properties of endothelial cells (Tsukada *et al.*, 1987; Tanaka *et al.*, 1987), the presence of T and B lymphocytes (concerned with both cellular and humoral immunity) and of Tac cells (with interleukin-2 receptors) in the perivascular infiltrate (Woodroofe *et al.*, 1986) and, lastly, the presence of perivenous lymphocytic infiltrates in active MS (Adams, 1977) and, particularly, in all 20 cases in a study on acute MS (Adams *et al.*, 1989; also see the 16 cases in Table 8). It is difficult to avoid the conclusion that the perivenous process sets up an initial 'bystander' inflammatory or autoimmune reaction, which then damages the myelin sheath at the periphery and activates macrophages to consume the altered myelin.

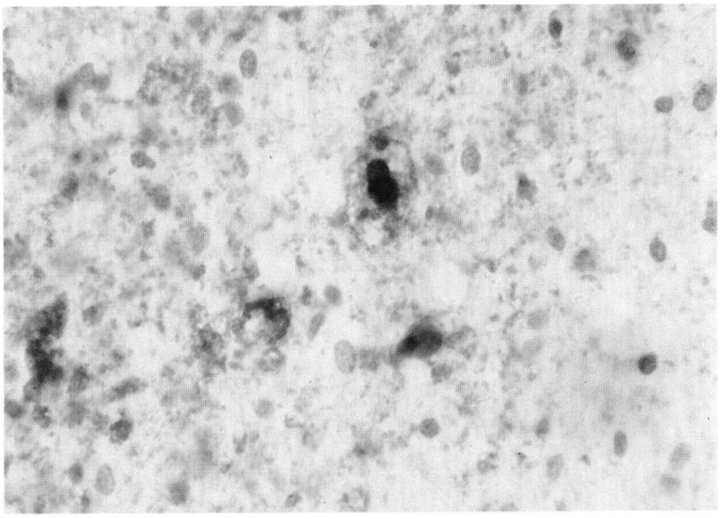
450

450 Uptake of IgG by astrocytes in periventricular region in multiple sclerosis. Anti-IgG-indirect peroxidase, × 300.

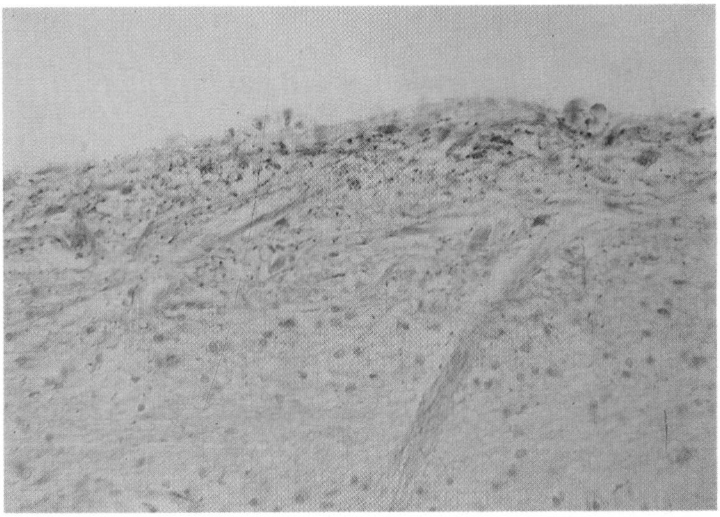
451

451 Uptake of IgG in subependymal gliosis of lateral ventricle in multiple sclerosis. Anti-IgG-indirect peroxidase, × 120.

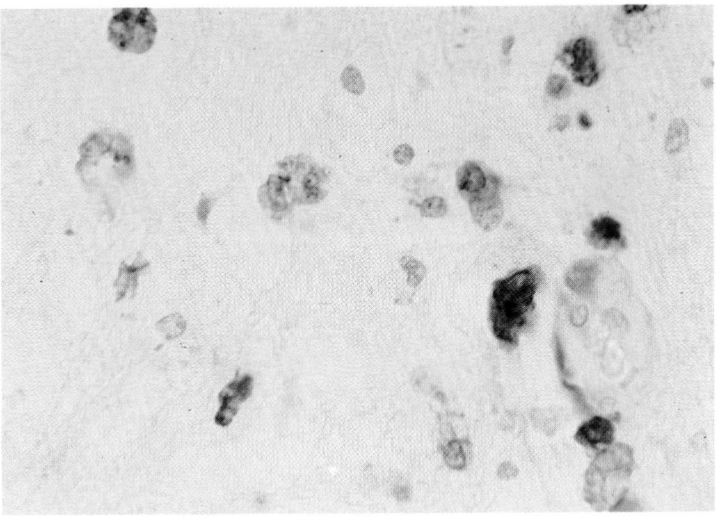
452

452 Haematogenous macrophages in parenchyma of an acute MS plaque stained by muramidase (anti-lysozyme)-peroxidase-antiperoxidase, × 300. *(Courtesy of Dr R.N. Poston)* (*see* Chapter 7).

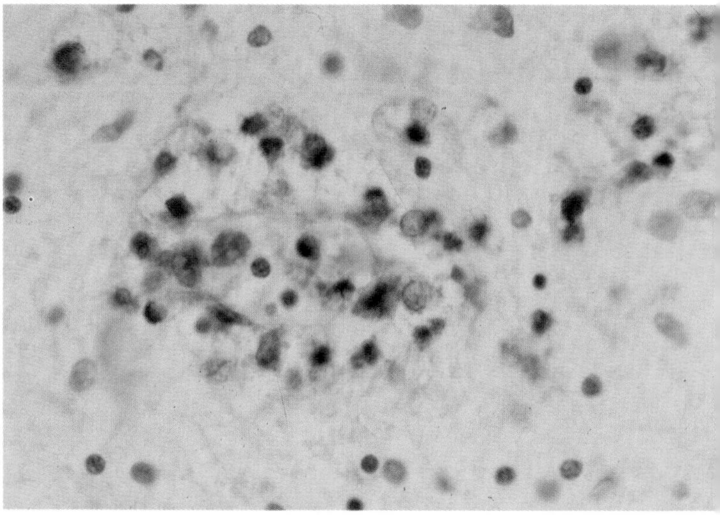

453 Haematogenous macrophages in parenchyma of an acute MS plaque stained by MAC-indirect peroxidase, × 200. *(Courtesy of Dr R.N. Poston)*

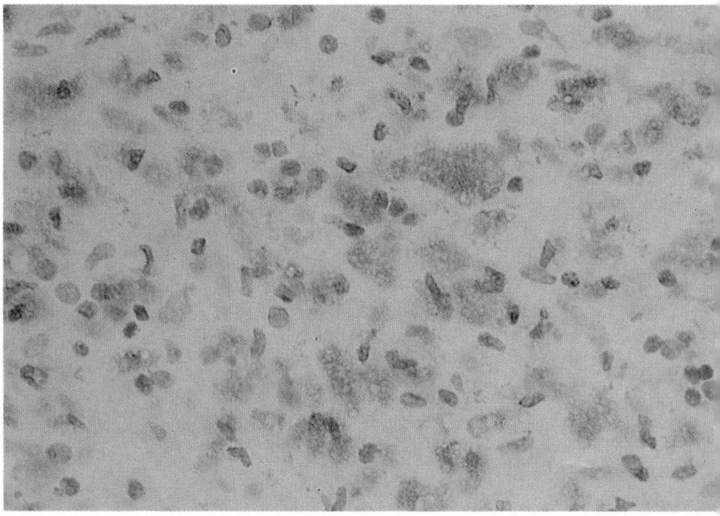

454 Macrophages and microglia in parenchyma of active MS plaque stained by the pan-macrophage marker, EBM11- indirect peroxidase, × 300. *(Courtesy of Drs M. Esiri and R.N. Poston)*

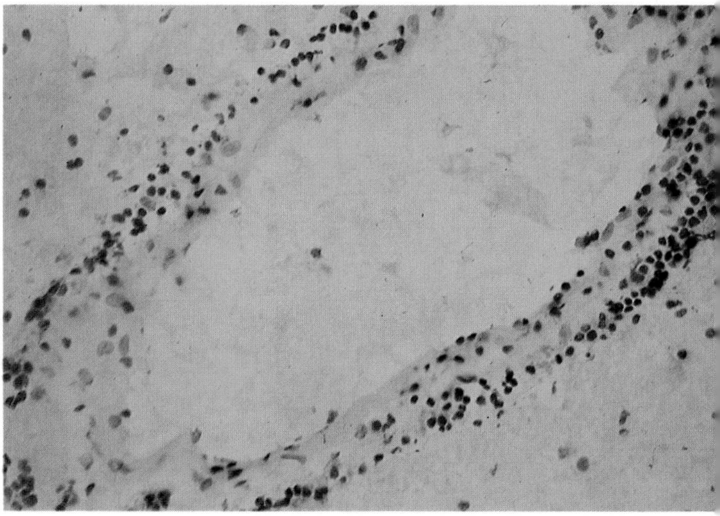

455 Perivascular lymphocytic infiltrate in active plaque of multiple sclerosis. Pan T marker, CD3, indirect peroxidase, × 80. *(Courtesy of Professor S. Leibowitiz)*

456

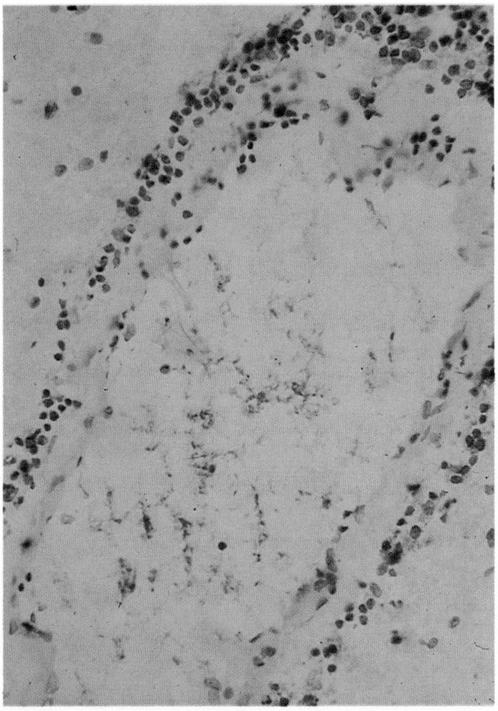

456 Perivascular infiltrate of suppressor T cells in active plaque of multiple sclerosis. CD8(T8)-indirect peroxidase, × 80. *(Courtesy of Professor S. Leibowitz)*

457

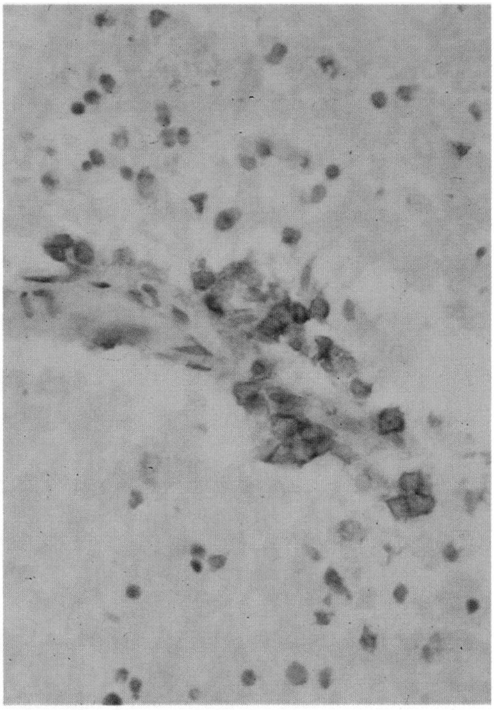

457 Moderate infiltration of suppressor T cells in active plaque of multiple sclerosis. CD8(T8)-indirect peroxidase, × 200. *(Courtesy of Professor S. Leibowitz)*

458

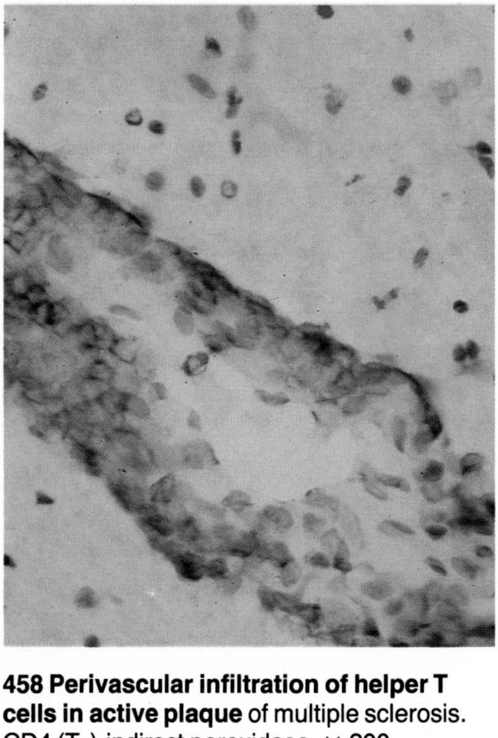

458 Perivascular infiltration of helper T cells in active plaque of multiple sclerosis. CD4 (T_4)-indirect peroxidase, × 200. *(Courtesy of Professor S. Leibowitz)*

459

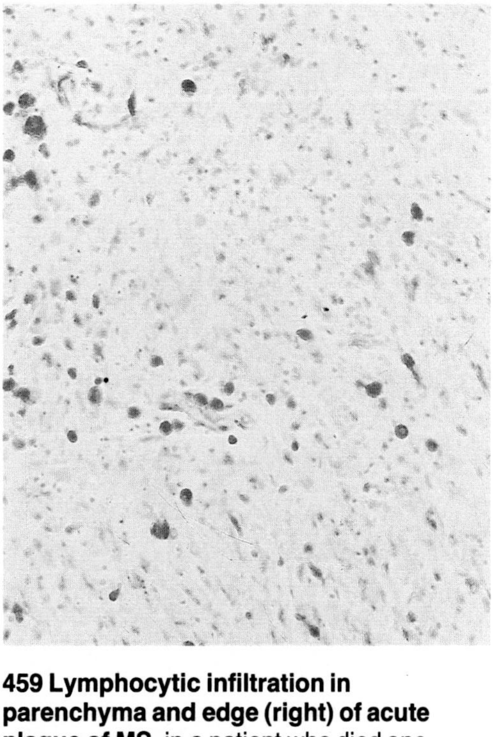

459 Lymphocytic infiltration in parenchyma and edge (right) of acute plaque of MS, in a patient who died one month after clinical onset. The extent of parenchymal lymphocytic infiltration is unusual. PD7/26 (CD45)-peroxidase, × 20.

10 Complications and causes of death in multiple sclerosis

Patients with MS rarely die from the direct effects of their disease on nerve conduction, except in the unusual circumstance of drowning in an overhot bath. It is now well known that impaired nerve conduction with increasing heat in MS (Uhthoff's phenomenon) may lead to such a regrettable accident. The young girl, whose case is illustrated in **305**, probably died in this way. By contrast, it is of much interest that lowering the body temperature in the MS patient improves nerve conduction, as assessed by visually-evoked potential and by improvement in the field of vision (Heider and Gottlob, 1987).

In our series of 176 cases with full pathological and clinical details, the average age at death was 54 years, with an average duration of 12 years. However, the stated duration only reflects the recorded time at which the patient first sought medical advice, and the true time-course may have been much longer (20-25 years, Kurtzke, 1983). Nevertheless, Lyon-Caen *et al.*, (1985) have observed that the duration of the disease is much shorter (8.6 years) in older subjects (onset after age of 45 years), contrasting with 29 years' survival with onset under 25 years (Izquierdo *et al.*, 1986). The average age in our series was well into the range for older subjects, and our shorter duration would be consistent with these French observations. Another factor is that our interest in the rapidly progressive (Marburg) form of MS may also have skewed our results towards a shorter survival time.

The immediate complications that seem to have caused death in 120 necropsy-proven cases studied by Allen *et al.*, (1978) and in the 176 necropsy cases studied by us (figures in parentheses) were:

a) 26 per cent died from unrelated conditions (24 per cent including 8 per cent with neoplasia); 74 per cent died from complications of MS (76 per cent).

b) the complications were bronchopneumonia 46 per cent (31 per cent); pyelonephritis and other urinary disorders 53 per cent (17 per cent); thrombosis and infarction 4 per cent (20 per cent including myocardial 16 per cent and cerebral 4 per cent); pulmonary embolism 5 per cent (8 per cent); choking and aspirating food into the airways (10 per cent); and suicide/road accident (4 per cent). In our series, pressure ulcers seem to have contributed through septicaemia towards death in 7 per cent, coma was the only cause of death in 2 per cent; while in 16 per cent MS was not diagnosed during life. (Some cases had more than one complication contributing towards death.) Our figures are comparable with those of a clinical study on 216 consecutive cases of MS by Phadke (1987), who found that 15 per cent died from myocardial infarction, 4 per cent from pulmonary embolism and 11 per cent from septicaemia.

Acute onset of MS is often associated with severe disease in the pons, medulla and brainstem. Because of the proximity of such lesions to brainstem and medullary nuclei (**247**, **251-256**), death is often sudden (bulbar or pseudobulbar palsy). The usual mode of death in these hyperacute cases (the Marburg form) seems to be asphyxia due to aspiration of food into the lungs, and lipid pneumonia (**460**) resulting from paralysis or inco-ordination of the muscles of the pharynx and upper airways tract ('masticatory spasm', Rindfleisch, 1873). Five (5) out of 8 of our hyperacute cases, dying within 4 weeks of clinical onset of disease, died in this way (see Table 7).

The usual causes of death in chronic MS seem to be attributable to interruption of the long tracts of the spinal cord, and the results of being chair-ridden or bedridden. Hence, bronchopneumonia of hypostatic nature (**461** and **462**), lung-abscess and empyema (**463**) are common causes of death. Pressure ulcers may occur over the sacrum, pelvis, heels and feet, particularly in patients with impaired pressure perception. Occasionally, patients die of septicaemia (**464**) as a result of these chronically infected ulcers that may penetrate down to bone. Pulmonary embolism due to deep vein thrombosis in the legs was a common cause of death in non-ambulatory patients confined to bed (**465** to **468**), but physiotherapy and other measures have now somewhat reduced its frequency. Muscle spasticity is very frequent as a result of interruption of the upper motor neurone in the cord or elsewhere, and may lead to flexion deformities of the legs, feet or wrists (**469**). Tenotomy or drugs may be used to correct muscle balance and tone.

Although most plaques in the cord are sited in its cervical part, urinary incontinence and disordered bladder function are extremely common in MS. The prime cause of this dysfunction would be expected to be interruption of the autonomic nuclei in the lateral or intermediate horn of the cord S_2-S_4 (Parsons, 1983), but the precise neuropathology is uncertain.

The corticospinal, reticulospinal and spinothalamic tracts are also important and subject to interruption by plaques in the cord (Parsons, 1983). The consequence of this bladder dysfunction in MS is a high frequency of cystitis and acute or chronic pyelonephritis (**470**). Pyelonephritis is a common finding in MS but it is not such an important factor in promoting renal hypertension as glomerulonephritis, where the renin-secreting juxta-glomerular apparatus is directly involved. It is a moot point whether or not the incidence of hypertension is increased in MS. Lumsden (1970) implied that it is, whereas Allen and colleagues (1978) and ourselves found no pathological evidence of a significant degree of hypertension. The low incidence of major primary cerebral haemorrhage (which is mainly caused by hypertension) in both Allen's and our MS series (2 cases in 283 MS patients) and in Lindegard's (1985) series (3 cases in 362 MS patients) strongly supports our view in disagreement with Lumsden's.

Thrombosis and platelet function have been investigated intermittently in MS since the 1930s' (*see* Chapter 8). However, no special incidence of thrombosis has been reported in the disease (see above). Our own series of MS cases shows a 16 per cent incidence of death from myocardial infarction. Such cases of sudden death in MS were more usually associated with coronary thrombosis (**471** and **472**) than with an acute electrical disturbance of the myocardium (for example, ventricular fibrillation). However, any supposed association of coronary disease with MS might be artefactual, as half such cases were obtained through the good offices of coroners' pathologists, and a medicolegal autopsy would commonly be required if death was caused other than by an obvious complication of MS. Moreover, the average age of death of these MS patients with myocardial infarction was 60 years, at which age coronary disease is common. There is no reason to suspect that MS patients should not suffer vascular disease as commonly as the rest of the population. Nevertheless, Lindegard (1985) includes myocardial infarction in a cluster of diseases associated with MS, and records a five-fold increase in its frequency in MS.

A view has been advanced that MS results from cerebral fat embolism (James, 1982), but this has been challenged (Adams and High, 1982). A fat embolus characteristically fills the embolised small artery or arteriole with sudanophilic lipid (**473**), but such embolism has never been seen in MS. Furthermore, a fat embolus is essentially composed of triglycerides (depot fat), whereas the accumulated lipid breakdown product in MS and other demyelinating diseases is mainly esterified cholesterol (*see* Chapter 1).

Neoplasia is quite frequent in MS subject (8 per cent in our series), but the 45-65 age range is a common time for both onset of neoplasia and death from MS. In this regard, Allen *et al.*, (1978) found no difference between MS patients and controls in the incidence of neoplasia. Nevertheless, an interesting rarity is the simultaneous occurrence of glioblastoma, ependymoma and multiple sclerosis in the case illustrated in **474** and **475**. Our series also showed four *subclinical* cases of MS associated with carcinoma, mainly of the breast (**476**). One case had complained of ataxia, but this had been regarded as paraneoplastic cerebellar disease. However, at autopsy a plaque was found in the middle cerebellar peduncle (**258** and **259**), accounting for the cerebellar signs.

Subclinical disease is common, accounting for at least 5 per cent of all autopsy cases of MS (Jellinger, 1969). Other authors have recorded an incidence of subclinical or benign MS as high as 20 per cent of all cases (brief reviews in Adams, 1983; Morariu and Klutzow, 1976). Nine coroner's cases in our series, where death was due to coronary thrombosis, showed unexpectedly multiple sclerosis at autopsy. Seventeen hospital cases also showed unexpected MS, making an incidence of 16 per cent of subclinical MS in our postmortem cases at the time of writing.

Vasculitis and haemosiderosis in MS are discussed in Chapter 8. The association of autoimmune disease with MS (for example, vasculitis and rheumatoid arthritis) may merely be fortuitous or may reflect some shared immune disorder. However, until proved otherwise, it is best to apply William Ockham's razor and adopt the simplest explanation.

Although Allen *et al.* (1978) could find no increase in thyroid atrophy in her MS series, there have been intermittent reports of an association between thyroiditis, myxoedema and MS (Roquer *et al.*, 1987; Nagashima *et al.*, 1984; and one case in our series). This could accord with the known role of thyroxine in controlling myelinogenesis (Dalal *et al.*, 1971; Anderson *et al.*, 1987; Shanker *et al.*, 1987; *see* Chapters 1 and 4).

In general, MS patients do not die from accidents resulting from their inco-ordination, ataxia and unreliability of muscular tone and power. Although bruising and fractures are exceedingly common, our series shows only one case where death was due to a fractured skull and two cases where MS may possibly have contributed to fatal motor car accidents.

460

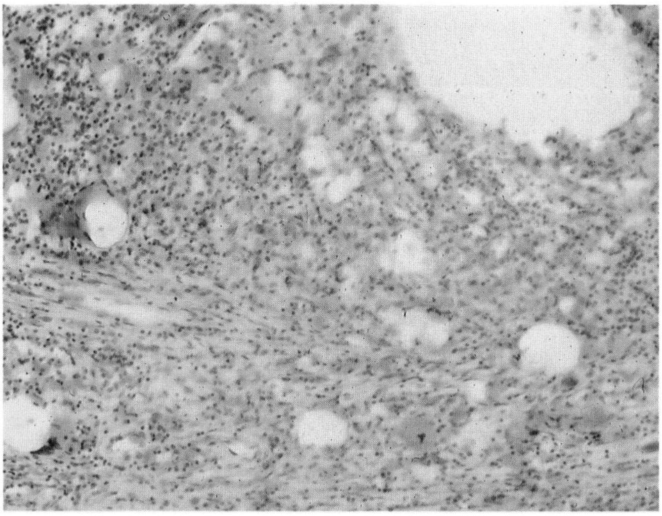

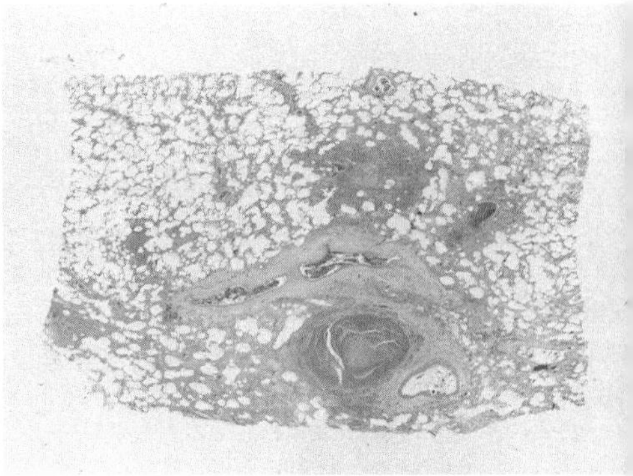

461 Bronchopneumonia. Note pus in a branch bronchus and inflammatory nodular infiltration of peribronchial tissues. Haematoxylin-eosin, × 2.

460 Lipid pneumonia due to aspiration of oily and fatty material, some of which is free-lying and some within macrophages. Oil red O, × 40.

462

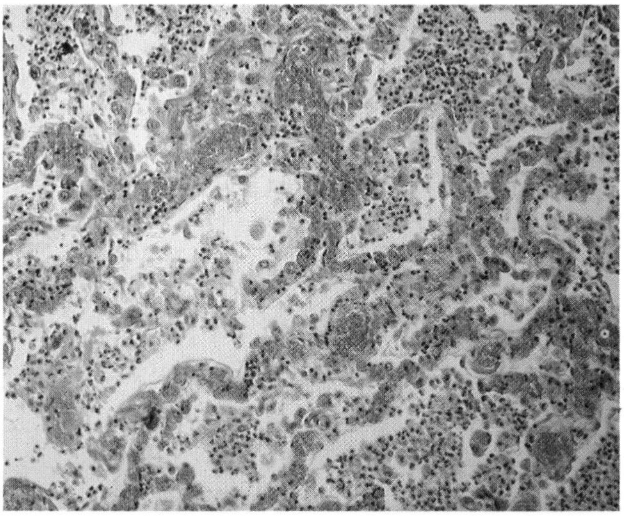

462 Bronchopneumonic infiltration of alveoli in lung with neutrophil polymorphonuclear leucocytes and fibrinous exudate. Haematoxylin-eosin, × 40.

463

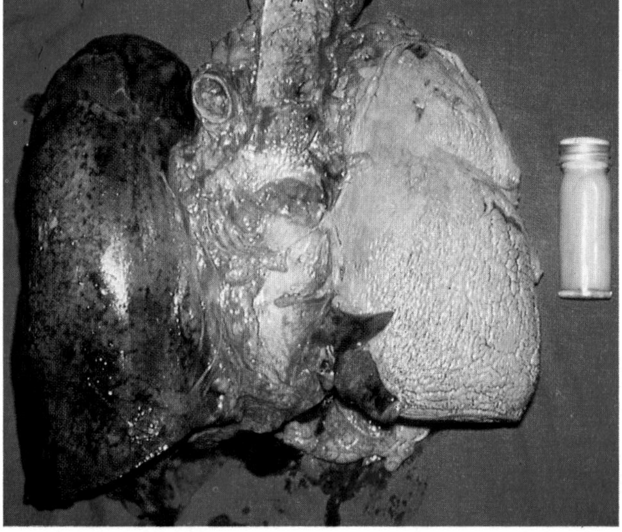

463 Staphylococcal fibrinopurulent empyema in a patient with multiple sclerosis.

464

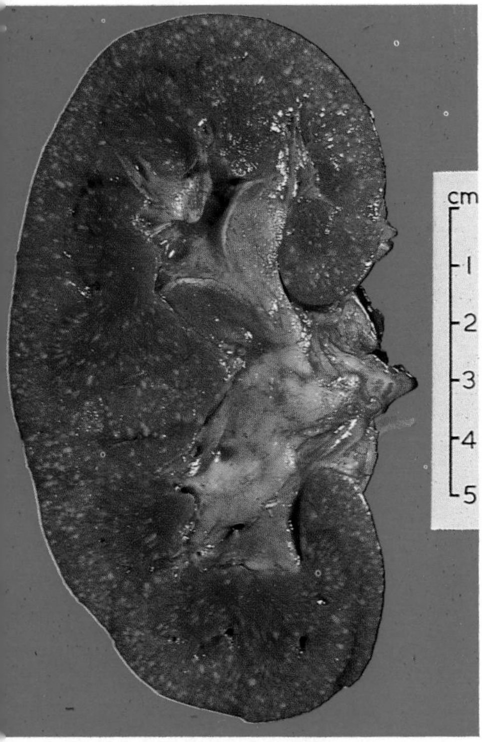

465

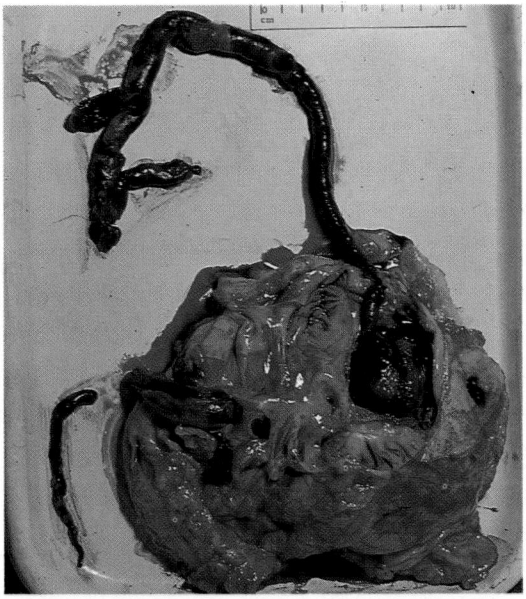

466

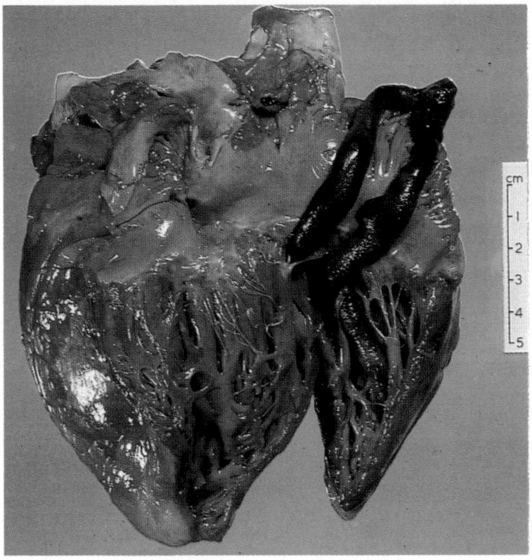

;4 Septicaemic kidney in MS. Note multiple
nall abscesses scattered over cortex and
edulla.

;5 Thromboembolism of heart. A
rombus of the saphenous vein is lodged in
e right atrium of the heart and in the
ılmonary artery.

;6 Thrombotic embolus from leg veins
ntangled in the tricuspid valve.

467

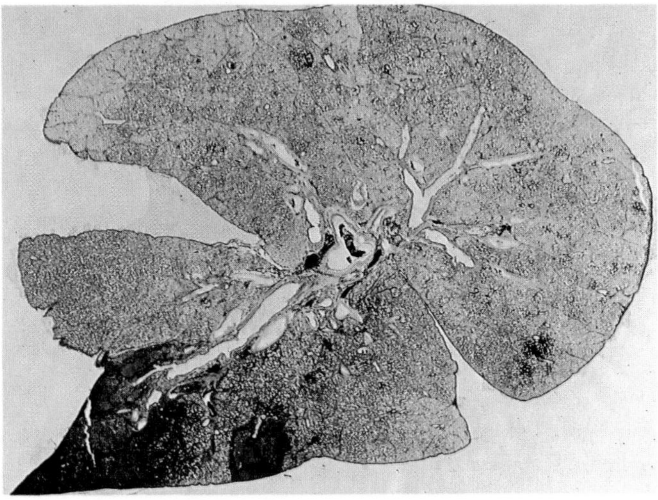

67 Lobular pulmonary infarction from
mall emboli lodged in branch pulmonary
eins. Perl's ferrocyanide, × 1/10.

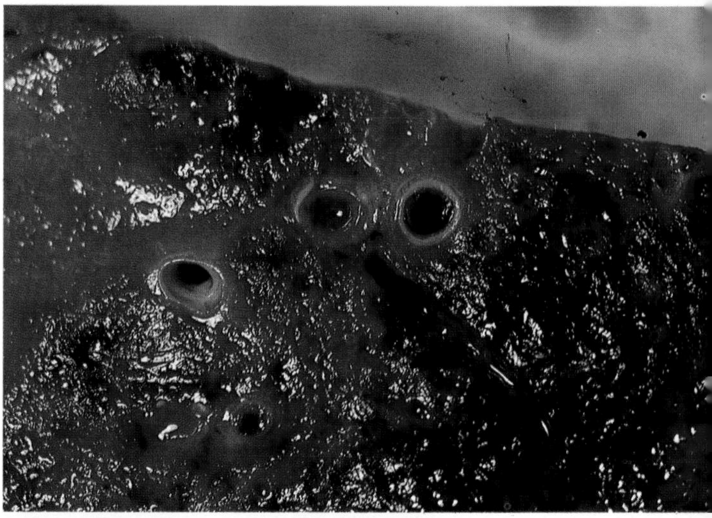

468 Red pulmonary infarction with thrombotic embolus in pulmonary artery (arrow) at centre.

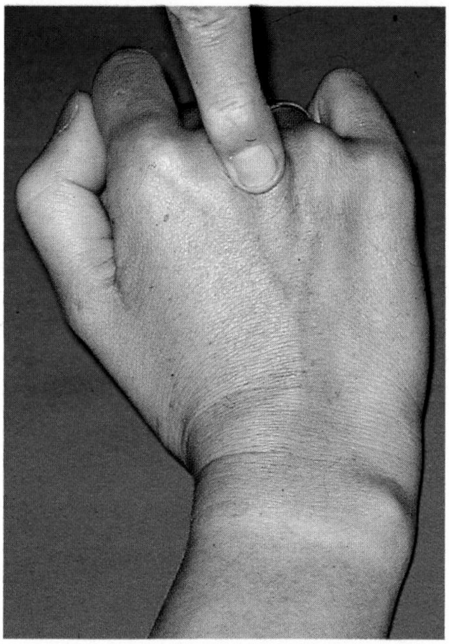

469

469 Flexion extension contractures caused by muscular spasticity in a patient with chronic multiple sclerosis.

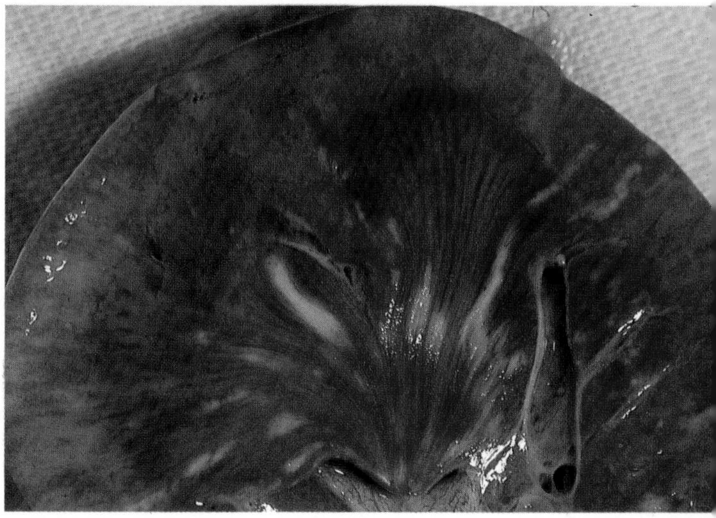

470 Acute purulent pyelonephritis. Note streaks of pus in the cortex, medulla and pyramid.

471

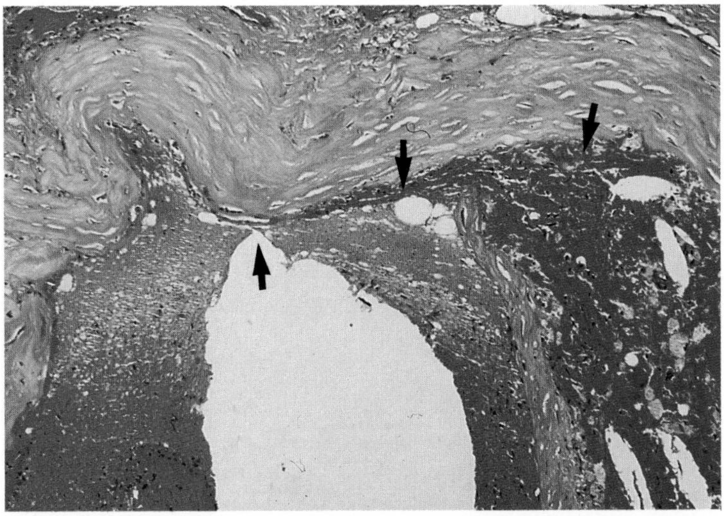

71 Coronary thrombosis, with racked intima (arrow) and subintimal aemorrhage (arrows). Cracking of the timal lining is thought to be an nportant predisposing cause of oronary thrombosis. Haemotoxylin-osin, × 40.

472

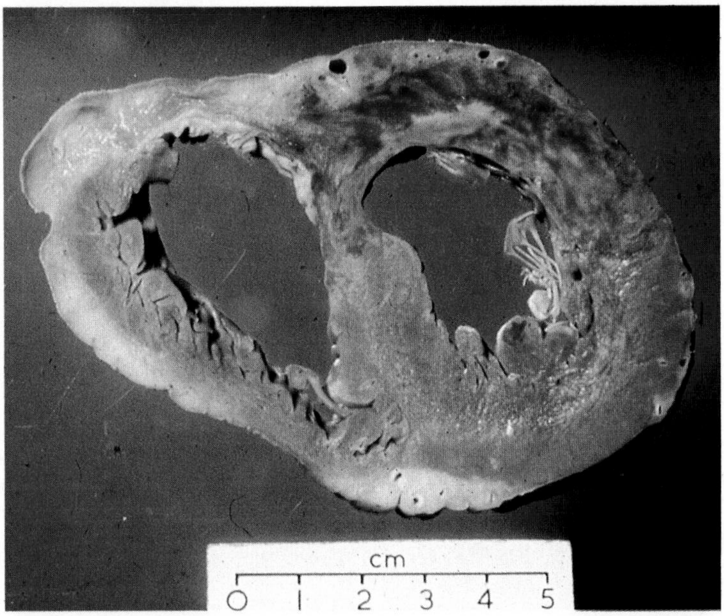

72 Recent infarction of posterior art of left ventricle (haemorrhagic), lder infarction of posterior right entricle (grey white). Thrombosis of osterior descending branch of right oronary artery, × ⅔.

473

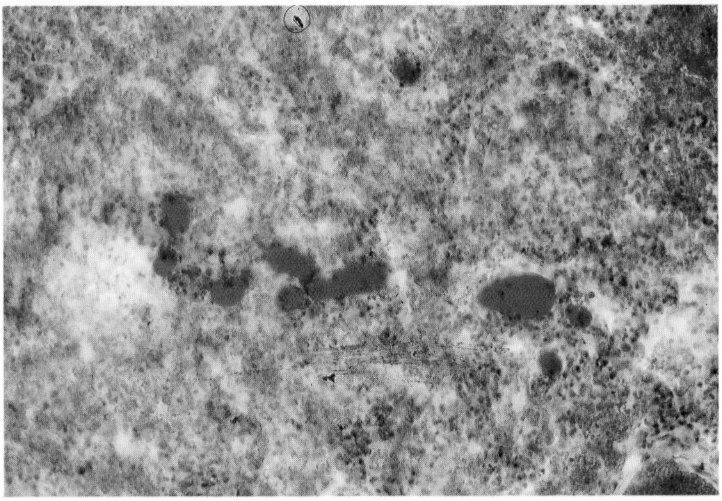

73 Fat embolus filling small ulmonary artery. Oil red O-aematoxylin, × 100.

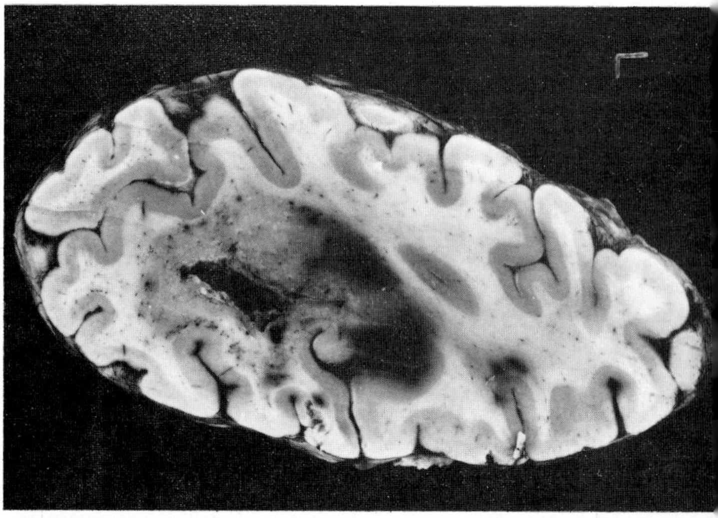

474 Glioblastoma multiforme complicating a case of multiple sclerosis, × ½.

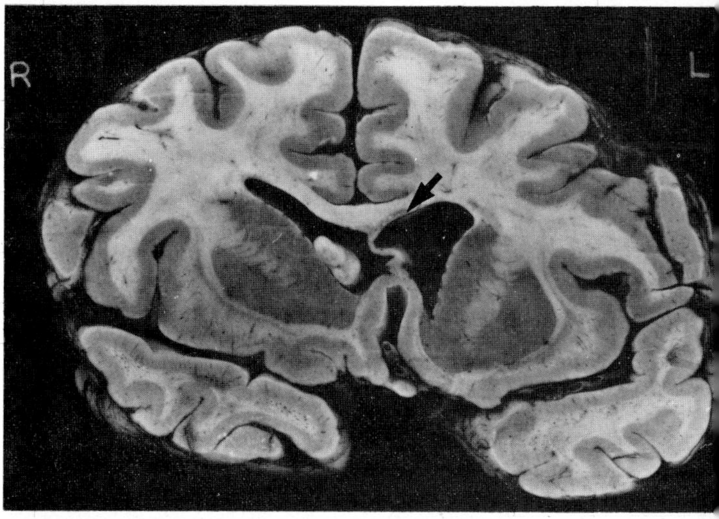

475 Ependymoma in right lateral ventricle in the same case as **474**. Note plaque of multiple sclerosis in left corpus callosum (arrow), × ½.

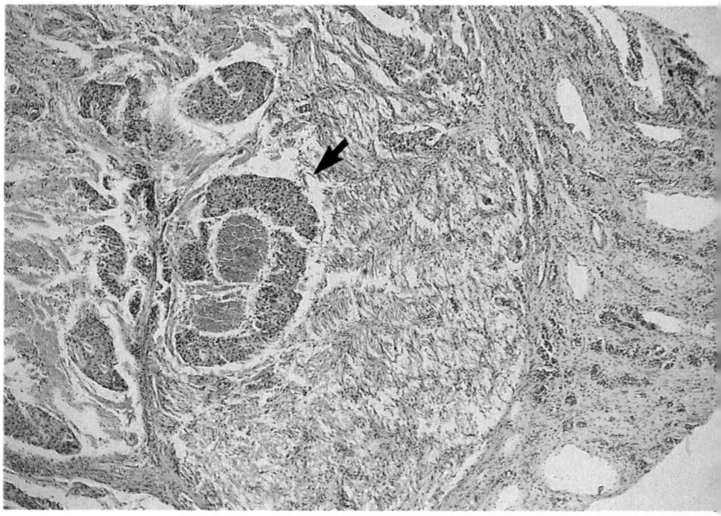

476 Metastic carcinoma (arrow) of breast in neurohypophysis (pituitary stalk) of a patient with multiple sclerosis. Haematoxylin-eosin, × 30.

References

Abramsky O., Lisak R.P., Silberberg G.H. and Pleasure D.E. 1977. Antibodies to oligodendroglia in patients with multiple sclerosis. *New Engl. J. Med.*, **297**, 1207-1208.

Acheson E.D. 1972. Part I. *Epidemiology*. In *Multiple Sclerosis: A reappraisal* by D. McAlpine, C.F. Lumsden and E.D. Acheson, Churchill Livingstone, pp 3-80.

Acheson E.D. 1977. Epidemiology of multiple sclerosis. *Brit. Med. Bull.*, **33**, 9-14.

Acheson E.D., Bachrach C.A. and Wright F.M. 1960. In Studies in Multiple Sclerosis III. *Acta Psychol. Neurol.*, Scand. Suppl. **147**, 132-147.

Adams C.W.M. 1958. Histochemical mechanisms of the Marchi reaction for degenerating myelin. *J. Neurochem.*, **2**, 178-186.

Adams C.W.M. 1959. A histochemical method for the simultaneous demonstration of normal and degenerating myelin. *J. Pathol. Bacteriol.*, **77**, 648-656.

Adams C.W.M. 1960. A perchloric acid-naphthoquinone method for the histochemical localization of cholesterol. *Nature*, **192**, 331-332.

Adams C.W.M. 1962a. The histochemisty of the myelin sheath. In *Neurochemistry*, ed. by K.A.C. Elliott, H. Page and J.H. Quastel, Thomas, Springfield, III., pp 85-112.

Adams C.W.M. 1962b. Histochemical aspects of myelination and demyelination. *Develop. Med. Child Neurol.*, **4**, 393-404.

Adams C.W.M. 1965. *Neurohistochemistry*. Elsevier, Amsterdam.

Adams C.W.M. 1968. The histochemistry of proteolytic enzymes and lipoproteins in the normal and diseased nervous system. In *Macromolecules and the Function of the Neurone*, ed. by Z. Lodin and S.P. Rose, Excerpta Medica, Amsterdam, pp 111-120.

Adams C.W.M. 1969. The general pathology of demyelinating diseases. In *The Structure and Function of Nervous Tissue*, ed. by G.W. Bourne, Academic Press, New York, pp 309-382.

Adams C.W.M. 1972. *Research on Multiple Sclerosis.* C.C. Thomas, Springfield, Ill.

Adams C.W.M. 1975. The onset and progression of the lesion in multiple sclerosis. *J. Neurol. Sci.*, **25**, 165-182.

Adams C.W.M. 1977. The pathology of the acute lesion in multiple sclerosis. *Brit. Med. Bull.*, **33**, 15-20.

Adams C.W.M. 1980. The pathology of the active lesion. In *Proceedings of the Göttingen Conference on Multiple Sclerosis* (ed. by H.J. Bauer, S. Poser and G. Ritter). Springer-Verlag, Berlin, pp 348-351.

Adams C.W.M. 1983. The general pathology of multiple sclerosis. In *Multiple Sclerosis*, ed. by J.F. Hallpike, C.W.M. Adams and W.W. Tourtellotte, Chapman and Hall, London, pp 203-240.

Adams C.W.M. 1988. Perivascular iron deposition and other vascular damage in multiple sclerosis. *J. Neurol. Neurosurg. Psychiat.*, **50**, 260-265.

Adams C.W.M. and Bayliss O.B. 1961. Histochemistry of myelin III. Peripheral nerve cathepsin. *J. Histochem. Cytochem.*, **9**, 473-476.

Adams C.W.M. and Bayliss O.B. 1975. Lipid Histochemistry. In *Techniques of Biochemical and Biophysical Morphology*, ed. by D. Glick and R. Rasenbaum, John Wiley, Baltimore, vol. 2, pp 99-156.

Adams C.W.M. and Davison A.N. 1959. The occurrence of esterified cholesterol in the developing nervous system. *J. Neurochem.*, **4**, 282-289.

Adams C.W.M. and Davison A.N. 1960. The form in which cholesterol occurs in the adult CNS. *J. Neurochem.*, **5**, 293-296.

Adams C.W.M. and Glenner G.G. 1962. Histochemistry of myelin IV. Aminopeptidase activity in CNS & PNS. *J. Neurochem.*, **9**, 233-239.

Adams C.W.M. and High O.B. 1982. Embolism and multiple sclerosis (letter). *Lancet*, **i**, 621.

Adams C.W.M. and Leibowitz S. 1969. The general pathology of demyelinating diseases. In *Structure and Function of Nervous Tissue*, Academic Press, New York, ed. by G. Bourne. vol. 3, pp 309-382.

Adams C.W.M. and Tuqan N.A. 1961. Histochemistry of myelin. II. Proteins, lipid-protein dissociation and proteinase activity in Wallerian degeneration. *J. Neurochem.*, **6**, 334-341.

Adams C.W.M., Csejtey J., Hallpike J.F. and Bayliss O.B. 1972. Histochemistry of myelin. XV. Changes in the myelin proteins of the peripheral nerve undergoing Wallerian degeneration – electrophoretic and microdensitometric observations. *J. Neurochem.*, **19**, 2043-2048.

Adams C.W.M., Bayliss O.B. and Turner D.R. 1975. Phagocytes, lipid-removal and regression of atheroma. *J. Pathol.*, **116**, 225-238.

Adams C.W.M., Poston R.N., Buk S.J., Sidhu Y.S. and Vipond H. 1985. Inflammatory vasculitis in multiple sclerosis. *J. Neurol. Sci.*, **69**, 269-283.

Adams C.W.M., Abdulla Y.H., Torres E.M. and Poston R.N. 1987. Periventricular plaques in multiple sclerosis: their perivenous origin and relationship to granular ependymitis. *Neuropath. Appl. Neurobiol.*, **13**, 141-152.

Adams C.W.M., Poston R.N. and Buk S.J. 1989. The pathology, histochemistry and immunocytochemistry of the lesions in 20 acute cases of multiple sclerosis. To be published.

Adams J.M. and Imagawa O.T. 1962. Measles antibodies in multiple sclerosis. *Proc. Soc. Exp. Biol. Med.*, **111**, 562-566.

Adams R.D. and Kubik C.S. 1952. The morbid anatomy of the demyelinative diseases. *Amer. J. Med.*, **12**, 510-546.

Adams R.D. and Richardson E.P., Jr. 1961. The demyelinative diseases of the human nervous system. A classification; a review of salient neuropathologic findings; comments on recent biochemical studies. In *Chemical Pathology of the Nervous System.* Ed. by Folch-Pi, J. Pergamon Press, New York, pp 162-196.

Adams R.D., Victor M. and Mancall E.L. 1959. Central pontine myelinoclasis. *Arch. Neurol. Psychiat.*, (Chicago) **81**, 154-172.

Alcolado R., Weller R. O., Parrish E. P. and Garrod D. 1988. The cranial arachnoid and pia mater in man: anatomical and ultrastructural observations. *Neuropathol. Appl. Neurobiol.*, **14**, 1-17.

Al Din H.S. 1986. Multiple sclerosis in Kuwait: Clinical and epidemiological study. *J. Neurol. Neurosurg. Psychiat.*, **44**, 928-931.

Alema G., and Bignami A. 1966. Involvement of the nervous system in Behcet's disease. In *Behcet's Disease*, ed. by M. Monacela and P. Nazzaro. Karger, Basel, pp 52-66.

Aleu F.P., Katzman R. and Terry R.D. 1963. Fine structure and electrolyte analyses of cerebral oedema induced by alkyltin intoxication. *J. Neuropath. Exp. Neurol.*, **22**, 403-413.

Alexander W.S. 1949. Progressive fibrinoid degeneration of fibrillary astrocytes associated with mental retardation in a hydrocephalic infant. *Brain*, **72**, 373-381.

Allen I.V. 1981. The pathology of multiple sclerosis. *Neuropath. Appl. Neurobiol.*, **7**, 169-182.

Allen I.V. and McKeown S.R. 1979. A histological histochemical and biochemical study of macroscopically normal white matter in multiple sclerosis. *J. Neurol. Sci.*, **42**, 81-91.

Allen, I.V., Millar J.H.D. and Hutchinson M.J. 1978. General disease in 120 necropsy-proven cases of multiple sclerosis. *J. Neuropath. Exp. Neurol.*, **4**, 279-284.

Allen I.V., Glover G., McKeown S.R. and McCormick D. 1979a. The cellular localization of enzymes in the plaque in multiple sclerosis. II. A histochemical study with combined demonstration of myelin and acid phosphatase. *Neuropath. Appl. Neurobiol.*, **5**, 197-210.

Allen I.V., Miller J.H.D., Kirk J. and Shillington R.K.A. 1979b. Systemic lupus erythematosis clinically resembling multiple sclerosis. *J. Neurol. Neurosurg. Psychiat.*, **42**, 392-401.

Alter M., Kahana E. and Loewenson R. 1978. Migration and risk of multiple sclerosis. *Neurology*, **28**, 1089-1093.

Alter M., Berman M. and Kahana E. 1979. The year of the dog. *Neurology*, **29**, 1023-1026.

Anders K.A., Guerra W.F., Tomiyasu Y., Verity M.A. and Vinters H.V. 1986. The neuropathology of AIDS. *Amer. J. Pathol.*, **124**, 537-558.

Anderson C.A., Higgins R.J., Smith M.E. and Osburn B.I. 1987. Border disease. Virus induced decrease in thyroid hormone levels with associated hypomyelination. *Lab. Invest.*, **57**, 168-175.

Andreoli F., Maffei F., Tonon G.C. and Zibetti A. 1973. Significance of plasma lysolecithin in patients with multiple sclerosis. *J. Neurol. Neurosurg. Psychiat.*, **36**, 661-667.

Ansari K.A., Hendrickson H., Sinha A.A. and Rand A. 1975. Myelin basic protein in frozen and unfrozen bovine brain: a study of autolytic changes *in situ*. *J. Neurochem.*, **25**, 193-195.

Ansari K.A., Hendrickson H. and Rand A. 1976. Electrophoretic and morphologic studies on normal human white matter obtained at surgery with special reference to its basic protein component. *J. Neuropath. Exp. Neurol.*, **35**, 606-612.

Antel J., Bania M., Noronha A. and Neely S. 1986. Defective suppressor cell function mediated by T8+ cell lines from patients with progressive multiple sclerosis. *J. Immunol.*, **137**, 3436-3439.

Arnason B.G.W. 1983. Abnormalities of immunocyte function in multiple sclerosis. *Acta Neuropathol.* (Berlin), Suppl. **9**, 7-20.

Arnon R., Crisp E., Kelly R., Ellison G.W., Myers L.W. and Tourtellotte W.W. 1980. Antiganglioside antibodies in multiple sclerosis. *J. Neurol. Sci.*, **46**, 179-186.

Arstila A.U., Riekkinen P. J., Rinne U.K. and Laitinen L. 1973. Studies of the pathogenesis of multiple sclerosis. Participation of lysosomes in demyelination in the CNS white matter. *Europ. Neurol.*, **9**, 1-21.

Asbury A.K. and Johnson P.C. 1978. *Pathology of Peripheral Nerve.* W.B. Saunders, Philadelphia, Pa.

Austin J.H., Balasubramanian A.S., Pattabiraman T.N., Saraswathi S., Basu D.K. and Bachhawat B.K. 1963. A controlled study of enzymatic activities in three human disorders of glycolipid metabolsm. *J. Neurochem.*, **10**, 805-816.

Austin J.H. and Lehfeldt D. 1965. Studies in globoid (Krabbe) leucodystrophy III. Significance of experimentally-produced globoid-like elements in rat white matter and spleen. *J. Neuropath. Exp. Neurol.*, **24**, 265-289.

Axelsson R., Roytta M., Sourander P., Akesson H.O. and Andersen O. 1984. Hereditary diffuse leucoencephalopathy with spheroids. *Acta Psychiat. Scand.*, **69** Suppl. No.314.

Bach M.A., Phan-Dinh-Tuy F., Tournier E., Chatenoud L., Bach J.F., Martin C. and Degos J.D. 1980. Deficit of suppressor T cells in active multiple sclerosis. *Lancet*, **ii**, 1221-1223.

Baker R.W.R., Thompson R.H.S. and Zilkha K.J. 1966. Changes in the amounts of linoleic acid in the serum of patients with multiple sclerosis. *J. Neurol. Neurosurg. Psychiat.*, **29**, 95-98.

Bailey P. 1934. Peculiarities of the intracranial venous system and their clinical significance. *Arch. Neurol. Psychiat.*, **32**, 1105.

Balo J. 1928. Encephalitis periaxialis concentrica. *Arch. Neurol. Psychiat.*, **19**, 242-264.

Balo J. 1950. The dural venous sinuses. *Anat. Rec.*, **106**, 319-325.

Barlow R.M. 1963. Further observation on swayback I. Transitional pathology. *J. Comp. Pathol.*, **73**, 51-61.

Barlow R.M. 1963. Further observations on Swayback II. Histochemical localisation of cytochrome oxidase activity in the central nervous system. *J. Comp. Pathol.*, **73**, 61-67.

Barlow R.M. 1969. The foetal sheep: morphogenesis of the nervous system and the histochemical aspects of myelination. *J. Comp. Neurol.*, **135**, 249-262.

Barlow R.M., Purves D., Butler E.J. and MacIntyre I.J. Swayback in Southeast Scotland II. Clinical, pathological and biochemical aspects. *J. Comp. Pathol.*, **70**, 411-428.

Barlow R.M. and Dickinson A.G. 1965. On the pathology and histochemistry of the central nervous system in border disease of sheep. *Res. Vet. Sci.*, **6**, 230-237.

Barron K.D. and Bernsohn J. 1965. Brain esterases and phosphatases in multiple sclerosis. *Ann. N.Y. Acad. Sci.*, **122**, 369-399.

Barron K.D., Dentinger M.P. and Csiza C.K. 1980. Ultrastructural observations on myelin deficiency (md), a dysmyelinating mutant in the Wistar rat. In *Neurological Mutations Affecting Myelination*, ed. by N. Baumann, Inserm Symp. No. 14, Elsevier/N. Holland, Amsterdam, pp 99-106.

Bass N.H., Netsky M.G. and Young E. 1970. Effect of neonatal malnutrition on developing cerebrum. *Arch. Neurol.*, **23**, 303-313.

Batchelor J.R., Compston A. and McDonald W.I. 1978. The significance of the association between HLA and multiple sclerosis. *Brit. Med. Bull.*, **34**, 279-284.

Bates D., Fawcett P.R.W., Shaw D.A. and Weightman D. 1978. Polyunsaturated fatty acids in treatment of acute remitting multiple sclerosis. *Brit. Med. J.*, **ii**, 1390-1391.

Bateson M.C., Hopwood D. and MacGillivray J.B. 1979. Jejunal morphology in multiple sclerosis. *Lancet*, **i**, 1108-1110.

Baumann N. (ed) 1980. *Neurological Mutations Affecting Myelination.* Inserm Symposium No. 14 Elsevier, Amsterdam.

Bayliss O.B. and Adams C.W.M. 1971. Cellular lipid inclusions in the white matter in multiple sclerosis. *Nature*, **233**, 264-265.

Bellamy A. S., Calder V. L., Feldman M. and Davison A. N. 1985. The distribution of interleukin – 2 receptor bearing lymphocytes in multiple sclerosis: evidence for a key role of activated lymphocytes. *Clin. Exper. Immunol.*, **61**, 248-258.

Besson J.A.O., Glen A.I.M., Foreman E.I., MacDonald A., Smith F.W., Hutchison J.M.S., Mallard J.R. and Ashcroft G.W. 1981. Nuclear magnetic resonance observations in alcoholic cerebral disorder and the role of vasopressin. *Lancet*, **ii**, 923-924.

Benetato G., Gabrielescu E. and Boros I. 1965. The histochemistry of cerebral proteases in experimental allergic encephalitis. *Rev. Human. Physiol.*, **2**, 379-384.

Benjamins J.A. and Smith M.E. 1984. Metabolism of myelin. In *Myelin*, ed. by P. Morell, Plenum Press, New York, 2nd edit. pp 225-258.

Benveniste E.N. and Merill J.E. 1986 Stimulation of oligodendroglial proliferation and maturation by interleukin 2. *Nature*, **32**, 610-613.

Berlet H.H., Ilzenhofer H. and Schulz G. 1984. Cleavage of basic protein in myelin by neutral protease activity of human white matter and myelin. *J. Neurochem.*, **43**, 627-633.

Bignami A. and Eng L.F. 1973. Biochemical studies of myelin in Wallerian degeneration of rat optic nerve. *J. Neurochem.*, **20**, 165-173.

Bignami A. and Rolston H.J. 1969. The cellular reaction to Wallerian degeneration in the CNS of the cat. *Brain Res.*, **13**, 444-461.

Birley J.L. and Dudgeon L.S. 1921. A clinical and experimental contribution to the pathogenesis of disseminated sclerosis. *Brain*, **44**, 150-212.

Blakemore W.F. 1973. Demyelination in the superior cerebellar peduncle in the mouse induced by cuprizone. *J. Neurol. Sci.*, **20**, 63-70.

Blakemore W.F. 1977. Remyelination of CNS axons by Schwann cells transplanted from the sciatic nerve. *Nature*, **266**, 68-69.

Blakemore W.F. 1978. Observations on remyelination in the rabbit spinal cord following demyelination induced by lysolecithin. *Neuropath. Appl. Neurobiol.*, **4**, 47-59.

Blakemore W.F., Crang A.J. and Evans R.J. 1983. The effect of chemical injury on oligodendrocytes. In *Viruses and Demyelinating Diseases*, ed. by C.A. Mims, M.L. Cuzner and R.E. Kelly. Academic Press, London, pp 167-190.

Boehme D.H., Umezawa H., Hashim G. and Marks N. 1978. Treatment of experimental allergic encephalomyelitis with an inhibitor of cathepsin D (Pepstatin). *Neurochem. Res.*, **3**, 185-194.

Boon A.P. and Potter A.E. 1987. Extensive extra pontine and central pontine myelinoclasis associated with correction of hyponatraemia. *Neuropath. Appl. Neurobiol.*, **13**, 1-9.

Booss J., Esiri M.M., Tourtellotte W.W. and Mason D.Y. 1983. Immunohistological analysis of T lymphocyte subsets in the CNS in chronic progressive multiple sclerosis. *J. Neurol. Sci.*, **62**, 219-232.

Bottaro D., Shepro D. and Hechtman H.B. 1986. Heterogeneity of intimal and microvessel endothelial cell barriers in vitro. *Microvasc. Res.*, **32**, 389-398.

Bowle J. 1982. *History of Europe*, Pan Books, London, pp 188-194.

Brady R.O. and Barranger J.A. 1981. Inborn lysomal enzyme deficiencies. In *The Molecular Basis of Neuropathology*, ed. by A.N. Davison and R.H. S. Thompson Arnold, London. pp 182-220.

Brady R.O., Gal A.E., Bradley R.M, Martensson E., Warchow A.L. and Laster L. 1967. Enzymatic defect in Fabry's disease: ceramide trihexosidase deficiency. *New Eng. J. Med.*, **276**, 1163-1167.

Broman T. 1947. Supravital analyses of disorders in cerebral vascular permeability; 2 cases of multiple sclerosis. *Acta psychiat. Scand.*, Suppl. **46**. 58-71.

Broman T. 1964. Blood-brain-barrier damage in multiple sclerosis. Supravital test observations. *Acta Neurologica Scand.*, **40**, Suppl. 10, 21-24.

Brosnan C.F., Cammer W., Norton W.T. and Bloom B.R. 1980. Proteinase inhibitors suppress the development of experimental allergic encephalomyelitis. *Nature*, **285**, 235-237.

Brostoff S. 1984. Immunological response to myelin and myelin components. In *Myelin*, ed. by P. Morell, Plenum Press, New York, 2nd edit., pp 405-439.

Bunge R.P. 1968. Glial cells and the central myelin sheath. *Physiological Reviews*, **48**, 197-251.

Bunge M.B., Bunge R.P. and Pappas G.D. 1962. Electron microscopic demonstration of connections between glia and myelin sheaths in the developing mammalian CNS. *J. Cell Biol.*, **12**, 448-453.

Bunge M.B., Bunge R.P. and Ris H. 1961. Ultrastructural study of remyelination in an experimental lesion in adult cat spinal cord. *J. Biochem. Biophys. Cytol*, **10**, 67-94.

Bunnell D.H., Visscher B.R. and Detels R. 1979. Multiple sclerosis and house dogs: a case control study. *Neurology*, **29**, 1027-1029.

Cammer W., Bloom B.R., Norton W.T. and Gordon S. 1978. Degradation of basic protein by neutral proteases secreted by stimulated macrophages: a possible mechanism of inflammatory demyelination. *Proc. Natl. Acad. Sci.*, **75**, 1154-1158.

Cammer W., Brosnan C.F., Bloom B.R. and Norton W.T. 1981. Degradation of Po, P_1 and Pr proteins in peripheral nervous system by plasmin: Implications regarding the role of macrophages in demyelinating diseases. *J. Neurochem.*, **36**, 1506-1514.

Campbell A.M.G., Danid P., Porter R.J., Russell W.R., Smith H.V. and Innes J.R.M. 1947. Disease of the nervous system occurring among research workers on swayback in lambs. *Brain*, **70**, 50-58.

Cancilla P.A. and Barlow R.M. 1968. An electronmicroscope study of the spinal cord in border disease of lambs. *Res. Vet. Sci.*, **9**, 88-90.

Carroll W.M., Jennings A.R. and Mastaglia F.L. 1985. Galactocerebroside antiserum causes demyelination of cat optic nerve. *Brain Res.*, **330**, 378-381.

Caspary E.A., Prineas J., Miller H. and Field E.J. 1965. Platelet stickiness in multiple sclerosis. *Lancet*, **ii**, 1108-1109.

Cervós-Navarro J. and Roggendorf W. 1983. Pathological changes in the vessel wall of intracerebral venules: an ultrastructural study. In *The Cerebral Veins. An Experimental and Clinical Update*, ed. by L.M. Auer and F. Heppner, Springer Verlag, Wien, pp 47-55.

Charcot J.M. 1868. Histologie de la sclerose en plaques. *Gazette des Hopitaux civils et militaires* (Paris), **41**, 554-566.

Charcot J.M. 1877. *Lectures on the Diseases of the Nervous System*, 1st series, transl. by G Sigerson, New Sydenham Society, London.

Chou B.H. 1986. Myelin-forming oligodendrocytes of developing mouse spinal cord: immunocytochemical and ultrastructural studies. *J. Neuropath. Exp. Neurol.*, **45**, 513-524.

Chou S.M. 1982. Acute haemorrhagic leucoencephalitis as vasculomyelinopathy (Abst.). *J. Neuropath. Exp. Neurol.*, **41**, 357.

Clayton P., Smith I., Harding B., Hyland K., Leonard J.V. and Leeming R.J. 1986. Subacute combined degeneration of the cord, dementia and Parkinsonism due to an inborn error of folate metabolism. *J. Neurol. Neurosurg. Psychiat.*, **49**, 920-927.

Cloys D.E. and Netsky M.G. 1970. Neuromyelitis optica. In *Handbook of Clinical Neurology*, ed. by P.J. Vinken and G.W. Bruyn, North Holland/Elsevier, Amsterdam, vol. 9, pp 426-435.

Collier J.R. 1967. Effect of diphtheria toxin on protein synthesis. *J. Molecul. Biol.*, **25**, 83-98.

Colover J. 1980. A new pattern of spinal-cord demyelination in guinea pigs with acute EAE mimicking multiple sclerosis. *Brit. J. Exp. Path.*, **61**, 390-400.

COMA Report (DHSS) 1984. *Diet and Cardiovascular Disease:* Report of the Panel on Diet in Relation to Cardiovascular Disease, HMSO, London.

Compston D.A.S., Vakaretis, B.N., Paul E., McDonald, W.I., Batchelor J.R. and Mims C.A. 1986. Viral infection in patients with multiple sclerosis and HLA-DR matched controls. *Brain*, **109**, 325-344.

Cone W. 1928. Acute pathologic changes in neuroglia and microglia. *Arch. Neurol. Psychiat. (Chicago)*, **20**, 34-68.

Connor J.R. and Fine R.E. 1987. Development of transferrin-positive oligodendrocytes in the rat central nervous system. *J. Neurosci. Res.*, **17**, 51-59.

Cook S.D., Natelson B.H., Levin B.E., Chavis P.S. and Dowling P.C. 1978a. House dogs and multiple sclerosis. *Annals of Neurology*, **3**, 141-143.

Cook S.D., Dowling P.C. and Russell W.C. 1978b. Multiple sclerosis and canine distemper. *Lancet*, **i**, 605-606.

Cook S. D., Cromarty J. I., Tapp W., Poskanzer D., Walker J. D. and Dowling P. C. 1985. Declining incidence of MS in the Orkney Islands. *Neurology*, **35**, 545-551.

Cook R.D., Flower R.L.P. and Dutton N.S. 1986. Light and electron microscopical studies of the immuno-peroxidase staining of multiple sclerosis plaques using antisera to a feline-derived agent and to galactocerebroside. *Neuropath. Appl. Neurobiol.*, **12**, 63-79.

Courville C. B. 1970. Concentric sclerosis. *Handbook of Clinical Neurology*, **9**, 437-451.

Coyle P. K. 1987. Detection and isolation of immune complexes in multiple sclerosis CSF *J. Neuroimmunol.*, **15**, 97-107.

Craelius W., Migdal M.W., Luessenhop C.P., Sugar A. and Mihalakis I. 1982. Iron deposits surrounding multiple sclerosis plaques. *Arch. Pathol.*, **106**, 397-399.

Cumings J.N. 1955. Lipid chemistry of the brain in demyelinating diseases. *Brain*, 78, 554-563.

Cummings J.F., Summers B.A., de Lahunta A. and Lawson C. 1986. Tremors in Samoyed pups with oligodendrocyte deficiencies and hypomyelination. *Acta Neuropathol.*, **71**, 267-277.

Currier R.D. and Eldridge R. 1982. Possible risk factors in multiple sclerosis as found in a national twin study. *Arch Neurol.*, **39**, 140-144.

Cuzner M.L. and Davison A.N. 1973. Changes in cerebral lysosome enzyme activity and lipids in multiple sclerosis. *J. Neurol. Sci.*, **19**, 29-36.

Cuzner M.L., Davison A.N. and Rudge P. 1978. Proteolytic enzyme activity of blood leucocytes and cerebrospinal fluid in multiple sclerosis. *Ann. Neurol.*, **4**, 337-344.

Dalal K. B., Valcana T., Timiras P. S. and Einstein E. R. 1971. Regulatory role of thyroxine on myelinogenesis in the developing rat brain. *Neurobiology*, **1**, 211-224.

Dal Canto M.C. and Barbano R.L. 1984. Remyelination during remission in Theiler's virus infection. *Amer. J. Pathol.*, **116**, 30-45.

Dal Canto M.C. and Lipton H.L. 1975. Primary demyelination in Theiler's virus infection – an ultrastructural study. *J. Lab. Invest.*, 626-637.

Dal Canto M.C. and Lipton H.L. 1977. Multiple sclerosis: animal model: Theiler's virus infection in mice. *Amer. J. Pathol.*, **88**, 497-500.

Dal Canto M.C. and Lipton H.L. 1980. Schwann cell remyelination. *Amer. J. Pathol.*, **98**, 101-122.

Dal Canto M.C., Wisniewski H.M., Johnson A.G., Brostoff S.W. and Raine C.S. 1975. Vesicular disruption of myelin in autoimmune demyelination. *J. Neurol. Sci.*, **24**, 313-319.

Dalgleish A.G., Fazakerley J.K. and Webb H.E. 1987. Do human T-lymphotrophic viruses (HTLV's) and other enveloped viruses induce autoimmunity in multiple sclerosis? *Neuropath. Appl. Neurobiol.*, **13**, 241-250.

Darriett D., Cassagne C. and Bourre J.M. 1978. Sciatic nerve contains alkanes: comparison between normal mice and neurological mutants – Jimpy, Quaking and Trembler. *J. Neurochem.*, **31**, 1541-1543.

Dastur D.K. and Singhal B.S. 1973. Two unusual neuropathologically proven cases of multiple sclerosis from Bombay. *J. Neurol. Sci.*, **20**, 397-414.

Davison A.N., Dobbing J., Morgan R.S. and Payling Wright G. 1959. Metabolism of myelin: the persistence of (4-14C) cholesterol in the mammalian central nervous system. *Lancet*, **i**, 658-660.

Dawson J.W. 1916a. The histology of disseminated sclerosis. *Trans. Roy. Soc. Edin.*, **50**, 517-725.

Dawson J.W. 1916b. The histology of disseminated sclerosis. Part II Histological study. *Edin. Med.J.*, NS**17**, 311-344.

Dawson J.W. 1916c. The histology of disseminated sclerosis. Part III Pathogenesis and Etiology: a critical discussion. *Edin. Med. J.*, NS**17**, 377-410.

Dawson R.M.C. and Richter D. 1950. Phosphorus metabolism in brain. *Proc. Roy. Soc.*, B. **137**, 253-267.

Day A.J. 1964. The macrophage system, lipid metabolism and atherosclerosis. *J. Atheroscler. Res.*, **4**, 117-130.

Dayan A.D. 1969. Subacute sclerosing panencephalitis: measles encephalitis of temperate evolution? *Postgrad. Med. J.*, **45**, 401-405.

Dean G. 1970. The multiple sclerosis problem. *Scientific American*, **223**, 40-46.

Dean G., McDougall E. I. and Elian M. 1985. Multiple sclerosis in research workers studying swayback in lambs – an updated report. *J. Neurol. Neurosurg. Psychiat.*, **48**, 859-865.

De Graaf J., Minderhoud J.M. and Teelken A.W. 1986. T-lymphocyte sub populations in peripheral blood of patients with multiple sclerosis, and patients with other neurological diseases. *Clin. Neurol. Neurosurg.*, **88**, 181-187.

De Rossi A., Gallo P., Tavolato B., Callegaro L. and Chieco-Banchi L. 1986. Search for HTLV-1 and LAV/HTLV-III antibodies in serum and CSF of multiple sclerosis patients. *Acta Neurol. Scand.*, **74**, 161-164.

Dick G., McAllister J.J., McKeown F. and Campbell A.M. 1965. Multiple sclerosis and scrapie. *J. Neurol. Neurosurg. Psychiat.*, **28**, 560-562.

Dickinson A.G. and Barlow R.M. 1967. The demonstration of the transmissibility of Border disease of sheep. *Vet Rec.*, **81**, 114-119.

Dipaolo R., Kanfer J.N. and Newberne P.M. 1974. Copper deficiency and the CNS: myelination in the rat. Morphological and biochemical studies. *J. Neuropath. Exp. Neurol.*, **33**, 226-236.

Dobbing J. 1968. Vulnerable periods in developing brain. In *Applied Neurochemistry*, ed. by A.N. Davison and J. Dobbing, Blackwell, Oxford, pp 287-316.

Done J.T. 1976. Developmental disorders of the nervous system in animals. *Adv. Vet. Sci. Comp. Med.*, 20, 69-113.

Dore-Duffy P., Donaldson J.O., Koff T., Longo M. and Perry W. 1986. Prostaglandin release in multiple sclerosis: correlation with disease activity. *Neurology*, **36**, 1587-1590.

Dow R.S. and Bergland G. 1942. Vascular pattern of lesions of multiple sclerosis. *Arch. Neurol. Psychiat.*, **47**, 1-18.

Dragenescu S., Petrescu A. and Anghelescu N. 1961. Histochemical investigations on lipid phagocytes in demyelinating lesions. *Proc. VII Internat. Congr. Neurology*, edited by G. Alema, Rome, pp 780-790.

Drayer B. P., Burger P., Hurwitz B., Dawson D., Cain J., Leong J., Herfkens R. and Johnson G. A. 1987. Magnetic resonance imaging in multiple sclerosis: decreased signal in the thalamus and putamen. *Annals of Neurology*, **22**, 546-550.

Duchen L.W., Eicher E.M., Jacobs J.M., Scaravilli F. and Teixera F. 1980. A globoid cell type of leucodystrophy in the mouse: the mutant twitcher. In *Neurological Mutations Affecting Myelination*, ed. by N. Baumann, Inserm Symp. No.14, Elsevier/N. Holland, Amsterdam, pp 107-114.

Duncan I.D., Hammang J.P. and Trapp B.D. 1987. Abnormal compact myelin in the myelin deficient rat: absence of proteolipid protein correlates with a defect in the intraperiod line. *Proc. Nat. Acad. Sci.*, **84**, 6287-6291.

Dupouey P., Zalc B., Lefroit-Joly M. and Gomes D. 1979. Localization of galactosylceramide and sulfatide of the surface of the myelin sheath. An immunofluorescence study in liquid medium. *Cell Molecul. Biol.*, **25**, 269-272.

Dyck P.J., Ellefson R.D., Lais A.C., Smith R.C., Taylor W.F. and Van Dyke R.A. 1970. Lipid abnormality in Dejerine-Sottas disease. *Mayo Clinic Proc.*, **45**, 286-327.

Dyck P.J., Lais A.C. and Offord K.P. 1974. The nature of myelinated nerve fibre degeneration in dominantly inherited hypertrophic neuropathy. *Mayo Clinic Proc.*, **49**, 34-39.

Einstein E.R. 1982. *Proteins of the Brain and CSF in Health and Disease.* C.C. Thomas, Springfield, Ill., pp 210-212.

Einstein E.R. and Adams C.W.M. 1988. Myelination: normal and abnormal. In *Handbook of Human Growth and Developmental Biology*, ed. by P.S. Timiras and E. Meisami. Vol. 1, Part A, in press.

Einstein E.R., Csejtey J. and Marks N. 1968. Degradation of encephalitogen by purified brain protease. *FEBS Letters* (Amsterdam), **1**, 191-195.

Einstein E.R., Dalal K.B. and Csejtey J. 1970. Increased protease activity and changes in basic proteins and lipids in multiple sclerosis plaques. *J. Neurol. Sci.*, **11**, 109-121.

Einstein E.R., Csejtey J., Dalal K.B., Adams C.W.M., Bayliss O.B. and Hallpike J.F. 1972. Proteolytic activity and basic protein loss in and around multiple sclerosis plaques – combined biochemical and histochemical observations. *J. Neurochem.*, **19**, 653-662.

Elian M. and Dean G. 1987. Multiple sclerosis among the United-Kingdom-born children of immigrants from the West Indies. *J. Neurol. Neurosurg. Psychiat.*, **50**, 327-332.

Engell T. 1986. Neurological disease activity in multiple sclerosis – patients with periphlebitis retinae. *Acta Neurol. Scand.*, **73**, 168-172.

Engell T. and Andersen P.K. 1982. The frequency of periphlebitis retinae in multiple sclerosis. *Acta Neurol. Scand.*, **65**, 601-608.

Engell T., Hvidberg A. and Uhrenholdt A. 1984. Multiple sclerosis: periphlebitis retinalis et cerebro-spinalis. *Acta Neurol. Scand.*, **69**, 293-297.

Engell T., Krogsaa B. and Lund-Andersen H. 1986. Breakdown of blood-retinal barrier in multiple sclerosis measured by vitreous fluorophotometry. *Acta Ophthalmol.* (Copenhagen), **64**, 583-587.

Esiri M.M. 1977. Immunoglobulin-containing cells in multiple sclerosis plaques. *Lancet*, **ii**, 478-479.

Esiri M.M. 1980. Multiple sclerosis: a quantitative and qualitative study of immunoglobulin-containing cells in the central nervous system. *Neuropathol. Appl. Neurobiol.* **6**, 9-21.

Esiri M.M. and McGee J. 1986. Monoclonal antibody to macrophages (EBM11) labels macrophages and microglial cells in human brain. *J. Clin. Pathol.*, **39**, 615-621.

Esiri M. M. and Reading M. C. 1987. Macrophage populations associated with multiple sclerosis plaques. *Neuropathol. Appl. Neurobiol.*, **13**, 451-465.

Feigin I. and Popoff N. 1966. Regeneration of myelin in multiple sclerosis: the role of mesenchymal cells in such regeneration and in myelin formation in the peripheral nervous system. *Neurology*, **16**, 364-372.

Feigin I. and Budzilovich G.N. 1980. The influence of the ground substance on the extra cellular water of normal and oedematous human brain: focal oedema and the demyelinating diseases, including multiple sclerosis. *J. Neuropath. Exp. Neurol.*, **39**, 13-21.

Field E.J. 1967. The significance of astroglial hypertrophy in scrapie, Kuru, multiple sclerosis and old age, together with a note on the possible nature of the scrapie agent. *Deutsche Zeit. Nervenheilkunde*, **192**, 265-274.

Finean J.B. 1957. The molecular structure of nerve myelin and its significance in relation to the nerve membrane. In *Metabolism of the Nervous System*, ed. by D. Richter, Pergamon Press, Oxford, pp 52-57.

Fisher M., Johnson M.H., Natale A.M. and Levine P.H. 1987. Linoleic acid levels in white blood cells, platelets and serum of multiple sclerosis patients. *Acta Neurol. Scand.*, **76**, 241-245.

Fog T. 1964. Vessel plaque relations, and cerebrospinal fluid and brain tissue changes in multiple sclerosis. *Acta Neurol. Scand.*, **40**, Suppl. 10, 9-15.

Fog T. 1965. The topography of plaques in multiple sclerosis with special reference to cerebral plaques. *Acta Neurol. Scand.*, **41**, Suppl. 15, 3-161.

Fontana A., Fierz W. and Wekerle H. 1984. Astrocytes present myelin basic protein to encephalitogenic T-cell lines. *Nature*, **307**, 273-276.

Forrester C. and Lascelles R.G. 1979. Association between polyneuritis and multiple sclerosis. *J. Neurol. Neurosurg. Psychiat.*, **42**, 864-866.

'orssman H., Kristensson K., Sourander P. and vennerholm L. 1967. Histological and chemical studies of case of phenylketonuria with long survival. *J. Ment. Defic. es.*, **11**, 195-206.

'rancis D.A., Compston D.A.S., Batchelor J.R. and IcDonald W.I., 1987. A reassessment of the risk of ıultiple sclerosis developing in patients with optic neuritis fter extended follow up. *J. Neurol. Neurosurg. Psychiat.*, **50**, 58-765.

'rederikson S., Link H. and Eneroth P. 1987. CSF eopterin as marker of disease activity in multiple sclerosis. *cta Neurol. Scand.*, **75**, 352-355.

'rick E. 1982. Cell mediated cytotoxicity by peripheral mphocytes against myelin basic protein. *J. Neurol. Sci.*, **7**, 55-56.

'riede R.L. 1961. Enzyme histochemical studies in ıultiple sclerosis. *Arch, Neurol.*, **5**, 433-443.

'riede R.L. 1964. Alexander's disease. *Arch. Neurol.*, **11**, 14-422.

'riede R. L. 1965. Enzyme histochemistry of neuroglia. *rogr. Brain Res.*, **15**, 35-47.

ɔabrielescu E. 1978. Neuroproteazele. Editura Academiei epublicii Socialiste Romania, Bucharest, Romania.

ɔadjusek D.C. 1967. Slow virus infections of the nervous ystem. *New Engl. J. Med.*, **276**, 392-400.

ɔallai-Hatchard J., Magee W.L., Thompson R.H.S. and Vebster G.R. 1962. The formation of lysophosphatides om diacyl phosphatides by brain preparations. *. Neurochem.*, **9**, 545-554.

ɔalli C., Kneebone G.M. and Paoletti R. 1969. An inborn rror of cerebroside biosynthesis as the molecular defect of ie Jimpy mouse brain. *Life Sci.*, **8**, 911-918.

ɔanser A.L. and Kirschner D.A. 1980. Myelin structure ı the absence of basic protein in the Shiverer mouse. ı *Neurological Mutations Affecting Myelination*, ed. by I. Baumann, Inserm Symposium 14, Elsevier/North Iolland, Amsterdam, pp 171-176.

ɔay D. and Dick G. 1986. Is MS caused by an oral pirochaete? *Lancet*, **ii**, 75-77.

ɔay D., Dick G. and Upton G. 1986. Multiple sclerosis ssociated with sinusitis. *Lancet*, **i**, 815-819.

ɔhatak N.R., Hirano A., Doron Y. and Zimmerman H.M. 973. Remyelination in multiple sclerosis with peripheral ype myelin. *Arch. Neurol. Psychiat.*, (Chicago) **29**, 262-267.

ɔilliatt R.W. 1975. Peripheral nerve compression and ntrapment. In *Eleventh Symposium on Advanced Medicine*, d. by A.F. Lant, Pitman Medical, London, pp 144-164.

ɔinalski H., Friede R.L., Cohen S.R. and Matthieu J.M. 980. Myelination in the MLD mouse: a neuro-athological and biochemical study. In *Neurological Iutations Affecting Myelination*, ed. by N. Baumann, Inserm ymposium No.14, Elsevier/North Holland, Amsterdam, p 147-152.

ɔoldstick L., Mandybur T.I. and Bode R. 1985. Spinal ord degeneration in AIDS. *Neurology*, **35**, 103-106.

Gonzales-Scarano F., Grossman R.I., Galetta S., Atlas S.W. and Silberberg D.H. 1987. Multiple sclerosis disease activity correlates with gadolinium-enhanced magnetic resonance imaging. *Annals Neurol.*, **21**, 300-306.

Goust M.J., Chenais F., Carnes J.E., Haines C.G., Fudenberg H.H. and Hogan E.L. 1978. Abnormal T-cell populations and circulating immune complexes in the Guillain-Barré syndrome and multiple sclerosis. *Neurology*, **28**, 421-425.

Govindarajan K.R., Rauch H., Clausen J. and Einstein E.R. 1974. Changes in cathepsins B-1 and D, neutral proteinase and 2′, 3′-cyclic nucleotide-3′-phosphohydrolase activities in monkey brain with experimental allergic encephalomyelitis. *J. Neurol. Sci.*, **23**, 295-306.

Graham D.I., Behan P.O. and More I.A.R. 1979. Acute haemorrhagic leucoencephalitis as a complication of the generalised Schwartzman reaction. *J. Neurol. Neurosurg. Psychiat.*, **42**, 19-28.

Gray F., Destee A., Bourre J-M., Gherardi R., Krivosic I., Warot P. and Poirier J. 1987. Pigmentary type of orthochromatic leukodystrophy (OLD): A new case with ultrastructural and biochemical study (Abst.). *J. Neuropathol. Exp. Neurol.*, **46**, 585-596.

Greenfield J.G. 1939. The histology of cerebral oedema associated with intracranial tumours. *Brain*, **62**, 129-155.

Gregson N.A. and Hall S.M. 1973. A quantitative analysis of the effects of the intraneural injection of lysophosphatidyl choline. *J. Cell Sci.*, **13**, 257-277.

Gregson N.A. and Leibowitz S. 1985. IgM paraproteinaemia, polyneuropathy and myelin associated glycoprotein (MAG). *Neuropathol. Appl. Neurobiol.*, **11**, 329-347.

Griffiths I.R., McCulloch M.C. and Abrahams S. 1987. Progressive axonopathy: an inherited neuropathy of Boxer dogs. 4. Myelin sheath and Schwann cell changes in the nerve roots. *J. Neurocytol.*, **16**, 145-153.

Guenet J.L. 1980. Mutants of the mouse with an abnormal myelination: a review for geneticists. In *Neurological Mutations Affecting Myelination*, ed. by N. Baumann, Inserm Symposium 14, Elsevier-North Holland, Amsterdam, pp 11-21.

Guseo A. and Jellinger A. 1975. The significance of perivascular infiltrations in multiple sclerosis. *J. Neurol.*, **211**, 51-60.

Haase A.T., Ventura P., Gibbs C.J. Jr. and Tourtellotte W.W. 1981. Measles virus nucleotide sequences: detection by hybridization in situ. *Science*, **212**, 672-675.

Hall S.M. and Williams P.L. 1970. Studies on the 'incisures' of Schmidt and Lanterman. *J. Cell Sci.*, **6**, 767-791.

Hall S. M. 1988. Lysophosphatidyl choline: its effects in the nervous system. In: *Monographs on Pathology of Laboratory Animals*, ed. by T. C. Jones. Springer-Verlag, Berlin. In press.

Hallpike J.F. 1972. Enzyme and protein changes in myelin

breakdown and multiple sclerosis. *Prog. Histochem. Cytochem.*, 3, 179-215.

Hallpike J.F. 1983. Clincial aspects of multiple sclerosis. In *Multiple Sclerosis*, ed. by J.F. Hallpike, C.W.M. Adams and W.W. Tourtellotte, Chapman & Hall, London, 1st edition, pp 129-161.

Hallpike J. F. 1988. Is there anything new for multiple sclerosis? *Current Therapeutics*, in press.

Hallpike J.F. and Adams C.W.M. 1969. Proteolysis and myelin breakdown – a review of recent histochemical and biochemical studies. *Histochem. J.*, **1**, 559-578.

Hallpike J.F., Adams C.W.M. and Bayliss O.B. 1970a. Histochemistry of myelin X. Proteolysis of normal myelin and release of lipid by extracts of degenerating nerve. *Histochem. J.*, **2**, 315-321.

Hallpike J.F., Adams C.W.M. and Bayliss O.B. 1970b. Histochemistry of myelin IX. Neutral and acid proteinases in early Wallerian degeneration. *Histochem. J.*, **2**, 209-218.

Hallpike J.F., Adams C.W.M. and Bayliss O.B. 1970c. Histochemistry of Myelin VIII. Proteolytic activity around multiple sclerosis plaques. *Histochem. J.*, **2**, 199-200.

Hammond S. R., de Wytt C., Maxwell I. C., Landy P. J., English D., McLeod J. G. and McCall, M. G. 1987. The epidemiology of multiple sclerosis in Queensland, Australia. *J. Neurol. Sci.*, **80**, 185-204.

Harrison B.M. 1983. Remyelination in the central nervous system. In *Multiple Sclerosis*, ed. by J.E. Hallpike, C.W.M. Adams and W.W. Tourtellotte, Chapman & Hall, London, pp 461-478.

Harrison B.M. and McDonald W.I. 1977. Remyelination after transient compression of the spinal cord. *Ann. Neurol.*, **1**, 542-551.

Harrison B.M., McDonald W.I. and Ochoa J. 1972. Central demyelination produced by diphtheria toxin. An electron microscope study. *J. Neurol. Sci.*, **17**, 281-291.

Hartman B.K., Agrawal H.C., Kalmbach S. and Shearer W.T. 1979. A comparative study of the immunohistochemical localisation of basic protein to myelin and oligodendrocytes in rat and chicken brain. *J. Comp. Neurol.*, **188**, 273-290.

Hauser S.L., Bhan A.K., Gilles F., Kemp M., Kerr C. and Weiner H.L. 1986. Immunohistochemical analysis of the cellular infiltrate in multiple sclerosis lesions. *Ann. Neurol.*, **19**, 578-587.

Hayashi H., Fukuda Y. and Kuwabara N. 1982. Pathological studies on neuro-Behcet's disease with special reference to leucocytic reaction. In *Behcet's Disease, Pathogenetic Mechanism and Clinical Features*, ed. by G. Inaba, University of Tokyo Press, pp 197-211.

Hayes G.M., Woodroofe M.N. and Cuzner M.L. 1987. Microglia are the major cell type expressing MHC Class II in human white matter. *J. Neurol. Sci.*, **80**, 25-37.

Heider W. and Gottlob I. 1987. A differential diagnostic test for optic neuritis. *Klin. Monat. Augenheilkd.*, **190**, 420-423.

Herndon R.M., Rubinstein L.J., Freeman J.M. and Mathieson G. 1970. Light and electron microscopic observations on Rosenthal fibres in Alexander's disease and in multiple sclerosis. *J. Neuropathol. Exp. Neurol.*, **29**, 524-551.

Herndon R.M., Price D.L. and Weiner L.P. 1977. Regeneration of oligodendroglia during recovering from demyelinating disease. *Science*, **195**, 643-644.

Hirsch H.E. and Parks M.E. 1975. Acid proteinases and other acid hydrolases in experimental allergic encephalomyelitis pinpointing the source. *J. Neurochem.*, **24**, 853-858.

Hirsch H.E., Duquette P. and Parks M.E. 1976. The quantitative histochemistry of multiple sclerosis plaques: acid proteinase and other acid hydrolases. *J. Neurochem.*, **26**, 505-512.

Hirsch H.E., Blanco C.E. and Parks M.E. 1981. Fibrinolytic activity of plaques and white matter in multiple sclerosis. *J. Neuropathol. Exp. Neurol.*, **40**, 271-280.

Hogan E.L. 1977. Animal models of genetic disorders of myelin. In *Myelin*, ed. by P. Morell, Plenum Press, New York, first edition, pp 489-520.

Hogan E.L. and Greenfield S. 1984. Animal models of genetic disorders of myelin. In *Myelin*, ed. by P. Morell, Plenum Press, New York, 2nd edition, pp 489-534.

Hortega P. Del Rio 1930. Concepts histogenique, morphologique et physio-pathologigue de la microglie. *Rev Neurol*, **37**, 956-986.

Howell J. McC. 1971. Disease affecting myelination in domestic animals. In *Myelination*, ed. by A.N. Davison and A. Peters, *Thomas, Springfield*, pp 199-226.

Howell J. McC. and Davison A.N. 1959. The copper content and cytochrome oxidase activity of tissues from normal and swayback lambs. *Biochem. J.*, **72**, 365-368.

Howell J. McC. and Palmer, A.C. 1971. Globoid cell leucodystrophy in two dogs. *J. Small Anim. Pract.*, **12**, 633-642.

Howell J. McC., Davison A.N. and Oxberry, J. 1964. Biochemical and neuropathological changes in swayback. *Res. Vet. Sci.*, **5**, 376-384.

Howell J. McC., Pass D.A. and Terlecki S. 1981. In Proceedings IVth Internat. Symposium on *Trace Element Metabolism in Man and Animals*, eds. J. McC. Howell, J.M. Gawthorne and C.L. White. *Austral. Acad. Science, Canberra*, pp 298-301.

Hughes R.A.C. 1985. Demyelinating Neuropathy. In *Handbook of Clinical Neurology*, ed. by P.J. Vinken, G.W. Bruyn and H.L. Klawans, Elsevier, Amsterdam, **vol.3**, 605-627.

Hughes R.A.C. and Mair W.G.P. 1977. Acute necrotic myelopathy with pulmonary tuberculosis. *Brain*, **100**, 223-228.

Hughes R.A.C., Russell W.C., Froude J.R.L. and Jarrett R.J. 1980. Pet ownership, distemper antibodies and multiple sclerosis. *J. Neurol. Sci.*, **47**, 429-432.

Hulberg B. and Olsson J-E. 1979. Lysosomal hydrolases in CSF of patients with multiple sclerosis. *Acta Neurol. Scand.*

59, 23-30.

Huszák I. 1972. Biochemical aspects of multiple sclerosis. In *Handbook of Neurochemistry*, ed. by A. Lajtha, Plenum Press, New York, pp 47-91.

Hutchings M. and Weller R.O. 1986. Anatomical relationship of the pia mater to cerebral blood vessels in man. *J. Neurosurg.*, **65**, 316-325.

Ibrahim M.Z.M. 1974. The mast cells of the mammalian CNS. Part 1: Morphology distribution and histochemistry. *J. Neurol. Sci.*, **21**, 431-478,

Ibrahim M.Z.M. and Adams C.W.M. 1963. The relationship between enzyme activity and neuroglia in plaques of multiple sclerosis. *J. Neurol. Neurosurg. Psychiat.*, **26**, 101-110.

Ibrahim M.Z.M. and Adams C.W.M. 1965. The relationship between enzyme activity and neuroglia in early plaques of multiple sclerosis. *J. Pathol. Bacteriol.*, **90**, 239-243.

Ibrahim M.Z.M. and Levine S. 1967. Effect of cyanide intoxication on the metachromatic material found in the CNS. *J. Neurol. Neurosurg. Psychiat.*, **30**, 545-555.

Ibrahim M.Z.M., Briscoe P.B. Jnr., Bayliss O.B. and Adams, C.W.M. 1963. The relationship between enzyme activity and neuroglia in the prodromal and demyelinating stages of cyanide encephalopathy in the rat. *J. Neurol. Neurosurg. Psychiat.*, **26**, 479-486.

Ibrahim M.Z.M., Morgan R.S. and Adams C.W.M. 1965. Histochemistry of the neuroglia and myelin in experimental cerebral oedema. *J. Neurol. Neurosurg. Psychiat.*, **28**, 91-98.

Innes J.R.M. and Shearer G.D. 1940. Swayback. A demyelinating disease of lambs with affinities to Schilder's disease in man. *J. Comp. Pathol.*, **53**, 1-42.

Inozuka T., Sato S., Baba H. and Miyatake T. 1987. Neutral protease in CSF from patients with multiple sclerosis and other neurological disease. *Acta Neurol. Scand.*, **76**, 18-23.

Ironsides R., Bosanquet F.D. and McMenemy W.H. 1961. Central demyelination of the corpus callosum (Marchiafava-Bignami Disease) with a report of a second case in Great Britain. *Brain*, **84**, 212-230.

Itoyama Y., Sternberger N.H., Webster H. de F., Quarles R.H., Cohen S.R. and Richardson E.P. Jr. 1980. Immunocytochemical observations on the distribution of myelin-associated glycoprotein and myelin basic protein in multiple sclerosis lesions. *Ann. Neurol.* **7**, 167-177.

Itoyama Y., Ohnishi A., Tateishi J., Kuroiwa Y. and Webster H. de F. 1985. Spinal cord MS lesions in Japanese patients: Schwann cell remyelination occurs in areas that lack glial fibrillary acidic protein (GFAP). *Acta Neuropathol.*, **65**, 217-223.

Izquierdo G., Lyon-Caen O., Marteau R., Martinez-Parra F., Lhermitte F., Castaigne P. and Hauw J.J. 1986. Early onset multiple sclerosis. Clinical study of 12 pathologically proven cases. *Acta Neurol. Scand.*, **73**, 493-497.

Jablensky A., Janota I. and Shepherd M. 1970. Neuropsychiatric illness and neuropathological findings in a case of Klinefelter's syndrome. *Psychol. Med.*, **1**, 18-29.

Jacobs Jean M., Cavanagh J.B. and Mellick R.S. 1966. Intraneural injection of diphtheria toxin. *Brit. J. exp. Path.*, **47**, 507-517.

James P.B. 1982. Evidence for subacute fat embolism as the cause of multiple sclerosis. *Lancet*, **i**, 380-382.

Jankovic J., Derman H. and Armstrong D. 1980. Haemorrhagic complications of multiple sclerosis. *J. Neurol. Neurosurg. Psychiat.*, **43**, 76-81.

Janzer R.C. and Raff M.C. 1987. Astrocytes induced blood-brain barrier properties in endothelial cells. *Nature*, **325**, 253-267.

Jellinger K. 1969. Einege morphologische Aspekte der Multiplen Sklerose. *Wiener Zeitschrift für Nervenheil Kunde*, Suppl., **II**, 12-37.

Johnson R.T. 1983. Persistent viral infections and demyelinating disease: an overview. In *Viruses and Demyelinating Diseases*, ed. by C.A. Mims, M.L. Cuzner and R.E. Kelly. Academic Press, London, pp 7-19.

Jones P.E., Pallis C. and Peters T.J. 1979. Morphological and biochemical findings in jejunal biopsies from patients with multiple sclerosis. *J. Neurol. Neurosurg. Psychiat.*, **42**, 402-412.

Kabat E.A., Wolf A. and Bezer A.E. 1947. The rapid production of acute disseminated encephalomyelitis in rhesus monkeys by injection of heterologous and homologous brain tissue with adjuvants. *J. Exp. Med.*, **85**, 117-129.

Kato T. 1987. Neuropathology of acquired immune deficiency syndrome (AIDS) in 53 autopsy cases with particular emphasis on microglial nodules and multinucleated giant cells. *Acta Neuropathol.*, (Berlin), **73**, 241-214.

Kennedy P.G.E., Narayan O., Ghotbi Z., Hopkins J., Gendelman H.E. and Clements J.E. 1985. Persistent expression of Ia antigen and viral genome in visna-maedi virus-induced inflammatory cells. Possible roles of lentivirus-induced interferon. *J. Exp. Med.*, **162**, 970-982.

Khalili-Shirazi A., Gregson N.A. and Webb H.E. 1986. Immunological relationship between a demyelinating RNA enveloped budding virus (Semliki Forest) and brain glycolipids. *J. Neurol. Sci.*, **76**, 91-103.

Kinney H.C., Brody B.A., Kloman A.S. and Gilles F.H. 1988. Sequence of central nervous system myelination in human infancy II. Patterns of myelination in autopsied infants. *J. Neuropath. Exp. Neurol.*, **47**, 217-234.

Kirk J. 1979. The fine structure of the CNS in multiple sclerosis. II. Vesicular demyelination in an acute case. *Neuropath. Appl. Neurobiol.*, **5**, 289-294.

Kirschner D.A. and Ganser A.L. 1984. Diffraction studies of molecular organization and membrane interaction. In *Myelin*, ed. by P. Morell, Plenum Press, New York, 2nd edit. pp 51-95.

Knobler R.L. and Oldstone M.B.A. 1983. The role of host genes and virus cell tropism in coronavirus-induced demyelination. In *Viruses and Demyelinating Disease*, ed. by C.A.C. Mims, M.L. Cuzner and R.E. Kelly, Academic Press, London, pp 53-65.

Knobler R.L., Rodriguez M., Lampert P.W. and Oldstone M.B.A. 1983. Virologic models of chronic relapsing demyelinating disease. *Acta Neuropathol.*, (Berlin), Suppl., **9**, 31-37.

Koeppen A.H. and Barron K.D. 1978. Marchiafava-Bignami disease. *Neurology*, **28**, 290-294.

Koeppen A.H. Ronca N.A., Greenfield E.A. and Hans M.B. 1987. Defective biosynthesis of proteolipid protein in Pelizaeus-Merzbacher disease. *Annal. Neurol.*, **21**, 159-170.

Koeppen A.H., Barron K.D., Csiza C.K. and Greenfield E.A. 1988. Comparative immunocytochemistry of Pelizaeus-Merzbacher disease, the jimpy mouse, and the myelin-deficient rat. *J. Neurol. Sci.*, **84**, 315-327.

Komoly S., Jeyasingham M.D., Pratt O.E. and Lantos P.E. 1987. Decrease in oligodendrocyte carbonic anhydrase activity preceding myelin degeneration in cuprizone-induced demyelination. *J. Neurol. Sci.*, **79**, 141-148.

Krabbe K. 1916. A new familial infantile form of diffuse brain sclerosis. *Brain*, **39**, 74-114.

Krakowka S. and Koestner A. 1978. Canine distemper virus and multiple sclerosis. *Lancet*, **i**, 1127-1128.

Kretzschmar H.A., Berg B.O. and Davis R.L. 1987. Giant axonal neuropathy. *Acta Neuropathol.*, (Berlin), **73**, 138-144.

Kurihara T., Nussbaum J.L. and Mandel P. 1970. 2′3′ cyclic nucleotide 3′ phosphohydrolase in brains of mutant mice with deficient myelination. *J. Neurochem.*, **17**, 993-997.

Kuroda Y. and Shibasaki H. 1987. CSF mononuclear cell subsets in active MS. *Neurology*, **37**, 497-499.

Kurtzke J.F. 1983. Epidemiology of multiple sclerosis. In *Multiple Sclerosis*, ed. by J.F. Hallpike, C.W.M. Adams and W.W. Tourtellotte, Chapman & Hall, London, pp 47-95.

Kurtzke J.F. and Priester W.A. 1979. Dogs, distemper and MS in the US. *Acta Neurol. Scand.*, **60**, 312-319.

Lake B.D. 1984. Lysosomal enzyme deficiencies. In *Greenfield's Neuropathology*, ed. by J.H. Adams, J.A.N. Corsellis and L.W. Duchen, pp 491-572.

Lampert P.W. 1969. Mechanism of demyelination in experimental allergic neuritis. Electron microscopic studies. *Lab. Invest.*, **20**, 127-138.

Lampert P.W. 1983. Fine structure of the demyelinating process. In *Multiple Sclerosis*, ed. by J.F. Hallpike, C.W.M. Adams and W.W. Tourtellotte, Chapman & Hall, London, pp 19-46.

Lancet Annotation, 1987. Lyme disease in Europe (conference report). *Lancet*, **ii**, 264-265.

Langley O.K. and Landon D.N. 1968. A light and electron histochemical approach to the node of Ranvier and myelin of peripheral nerve fibres. *J. Histochem. Cytochem.*, **15**, 722-731.

Lassmann H. and Wisniewski H.M. 1978. Chronic relapsing EAE. Time course of neurological symptoms and pathology. *Acta Neuropathol.* (Berlin), **43**, 35-42.

Lassmann H., and Wisniewski H.M. 1979. Chronic relapsing experimental allergic encephalomyelitis – clinicopathological comparison with multiple sclerosis. *Arch. Neurol.*, **36**., 490-497.

Lassmann H., Budka H. and Schnaberth G. 1981. Inflammatory demyelinating polyradiculitis in a patient with multiple sclerosis. *Arch. Neurol.*, **38**, 99-102.

Laureno R., and Karp B.I. 1988. Pontine and extra pontine myelinolysis following rapid correction of hyponatraemia. *Lancet*, **i**, 1439-1441.

Lazorthes G. 1961. La circulation veineuse cerebrale. In *Vascularisation et Circulation Cerebrales*, Masson, Paris, pp 236-239.

Lees M.B. and Chan D.S. 1975. Proteolytic digestion of bovine brain white matter proteolipid. *J. Neurochem.*, **25**, 595-600.

Le Gros Clark W.E. 1940. A vascular mechanism related to the great vein of Galen. *Brit. Med. J.*, **i**, 476.

Lehmann W., Cho E-S., Nielsen S. and Petito C. 1985. Neuropathological findings in 104 cases of acquired immunodeficiency syndrome (AIDS): an autopsy study. *J. Neuropathol. Exp. Neurol.*, **44**, 349 (Abst).

Lehner T. and Adams C.W.M. 1968. Lipid histochemistry of Fabry's disease. *J. Pathol. Bacteriol.*, **95**, 411-415.

Leibowitz S. 1983. The Immunology of MS. In *Multiple Sclerosis*, ed. by J.F. Hallpike, C.W.M. Adams and W.W. Tourtellotte, Chapman & Hall, London, pp 379-412.

Leibowitz S. and Kennedy L. 1972. Cerebral vascular permeability and cellular infiltration in experimental allergic encephalomyelitis. *Immunology*, **22**, 859-869.

Leibowitz S., Morgan R.S, Berkinshaw-Smith E.M.I. and Payling Wright G. 1961. Cerebral vascular damage in guineapigs induced by various heterophil antisera injected by the Forsmann intracarotid technique. *Brit. J. Exp. Pathol.*, **42**, 455-463.

Lendrum A.C. 1963. The hypertensive kidney as a model of the so-called collagen diseases. *Canad. Med. Assoc. J.*, **88**, 442-452.

Lhermitte F., Escourolle R., Hauw J.J., Gray F., Sedaru M. and Lyon-Caen O. 1981. Les formes cavitaires de la sclerose en plaques et de la maladie de Schilder. *Rev. Neurol.*, **137**, 589-600.

Lightman S., McDonald W.I, Bird A.C., Francis D.A., Hoskins A., Batchelor J.R. and Halliday A.M. 1987. Retinal venous sheathing in optic neuritis: its significance for the pathogenesis of multiple sclerosis. *Brain*, **110**, 405-414.

Lindegard B. 1985. Diseases associated with multiple sclerosis and epilepsy. *Acta Neurol. Scand.*, **71**, 267-277.

Liversedge L.A. 1977. Treatment and management of multiple sclerosis. *Brit. Med. Bull.*, **33**., 78-83.

Lubínska L. 1963. Demyelination and remyelination in the

proximal parts of regenerating nerve fibres. *J. Comp. Neurol.*, **117**, 275-289.

Ludwin S.K. 1978. CNS demyelination and remyelination in the mouse. An ultrastructural study of cuprizone toxicity. *Lab. Invest.*, **39**, 597-612.

Ludwin S.K. 1979. The perineuronal satellite and oligodendrocyte. A role in remyelination. *Acta Neuropath.* (Berlin), **47**, 49-53.

Ludwin S.K. 1981. Demyelination and remyelination. In *Demyelinating Disease: Basic and Clinical Electrophysiology*, ed. by Waxman S.G. and Ritchie J.M., Raven Press, New York, pp 123-168.

Ludwin S.K. 1987. Remyelination in demyelinating diseases of the central nervous system. *Critical Rev. Neurobiol.*, **3**, 1-28.

Lumsden C.E. 1951. Fundamental problems in the pathology of multiple sclerosis and allied demyelinating diseases. *Brit. Med. J.*, **i**, 1035-1043.

Lumsden C.E. 1957. The problem of correlation of quantitative methods and tissue morphology in the CNS. The distribution of cholinesterases. In *Metabolism of the Nervous System*, ed. by D. Richter, Pergamon Press, London, pp 91-100.

Lumsden C.E. 1970. The pathology of multiple sclerosis. In *Handbook of Clinical Neurology*. ed. by P.J. Vinken and G.W. Bruyn, North-Holland, Amsterdam, vol.9, pp 217-309.

Lyon G. and Goffinet A. 1980. Genetics and pathology of dysmyelinating disorders of the central nervous system. In *Neurological Mutations Affecting Myelination*, ed. by N. Baumann, Inserm Symposium No. 14, Elsevier/North Holland, Amsterdam, pp 33-46.

Lyon-Caen O., Izquierdo G., Marteau R., Lhermitte F., Castaigne P. and Hauw J.J. 1985. Late onset multiple sclerosis. A clinical study of 16 pathologically proven cases. *Acta Neurol. Scand.*, **72**, 56-60.

McCallum K., Esiri M.M., Tourtellotte W.W. and Booss J. 1987. T-cell subsets in multiple sclerosis: gradients at plaque borders and differences in non-plaque regions. *Brain*, **110**, 1297-1308.

McCaman R.E. and Robins, E. 1959. Quantitative biochemical studies of Wallerian degeneration in the peripheral and central nervous system. Part 1. Chemical constituents. *J. Neurochem.*, **5**, 18-31.

Macchi G. 1954. The pathology of blood vessels in multiple sclerosis. *J. Neuropath. Exp. Neurol.*, **13**, 378-384.

McDonald, W.I. 1974. Remyelination and clinical lesions of the central nervous system. *Brit. Med. Bull.*, **30**, 186-189.

McKeown S.R. and Allen I.V. 1978. The cellular origin of lysosomal enzymes in the plaque in multiple sclerosis: a combined histological and biochemical study. *Neuropathol. Appl. Neurobiol.*, **4**, 471-482.

McKeown S.R. and Allen I.V. 1979. The fragility of cerebral lysosomes in multiple sclerosis. *Neuropathol. Appl. Neurobiol.*, **5**, 405-415.

McKhann G. 1982. Multiple Sclerosis. *Ann. Rev. Neurosci.*, **5**, 219-239.

McLardy, T. 1951. Case of Marchiafava's disease. Primary degeneration of the corpus callosum. *Proc. Roy. Soc. Med.*, **44**, 685-686.

Madden D.L., Wallen W.C., Houff S.A., Shekarchi I.C., Lenikki P.O., Castellano G.A., and Sever J.L. 1981. Measles and canine distemper antibody. Presence in sera from patients with multiple sclerosis and matched control subjects. *Arch. Neurol.*, **38**, 13-15.

Madrid, R.E. and Wisniewski H.M. 1977. Axonal degeneration in demyelinating disorders. *J. Neurocytol.*, **6**, 103-117.

Mandelbrote B.M., Stanier M.W., Thompson R.H.S. and Thruston M.N. 1948. Studies on copper metabolism in demyelinating disease of central nervous system. *Brain*, **71**, 212-218.

Mander A.J., Smith M.A., Kean D.M., Chick J., Douglas R.H.B., Rehman A.U., Weppner G.J. and Best J.J.K. 1985. Brain water measured in volunteers after alcohol and vasopressin. *Lancet*, **ii**, 1075.

Marchiafava E. and Bignami A. 1903. Sopra un'alterazione del corpo calloso osservata in soggetti alcoohisti. *Riv. Patol. Nerv. Ment.*, **8**, 544-549.

Marks N., Grynbaum A. and Benuck M. 1976. On the sequential cleavage of myelin basic protein by cathepsins A & D. *J. Neurochem.*, **27**, 765-768.

Marples E.A., Thompson R.H.S. and Webster, G.R. 1959. The liberation of active enzymes from brain tissue by lysolecithin. *J. Neurochem.*, **4**, 62-70.

Martin J.B. 1984. Neurological disease: of mice and men. *Nature*, **307**, 10.

Mastin-Mondiere C., Jacque C., Delasalle A., Cesaro P., Carydakis C. and Degos J.D. 1987. Cerebrospinal myelin basic protein in multiple sclerosis. Identification of two groups of patients with acute exacerbation. *Arch. Neurol.*, **44**, 276-278.

Matthews J.B. 1983. The immunoglobulin nature of Russell bodies. *Brit. J. Exp. Pathol.*, **64**, 331-335.

Medaer R. 1979. Does the history of MS go back as far as the 14th Century. *Acta Neurol. Scand.*, **60**, 189-192.

Mehl E. and Jatzkewitz H. 1965. Evidence for the genetic block in metachromatic leucodystrophy (ML). *Biochem. Biophys. Res. Comm.*, **19**, 407.

Meloff K. 1980. Multiple sclerosis and polyarteritis. *Arch. Neurol.*, **37**, 786 (letter).

Menton I.S., Dewar H.A. and Newell D.J. 1969. Fibrinolytic activity in venous blood in patients with multiple sclerosis. *Neurology*, **19**, 101-104.

Mertin J. and Meade C.J. 1977. Relevance of fatty acids in multiple sclerosis. *Brit. Med. Bull.*, **33**, 67-71.

Messert B., Orrison W.W., Hawkins M.J. and Quaglieri C.E. 1979. Central pontine myelinolysis. *Neurology*, **29**, 147-160.

Millar J.H.D., Zilkha K.J., Langman M.J.S., Payling

Wright H., Smith A.D., Belin J. and Thompson R.H.S. 1973. Double blind trial of linoleate supplementation of the diet in multiple sclerosis. *Brit. Med. J.*, **i**, 765-768.

Millar J.H.D., Zilkha K.J., Langman M.J.S., Wright, H.P., Smith A.B., Belin J. and Thompson R.H.S. 1975. Double blind trial of linoleate supplementation of the diet in multiple sclerosis. In *Multiple Sclerosis Research*, ed. by A.N. Davison, J.H. Humphrey, A.L. Liversedge, W.I. McDonald and J.S. Porterfield, HMSO, London, pp 218-225.

Miller D.H., Newton M.R., Rudge P. and Cruickshank K. 1987. Magnetic resonance imaging in HTLV-1 antibody positive patients. *Lancet*, **ii**, 514.

Miller R.F. and Semple S.J.G. 1987. Autonomic neuropathy in AIDS. *Lancet*, **ii**, 343-344.

Möller J.R., Yanagisawa K., Brady R.O., Tourtellotte W.W. and Quarles R.H. 1987. Myelin-associated glycoprotein in multiple sclerosis lesions. *Annals of Neurology*, **22**, 469-474.

Morariu M. and Klutzow W.F. 1976. Subclinical multiple sclerosis. *J Neurol.*, **213**, 71-76.

Morello D., Dantigny A., Pham-Dinh D. and Jolles P. 1986. Myelin proteolipid proteins (PLP and DM-20) transcripts are deleted in Jimpy mutant mice. *EMBO J.*, **5**, 3489-3493.

Morimoto C., Hafler D.A., Weiner H.L., Letvin N.L. Hagan M., Daley J., and Schlossman S.F. 1987. Selective loss of the suppressor-inducer T cell subset in progressive multiple sclerosis. *New Engl. J. Med.*, **316**, 67-72.

Moser H.W., Moser A.B., Frayer K.K., Chen W., Schulman J.D., O'Neill B. and Kishimoto Y. 1981. Adrenoleucodystrophy: increased plasma content of saturated very long chain fatty acids. *Neurology*, **31**, 1241-1249.

Moskowitz L.B., Hensley G.T., Chan J.C., Gregorios J. and Conley F.K. 1984. The neuropathology of the acquired immune deficiency syndrome. *Arch. Pathol.*, **108**, 867-872.

Moxon, W. 1875. Eight cases of insular sclerosis of the brain and spinal cord. *Guy's Hosp. Rep.*, **35**, 437-478.

Nagashima T., Yamada K., Uono M. and Nagashima K. 1984. Multiple sclerosis co-existent with myxedema – an autopsy report. *J. Neurol. Sci.*, **66**, 217-221.

Narayano S., Trandberg J.D., Griffin D.E., Clements J.E. and Adams R.J. 1983. Aspects of the pathogenesis of visna in sheep. In *Viruses and Demyelinating Diseases*, ed. by C.A. Mims, M.L. Cuzner and R.E. Kelly, Academic Press, London, pp 125-140.

Nathanson N., Georgsson G., Lutley R., Palsson P.A. and Petursson G. 1983. Pathogenesis of visna in Icelandic sheep. In *Viruses of Demyelinating Diseases*, ed. by C.A. Mims, M.L. Cuzner and R.E. Kelly, Academic Press, London, pp 111-124.

Nelson J.S., Filch C.D., Fischer V.W., Broun G.O. and Chou A.C. 1981. Progressive neuropathologic lesions in vitamin E-deficient Rhesus monkeys. *J. Neuropath. Exp. Neurol.*, **40**, 166-186.

Niebrój-Dobosz I., Fidzańska A., Rafalowska J. and Sawicka E. 1980. Correlative biochemical and morphological studies of myelination in human ontogenesis. *Acta Neuropathol.*, (Berlin), **49**, 145-152.

Nilsson O., Larsson E.M. and Holtås S. 1987. Myelopathy patients studied with magnetic resonance for multiple sclerosis plaques. *Acta Neurol. Scand.*, **76**, 272-277.

Norenberg M.D., Leslie K.O. and Robertson A.S. 1982. Association between rise in serum sodium and central pontine myelinoclasis. *Annal. Neurol.*, **11**, 128-135.

Norenberg M.D. and Papendick R.E. 1984. Chronicity of hyponatremia as a factor in experimental myelinolysis. *Annal. Neurol.*, **15**, 544-547.

Norton W.T. 1982. Biochemistry of myelin. In *Basic and Clinical Electrophysiology*, ed. by S.G. Waxman and J.M. Ritchie, Raven Press, New York, pp 93-121.

Norton, W.T. and Cammer W. 1984. Chemical pathology of diseases involving myelin. In *Myelin*, 2nd edit. ed. by P. Morell, Plenum Press, New York, pp 369-403.

Norton W.T. and Poduslo S.E. 1982. Biochemical studies of metachromatic leukodystrophy in three siblings. *Acta Neuropathol.*, (Berlin) **57**, 188-196.

Norton W.T., Cammer W., Bloom B.R. and Gordon S. 1978. Neutral proteinases secreted by macrophages degrade basic protein: a possible mechanism of inflammatory demyelination. In *Myelination and Demyelination*, ed. by J. Palo, Plenum Press, New York, pp 365-381.

Nussbaum J.L., Neskovic N. and Mandel P. 1969. A study of the lipid components in brain of the 'Jimpy' mouse, a mutant with myelin deficiency. *J. Neurochem.*, **16**, 927-934.

Ogata J. and Feigin I. 1975. Schwann cells and regenerated peripheral myelin in multiple sclerosis in an ultrastructural study. *Neurology*, **25**, 713-716.

Oliver M.F., Heady J.A., Morris J.N. and Cooper J. (Committee of Principal Investigators). 1978. A cooperative trial in the primary prevention of ischaemic heart disease using clofibrate. *Brit. Heart J.*, **40**, 1069-1118.

Olsson Y., Sourander P. and Svennerholm L. 1966. Experimental studies on the pathogenesis of leucodystrophies. I. The effect of intracerebrally injected sphingolipids in the rat's brain. *Acta Neuropathol., (Berlin)*, **6**, 153-163.

Olsson Y. 1968. Mast cells in the nervous system. *Internat. Rev. Cytol.*, **24**, 27-70.

Olsson Y. 1974. Mast cells in plaques of multiple sclerosis. *Acta Neurol.*, Scand. **50**, 611-618.

Ormerod I.E.C., Miller D.H., McDonald W.I. et al., 1987. The role of NMR imaging in the assessment of multiple sclerosis and isolated neurological lesions. *Brain*, **110**, 1579-1616.

Padget D.H. 1956. The cranial venous system in man in reference to development, adult configuration, and relation to the arteries. *Amer. J. Anat.*, **98**, 307-355.

Parsons C.L. 1983. The bladder in multiple sclerosis. In *Multiple Sclerosis*, ed. by J.F. Hallpike, C.W.M. Adams and W.W. Tourtellotte, Chapman & Hall, London, 1st edition, pp 579-602.

Partridge S.M. 1969. Elastin, biosynthesis and structure. *Gerontologia*, **15**, 85-100.

Pearce W.J, and Bevan J.A. 1983. Influence of sympathetic extra cranial veno constriction on canine cerebral veins, sigmoid sinus, and mean arterial pressures. In *The Cerebral Veins. An Experimental and Clinical Update*, ed. by L.M. Auer and F. Heppner, Springer-Verlag, Wien, pp 239-247.

Perry V.H., Brown M.C. and Gordon S. 1987. The macrophage response to central and peripheral nerve injury. A possible role for macrophages in regeneration. *J. Exp. Med.*, **165**, 1218-1223.

Peters A. and Vaughan J.E. 1970. Morphology and development of the myelin sheath. In *Myelination*, ed. by A.N. Davison and A. Peters, C.C. Thomas, Springfield, Ill., pp 3-79.

Petito C.K., Navia B.A., Cho E-S., Jordan B.D., George D.C. and Price R.W. 1985. Vacuolar myelopathy resembling subacute combined degeneration in patients with the acquired immune deficiency syndrome. *New Eng. J. Med.*, **312**, 875-879.

Petito C.K., Cho E-S., Lemann W., Navia B.A. and Price R.W. 1986, Neuropathology of AIDS: an autopsy review. *J. Neuropathol. Exp. Neurol.*, **45**, 635-646.

Petrescu A. 1966. Contributions histochimiques a l'etude des lipides dans les lesions demyelinisantes. *Ann. Histochim.*, **11**, 237-252.

Petrescu A. 1969. Histochemical identification of two types of lysomacrophages in demyelinating lesions of sudanphilic type. *Rev. Roum. Neurol.*, **6**, 165-168.

Petrescu A. 1981. Progressive oil-spot-like lesion in multiple sclerosis. *Acta Neuropathol.*, (Berlin), Suppl. **VII**, 182-184.

Petrescu A. 1982. Correlations between neurochemical, histochemical and electronmicroscopic data in demyelinating diseases. *Acta Morphologica*, **3**, 60-66.

Petrescu A. and Marcovici G. 1971. Correlation between demyelination stages and vascular reticulin proliferation in multiple sclerosis. *Rev. Roum. Neurol.*, **8**, 61-67.

Petrescu A., Patriche-Macovei M., Wender M. and Adamczewska Z. 1975. Histochemical and biochemical data in a case of Marchiafava-Bignami disease. In *Proc. VII Internat. Congress of Neuropathology*, ed. by S. Kornyey, S. Tariska and G. Gosztonyi, Akademiai Kiado, Budapest, vol. 2, pp 171-174.

Phadke J.G. 1987. Survival pattern and cause of death in patients with multiple sclerosis. *J. Neurol. Neurosurg. Psychiat.*, **50**, 523-531.

Pollock M., Calder C. and Allpress S. 1977. Peripheral nerve abnormalities in multiple sclerosis. *Ann. Neurol.*, **2**, 41-48.

Porcellati G. and Curti B. 1960. Proteinase activity of peripheral nerves during Wallerian degeneration. *J. Neurochem.* **5**, 277-282.

Portnoy, H.D. Chopp M., Branch C. and Shannon M. 1983. CSF and venous pulse waves; a look at myogenic autoregulation. In *The Cerebral Veins*, ed. by L.M. Auer and F. Heppner, Springer-Verlag, Wien, pp 213-221.

Poser C.M. 1987. The peripheral nervous system in multiple sclerosis. *J. Neurol. Sci.*, **79**, 83-90.

Poskanzer D.C., Schapira K. and Miller H. 1963. *Multiple sclerosis and poliomyelitis. Lancet*, **ii**, 917-921.

Poskanzer D.C., Prenney L.B., Sheridan J.L. and Yonkondy J. 1980. Multiple sclerosis in the Orkney and Shetland Islands. 1. Epidemiology, clinical factors and methodology. *Journal of Epidemiology and Community Health*, **34**, 240-252.

Powers J.M., Moser H.W., Moser A.B., Ma C.K., Elias S.B. and Norman R.A. 1987. Pathologic findings in adrenoleucodystrophy heterozygotes. *Arch. Pathol.*, **111**, 151-153.

Price P. and Cuzner M.L. 1979. Proteinase inhibitions in CSF in MS. *J. Neurol. Sci.*, **42**, 251-259.

Prineas J.W. 1975. Pathology of the early lesion in multiple sclerosis. *Human Pathol.*, **6**, 531-554.

Prineas J.W. 1979. Multiple sclerosis: presence of lymphatic capillaries and lymphoid tissue in the brain and spinal cord. *Science*, **203**, 1123-1125.

Prineas J.W. 1985. The neuropathology of multiple sclerosis. In *Handbook of Clinical Neurology*, ed. by P.J. Vinken, G.W. Bruyn, and H.L. Klawans. Elsevier Science Publishers, Amsterdam, vol. 47, pp 213-257.

Prineas J.W. and Connell F. 1979. Remyelination in multiple sclerosis. *Ann. Neurol.*, **5**, 22-31.

Prineas J.W. and Graham J.S. 1981. Multiple sclerosis: capping of surface immunoglobulin G on macrophages engaged in myelin breakdown. *Ann. Neurol.*, **10**, 149-158.

Prineas J.W. and Wright R.G. 1978. Macrophages, lymphocytes and plasma cells in the perivascular compartment in chronic multiple sclerosis. *Lab. Invest.*, **38**, 409-421.

Prineas J.W., Kwon E.E., Cho E-S. and Sharer L.R. 1984. Continual breakdown and regeneration of myelin in progressive multiple sclerosis plaques. *Ann. N.Y. Acad. Sci.*, **436**, 11-32.

Putnam T.J. 1937. Evidences of vascular occlusion in multiple sclerosis and 'encephalomyelitis'. *Arch. Neurol. Psychiat.*, **37**, 1298-1321.

Putnam T.J. and Adler A. 1937. Vascular architecture of the lesion of multiple sclerosis. *Arch. Neurol. Psychiat.*, **38**, 1-15.

Raff M.C., Fields K.L., Hakomori S., Mirsky R., Pruss R.M. and Winter J. 1979. Cell-type specific markers for distinguishing and studying neurons and the major classes of glial cells in culture. *Brain Res.*, **174**, 283-308.

Raff M.C., Miller R.H. and Noble M. 1983. A glial progenitor cell that develops in vitro into an astrocyte or an oligodendrocyte depending on culture medium. *Nature*, **303**, 390-396.

Raine C.S. 1976. On the development of CNS lesions in natural canine distemper encephalomyelitis. *J. Neurol. Sci.*, **30**, 13-28.

Raine C.S. 1983. Multiple sclerosis and relapsing EAE. Comparative ultrastructural neuropathology. In *Multiple Sclerosis*, ed. by J.F. Hallpike, C.W.M. Adams and W.W. Tourtellotte, Chapman & Hall, London, pp 413-460.

Raine C.S. 1984. The neuropathology of myelin diseases. In *Myelin* ed. by P. Morell, Plenum Press, New York, 2nd ed., pp 259-310.

Raine C.S., Scheinberg L. and Waltz J.M. 1981. Multiple sclerosis. Oligodendrocyte survival and proliferation in an active established lesion. *Lab. Invest.*, **45**, 534-546.

Rake M. and Saunders M. 1966. Refsum's disease. *J. Neurol. Neurosurg. Psychiat.*, **29**, 417-422.

Rhodes R.H. 1987. Histopathology of the central nervous system in the acquired immunodeficiency syndrome. *Human Pathol.*, **18**, 636-643.

Riekkinen P.J., Clausen J., Frey H.J., Fog T. and Rinne U.K. 1970. Acid proteinase activity of white matter and plaques in multiple sclerosis. *Acta Neurol. Scand.*, **46**, 349-353.

Riekkinen P.J, Palo J., Arstila A.U., Savolainen H.J., Rinne U.K. Kivalo E.K. and Frey H. 1971. Protein composition of multiple sclerosis myelin. *Arch. Neurol.*, **24**, 545-549.

Riggs J.E., Scochet S.S., Kopitnek T.A. and Gutmann L. 1986. Target fibres in multiple sclerosis implications for pathogenesis. *Neurology*, **36**, 297-298.

Rindfleisch E. 1863. Histologische Detail zu der grauen Degeneration von Gehirn und Ruckenmark. *Arch. Path. Anat.*, **26**, 474-488.

Rindfleisch E. 1873. 'Grey Degeneration' In *Pathological Histology*. Engl. Trans. The New Sydenham Society, London, vol. 2, pp 344-351.

Rivers T.M. and Schwentker F.F. 1935. Encephalomyelitis accompanied by myelin destruction experimentally produced in monkeys. *J. Exp. Med.*, **61**, 689-702.

Roach A., Boylan K., Horvath S., Prusiner S.B. and Hood L.E. 1983. Characterisation of cloned DNA representing rat myelin basic protein: absence of expression in Shiverer mutant mice. *Cell*, **34**, 799-806.

Rodgers-Johnson P., Gajdusek D.C., Morgan O. St. C., Zaninovic V., Sarin P.S. and Graham D.S. 1985. HTLV-1 and HTLV-III antibodies and tropical spastic paraparesis. *Lancet*, **ii**, 247-248.

Rodriguez M., Lafuse W.P., Leibowitz J. and David C.S. 1986. Partial suppression of Theiler's virus-induced demyelination in vivo by administration of monoclonal antibodies to immune-response gene products (Ia antigens). *Neurology*, **36**, 964-970.

Rodriguez M., Lennon V., Benveniste E.N. and Merrill J.E. 1987. Remyelination by oligodendrocytes stimulated by antiserum to spinal cord. *J. Neuropath. Exp. Neurol.*, **46**, 84-95.

Roessmann U. and Friede R.L. 1966. Changes in butyryl cholinesterase activity in reactive glia. *Neurology*, **16**, 123-129.

Rojiani A.M., Prineas J.W. and Cho E-S. 1987. Protective effect of steroids in electrolyte-induced demyelination. *J. Neuropathol. Exp. Neurol.*, **46**, 495-504.

Roman G.C., Schoenberg B.S., Madden D.L., Sever J.L., Hugon J., Ludolph A. and Spencer P.S. 1987. Human T-lymphocyte virus type 1 antibodies in the serum of patients with tropical spastic paraparesis in the Seychelles. *Arch. Neurol.*, **44**, 605-608.

Roquer J., Escudero D., Herraiz J., Maso E. and Cano F.J. 1987. Multiple sclerosis and Hashimoto's thyroiditis. *J. Neurol.*, **234**, 23-24.

Rosati G., Aiello I., Pirastru M.I., Mannu L., Demontis G., Beccio S., Sau G. and Zoccheddu A. 1987. Sardinia. A high risk area for multiple sclerosis. *Ann. Neurol.*, **21**, 190-194.

Rose L.M., Ledbetter J.A., Ginsberg A.H., Clark E.A. and Rothstein T.L. 1987. Suppressor-induced T cells in multiple sclerosis. *New Engl. J. Med.*, **317**, 118-119.

Röyttä M., Frey H., Riekkinen P.J., Laaksonen H. and Rinne U.K. 1974. Myelin breakdown and basic protein. *Exp. Neurol.*, **45**, 174-185.

Rubin M., Karpati G. and Carpenter S. 1987. Combined central and peripheral myelinopathy. *Neurology*, **37**, 1287-1290.

Saida T., Saida K., Dorfman S., Silberg D.H., Sumner A., Manning M., Lisak R.P. and Brown M.J. 1979a. Experimental allergic neuritis induced by sensitisation with galactocerebroside. *Science*, **204**, 1103-1106.

Saida T., Saida K., Brown M.J. and Silberberg D.H. 1979b. In vivo demyelination produced by intraneural injection of antigalactocerebroside serum. A morphologic study. *Amer. J. Pathol.*, **95**, 99-110.

Salmi A., Arnadottir T., Reunanen M. and Ilonen J. 1983. The significance of virus antibody synthesis in the central nervous system of multiple sclerosis patients. In *Viruses of Demyelinating Diseases*, ed. by C.A.C. Mims, M.L. Cuzner and R.E. Kelly, Academic Press, London, pp 141-152

Sanders E.A.C.M. and Lee K.D. 1987. Acute Guillain-Barré syndrome in multiple sclerosis. *J. Neurol.*, **24**, 128.

Scaravilli F. and Jacobs J.M. 1982. Improved myelination in nerve grafts from the leucodystrophic twitcher into trembler mice: evidence for enzyme replacement. *Brain Res.*, **237**, 163-172.

Scaravilli F. and Suzuki K. 1983. Enzyme replacement in grafted nerve of Twitcher mouse. *Nature*, **305**, 713-715.

Schauf C.L., Schauf V., Davis F.A. and Mizer M.R. 1978. Complement dependent serum neuroelectric blocking activity in multiple sclerosis. *Neurology*, **28**, 426-430.

Scheinker M. 1949. Histogenesis of the early lesions of multiple sclerosis. 1. Significance of vascular changes. *Arch. Neurol. Psychiat.*, **49**, 178-185.

Schelling F. 1986. Damaging venous reflux into the skull or spine: relevance to multiple sclerosis. *Medical Hypotheses*, **21**, 141-148.

Schelper R.L. and Adrian E.K. Jr. 1986. Monocytes become macrophages: they do not become microglia. A light and electron microscopic autoradiographic study. *J. Neuropathol. Exp. Neurol.*, **45**, 1-19.

Schlaepfer W.W. 1977. Vesicular disruption of myelin simulated by exposure of nerve to calcium ionophore. *Nature*, **265**, 734-736.

Schlesinger B. 1939. The venous drainage of the brain with special reference to the Galenic system. *Brain*, **62**, 274-291.

Schoene W.C., Carpenter S., Behan P.O. and Geschwind, N. 1977. 'Onion bulb' formations in the central and peripheral nervous systems in association with multiple sclerosis and hypertrophic polyneuropathy. *Brain*, **100**, 755-773.

Schroder J.M. and Krücke W. 1970. Ultrastructure of experimental allergic neuritis in the rabbit. *Acta Neuropathol.* **14**, 261-283.

Schutzhard E., Polhl P. and Stanek G. 1987. Lyme disease in Europe. *Lancet*, **ii**, 264-265.

Seitelberger F. 1970. Pelizaeus-Merzbacher disease. In *Handbook of Clinical Neurology*, vol. 10. ed. P.J. Vinken and G.W. Bruyn, Elsevier/North Holland, Amsterdam, pp 150-202.

Sergott R.C., Brown M.J., Lisak R.P. and Miller S.L. 1988. Antibody to myelin-associated glycoprotein produces central nervous system demyelination. *Neurology*, **38**, 422-426.

Shah S.N. and Johnson R.C. 1980. Activity levels of cholesterol ester metabolizing enzymes in brain in multiple sclerosis: correlation with cholesterol ester concentration. *Exp. Neurol.*, **68**, 601-604.

Shanker G., Campangnoni A.T. and Pieringer R.A. 1987. Investigations on myelinogenesis in vitro: developmental expression of myelin basic protein in RNA and its regulation by thyroid hormone in primary cerebral cell cultures from embryonic mice. *J. Neurosci. Res.*, **17**, 220-224.

Shaw P.J., Smith N.M., Ince P.G. and Bates D.J. 1987. Chronic periphlebitis retinae in mutliple sclerosis. A histopathological study. *J. Neurol. Sci.*, **77**, 147-152.

Sibley W.A., Bamford C.R. and Clark K. 1985. Clinical viral infections and multiple sclerosis. *Lancet*, **i**, 1313-1315.

Sidman R.L., Dickie M.M. and Appel S.H. 1964. Mutant mice (Quaking and Jimpy) with deficient myelination in the central nervous system. *Science*, **144**, 309-311.

Simon J.H., Hottas S.L., Schiffer R.B., Rudick R.A., Herndon R.M, Kido D.K., Utz R. 1986. Corpus callosum and subcallosal-periventricular lesions in multiple sclerosis: detection with MRI. *Radiology*, **160**, 363-367.

Simpson J.F. Tourtellotte W.W., Kokmen E., Parker J.A. and Itabashi H.H. 1969. Fluorescent protein tracing in multiple sclerosis brain tissue. *Arch. Neurol.*, **20**, 373-377.

Singh, I., Moser H.W. and Kishimoto Y. 1981. Adrenoleucodystrophy: impaired oxidation of long chain fatty acids in cultured skin fibroblasts and adrenal cortex. *Biochem. Biophys. Res. Comm.*, **102**, 1223-1229.

Sloan J.B., Berk M.A. Gebel H.M. and Fretzin D.F. 1987. Mutliple sclerosis and systemic lupus erythematosis. Occurrence in two generations of the same family. *Arch. Intern. Med.*, **147**, 1317-1320.

Small J.A., Scangos G.A., Cork L., Jay G. and Khoury, G. 1986. The early region of human papovavirus JC induces dysmyelination in transgenic mice. *Cell*, **46**, 13-18.

Smith M.E. 1977. Studies on the mechanism of demyelination: myelin autolysis in normal and oedematous central nervous system tissue. *J. Neurochem.*, **28**, 341-348.

Smith M.E. 1979. Neutral protease activity is lymphocytes of Lewis rats with acute experimental allergic encephalomyelitis. *Neurochem. Res.*, **4**, 687-694.

Smith M.E. 1980. Proteinase inhibitors and the suppression of EAE. In *Suppression of Experimental Allergic Encephalomyelitis and Multiple Sclerosis*. ed. by A.N. Davison and M.L. Cuzner, Academic Press, London, pp 211-222.

Smith M.E. and Amaducci L.A. 1982. Observations on the effects of protease inhibitors on the suppression of experimental allergic encephalomyelitis. *Neurochem. Res.*, **7**, 541-544.

Smith M.E. and Benjamins J.A. 1984. Model systems for study of perturbations of myelin metabolism. In *Myelin*, ed. by P. Morell, Plenum Press, New York, pp 441-487.

Smith M.E. and Hasinoff C.M. 1971. Biosynthesis of myelin proteins in vitro. *J. Neurochem.*, **18**, 739-747.

Smith M.E. and Sedgewick L.M. 1975. Studies of the mechanism of demyelination: regional differences in myelin stability in vitro. *J. Neurochem.*, **24**, 763-770.

Smith M.E., Sedgewick L.M. and Tagg J.S. 1974. Proteolytic enzymes and experimental demyelination in the rat and monkey. *J. Neurochem.*, **23**, 965-971.

Smith K.J., Blakemore W.F. and McDonald, W.I. 1981. The restoration of conduction by central remyelination. *Brain*, **104**, 383-404.

Smith K.J., Hall S.M. and Schauf C.L. 1985. Vesicular demyelination induced by raised intracellular calcium. *J. Neurol. Sci.*, **71**, 19-37.

Smith M.A., Chick J., Kean D.M., Douglas R.H.B., Singer A., Kendell R.E. and Best J.J.K. 1985. Brain water in chronic alcoholic patients measured by magnetic resonance imaging. *Lancet*, **i**, 1273-1274.

Smith I., Howells D.W. and Hyland K. 1986. Pteridines and monamines: relevance to neurological damage. *Postgrad. Med. J.*, **62**, 113-123.

Smith I., Howells D.W., Kendall B., Levinsky R. and Hyland K. 1987. Folate deficiency and demyelination in AIDS. *Lancet*, **ii**, 215.

Snyder D.H., Hirano A. and Raine C.S. 1975. Fenestrated CNS blood vessels in chronic experimental encephalomyelitis. *Brain Res.*, **100**, 645-649.

Sorensen O., Collins A., Flintoff W., Ebers G. and Daler S. 1986. Probing for the human coronavirus OC43 in multiple sclerosis. *Neurology*, **36**, 1604-1606.

Sosa A., DeMora A.F., Navarro M.C., Reyes M.P., Garcia J.R. and Betancor P. 1987. Multiple sclerosis on Islands (letter), *Lancet*, **i**, 119.

Sourander P. and Olsson Y. 1968. Peripheral neuropathy in globoid cell leucodystrophy (Morbus Krabbe). *Acta Neuropathol.* (Berlin), **11**, 69-81.

Spencer P.S., Weinberg H.J., Raine C.S. and Prineas J.W. 1975. The perineurial window – a new model of focal demyelination and remyelination. *Brain Res.*, **96**, 323-329.

Spillert C.R., Hafstein M.P., Lanka V. and Lazaro E.J. 1986. Increased thromboplastin production in multiple sclerosis: an immunologic defect. *Annal. N.Y. Acad. Sci.*, **475**, 345-346.

Sterman A.B., Coyle P.K., Panasci D.J. and Grimson R. 1985. Disseminated abnormalities of cardiovascular autonomic functions in multiple sclerosis. *Neurology*, **35**, 1665-1668.

Stewart G.J. and Kirk R.L. 1983. The genetics of multiple sclerosis: the HLA system and other genetic markers. In *Multiple Sclerosis*, ed. by J.F. Hallpike, C.W.M. Adams and W.W. Tourtellotte, Chapman & Hall, first edition, pp 97-128.

Stewart J.M., Houser O.W., Baker H.L., O'Brien P.C. and Rodriguez M. 1987. Magnetic resonance imaging and clinical relationships in multiple sclerosis. *Mayo Clinic Proc.*, **62**, 174-184.

Summers B.A., Greisen H.N. and Appel M.J.G. 1979. Early events in canine distemper demyelinating encephalomyelitis. *Acta Neuropathol.* (Berlin), **46**, 1-10.

Suzuki Y. and Grover W.D. 1970a. Ultrastructural and biochemical studies of Schilder's disease. I. Ultrastructure. *J. Neuropath. Exp. Neurol.*, **29**, 392-404.

Suzuki K., Andrews J.M., Waltz J.M. and Terry R.D. 1969. Ultrastructural studies of multiple sclerosis. *Lab. Invest.*, **20**, 444-454.

Suzuki K. and Grover W.D. 1970b. Krabbe's leucodystrophy (globoid cell leucodystrophy). *Arch. Neurol.*, **22**, 385-396.

Suzuki K. and Suzuki Y. 1970. Globoid cell leukodystrophy (Krabbe's disease): deficiency of galactocerebroside β-galactosidase. *Proc. Nat. Acad. Sci.*, (Wash.), **66**, 302-309.

Suzuki Y., Austin J., Armstrong D., Suzuki K., Schlenker J. and Fletcher T. 1970. Studies in globoid leucodystrophy: enzymatic and lipid findings in the canine form. *Exp. Neurol.*, **29**., 65-75.

Swank R.L. 1961. *A Biochemical Basis of Multiple Sclerosis.* Thomas, Springfield, Ill., pp 31.

Swank R.L. 1970. Multiple sclerosis: twenty years on a low fat diet. *Arch. Neurol.*, **23**, 460-474.

Swank R.L., Lerstad O., Strom A. and Backer J. 1952. Multiple sclerosis in rural Norway: its geographic and occupational incidence in relation to nutrition. *New Eng. J. Med.*, **246**, 721-728.

Swingler R.J. and Compston D. 1986. The distribution of multiple sclerosis in the United Kingdom. *J. Neurol. Neurosurg. Psychiat.*, **49**, 1115-1124.

Swingler R.J., Hughes P.J., Munro J.A. and Compston D.A.S. 1987. Human T-Cell lymphotrophic viruses in patients with multiple sclerosis. *J. Neurol.*, **234**, 448.

Symonds C.P. 1924. The pathological anatomy of disseminated sclerosis. *Brain*, **47**, 37-56.

Tanaka R., Iwasaki Y. and Koprowski H. 1975. Ultrastructural studies of perivascular cuffing cells in multiple sclerosis brain. *Amer. J. Pathol.*, **81**, 467-478.

Tanaka Y., Tsukada N., Koh Ch-S. and Yanagisawa N. 1987. Antiendothelial cell antibodies and circulating immune complexes in the sera of patients with MS. *J. Neuroimmunol.*, **17**, 49-59.

Tanphaichitr K. 1980. Multiple sclerosis associated with eosinophilic vasculitis, pericarditis and hypocomplementemia. *Arch. Neurol.*, **37**, 314-315.

ter Meulen V. and Stephenson J.R. 1983. The possible role of viral infections in multiple sclerosis and other related demyelinating diseases. In *Multiple Sclerosis*, ed. by J.F. Hallpike, C.W.M. Adams and W.W. Tourtellotte, Chapman & Hall, London, first edition, pp 241-274.

Thomas P.K. Walker R.W.H., Rudge P., Morgan-Hughes J.A., King R.H.M., Jacobs J.M., Mills K.R., Ormerod I.E.C., Murray N.M.F. and McDonald W.I., 1987. Chronic demyelinating peripheral neuropathy associated with multifocal central nervous system demyelination. *Brain*, **110**, 53-76.

Thompson E.J., Kaufmann P., Shortman R.C., Rudge P. and McDonald W.I. 1979. Oligoclonal immunoglobulins and plasma cells in spinal fluid of patients with multiple sclerosis. *Brit. Med. J.*, **i**, 16-17.

Thompson R.H.S. 1961. Myelinolytic mechanisms. *Proc. Roy. Soc. Med..*, **54**, 30-33.

Triarhou L.C. and Herndon R.M. 1985. Effect of macrophage inactivation on the neuropathology of lysolecthin induced demyelination. *Brit. J. Exp. Pathol.*, **66**, 293-301.

Toro G. and Román G., 1978. Cerebral malaria is a disseminated vasculomyelinopathy. *Arch. Neurol.*, **35**, 271-275.

Tournier-Lasserve E., Gout O., Gessain A., Iba-Zizen M.T., Lyon-Caen O., Lhermitte F. and De-The G. 1987. HTLV1, brain abnormalities on magnetic resonance imaging and relation with multiple sclerosis. *Lancet*, **ii**, 49-50.

Tourtellotte W.W. and Baumhefner R.W. 1983. Comprehensive management of multiple sclerosis. In *Multiple Sclerosis*, ed. by J.F. Hallpike, C.W.M. Adams and W.W. Tourtellotte, Chapman & Hall, London, pp 513-578.

Towfigi J., Young R.S., Sassami J., Ramer J. and Horoupian D.S. 1983. Alexander's disease: further light and electron microscopic findings. *Acta Neuropathol.*

Berlin), **61**, 36-42.

Trapp B.D. and Quarles R.H. 1984. Immunocytochemical localisation of the myelin associated glycoprotein: fact or artefact. *J. Neuroimmunol.*, **6**, 231-249.

Traugott U. and Raine C.S. 1982. T and B cell distribution in MS lesions (Abst.), *J. Neuropath. Exp. Neurol.*, **41**, 382.

Traugott U. and Raine C.S. 1985. Multiple sclerosis; evidence for antigen presentation in situ by endothelial cells and astrocytes. *J. Neurol. Sci.*, **69**, 365-370.

Traugott U., Snyder D.S. and Raine C.S. 1979. Oligodendrocyte staining by mutliple sclerosis serum is non-specific. *Ann. Neurol.*, **6**, 13-20.

Traugott U., Reinherz E.L. and Raine C.S. 1983. Distribution of T cells, T-cell subsets and Ia positive macrophages in lesions of different ages. *J. Neuroimmunol.*, **4**, 201-221.

Traugott U., McFarlin D.E., Raine C.S. 1986. Immunopathology of the lesion in chronic relapsing autoimmune encephalomyelitis in the mouse. *Cellular Immunology*, **99**, 395-410.

Tsukada N., Koh C-S., Yanagisawa N., Okano A., Behan W.M.H. and Behan P.O. 1987. A new model for multiple sclerosis: CEAE induced by immunization with cerebral endothelial membrane. *Acta Neuropathol.* (Berlin), **73**, 259-266.

Tuqan N.A. and Adams C.W.M. 1961. Histochemistry of myelin I. Proteins and lipid-protein complexes in the normal sheath. *J. Neurochem.* **6**, 327-333.

Turnbull H.M. and McIntosh J. 1926. Encephalomyelitis following vaccination. *Brit. J. Exp. Pathol.*, **7**, 181-222.

Uchimura I. and Shiraki H. 1957. A contribution to the classification and pathogenesis of demyelinating encephalomyelitis, with special reference to the CNS lesions caused by preventative inoculation against rabies. *J. Neuropath. Exp. Neurol.*, **16**, 139-203.

Ulrich J. and Groebke-Lorenz W. 1983. The optic nerve in multiple sclerosis. A morphological study with retrospective clinicopathological correlations. *Neuro-ophthalmology*, **3**, 149-159.

Vandenheuvel F.A. 1965. Structural studies of biological membranes: the structure of myelin. *Ann. N.Y. Acad. Sci.*, **122**, 57-76.

Van der Veen R., Brinkman C.J.J., Hommes O.R. and Lamers K.J. B. 1985. The effect of myelin basic protein on the protease inhibitors alpha1 antitrypsin and alpha2 macroglobulin. *Acta Neurol. Scand.*, **71**, 199-205.

Vassallo L., Elian M. and Dean G. 1979. Multiple sclerosis in Southern Europe II. Prevalence in Malta since 1978. *J. Epidemiol. Commun. Health*, **33**, 111-113.

Vinters H.V., Anders K.H. and Barach P. 1987. Focal pontine leucoencephalopathy in immunosuppressed patients. *Arch. Pathol.*, **111**, 192-196.

Visscher B.R., Sullivan C.B., Detels R., Madden D.L., Sever J.L., Terasaki P.I., Park M.S. and Dudley J.P. 1981. Measles antibody titres in multiple sclerosis and HLA-matched and unmatched siblings. *Neurology*, **31**, 1142-1145.

Wagner H-J., Pilgrim Ch. and Brandl J., 1974. Penetration and removal of horseradish peroxidase injected into the CSF: role of cerebral perivascular spaces, endothelium and microglia. *Acta Neuropathol.* (Berlin), **27**, 299-315.

Waksman B.H. and Adams R.D. 1962. Infectious leucoencephalitis. A critical comparison of certain experimental and naturally occurring viral leucoencephalitis with experimental allergic encephalomyelitis. *J. Neuropath. Exp. Neurol.*, **21**, 491-518.

Walsh M.J. and Tourtellotte W.W. 1983. The cerebrospinal fluid in multiple sclerosis. In *Multiple Sclerosis*, ed., by J.F. Hallpike, C.W.M. Adams and W.W. Tourtellotte, Chapman & Hall, London, first edition, pp 275-358.

Walton J.C. and Kaufman J.C.E. 1984. Iron deposits and multiple sclerosis. *Arch. Pathol.*, **108**, 755-756.

Wayne Moore G.R., McCarron R.M., McFarlin D.E. and Raine C.S. 1987. Chronic relapsing necrotising encephalomyelitis produced by myelin basic protein in mice. *Lab. Invest.* **57**, 157-167.

Webb H.E., Mehta S., Leibowitz S. and Gregson N.A. 1984. Immunological reaction of the demyelinating Semliki Forest virus with immune serum to glycolipids and its possible importance to central nervous system viral autoimmune disease. *Neuropathol. Appl. Neurobiol.*, **10**, 77-84.

Webster, G.R. 1957. Clearing action of lysolecithin on brain homogenates. *Nature*, (London), **180**, 660-661.

Webster, G.R. 1965. The acylation of lysophosphatides with long-chain fatty acids by rat brain and other tissues. *Biochem. Biophys. Acta.*, 98, 512-519.

Weller R.O. 1967. An electron microscopic study of hypertrophic neuropathy of Dejerine and Sottas. *J. Neurol. Neurosurg. Psychiat.*, **30**, 111-125.

Weller R.O. and Cervos-Navarro J. 1977. *Pathology of the Peripheral Nerve*. Butterworth, London, pp 102-108.

Wender M. and Kozik M. 1969. Contribution to the histoenzymic changes in multiple sclerosis. *Acta Neuropath.*, **13**, 143-148.

Wender M., Filipek-Wender H. and Stanislawska B. 1973. Cholesterol esters in apparently normal white matter in multiple sclerosis. *Europ. Neurol.*, **10**, 340-348.

White F.V., Burroni D., Ceccarini C., Matthieu J.M., Manetti R. and Ceccarini E.C. 1986. Trembler mouse Schwann cells in culture: anomalies in the synthesis of lipids and proteins. *Brain Res*, **27**, 85-92.

Williams E.S. and McKeran R.O. 1986. Prevalence of multiple sclerosis in a South London borough. *Brit. Med. J.*, **293**, 237-239.

Wisniewski H.M. 1977. Immunopathology of demyelination in autoimmune diseases and virus infections. *Brit. Med. Bull.*, **33**, 54-59.

Wisniewski H.M. and Bloom B.R. 1975. Primary demyelination as a non-specific consequence of a cell-mediated immune reaction. *J. Exp. Med.*, **141**, 346-359.

Wisnieski H.M. and Raine C.S. 1971. An ultrastructural study of experimental demyelination and remyelination V. Central and peripheral nervous system lesions caused by diphtheria toxin. *Lab. Invest.*, **25**, 73-80.

Wisniewski H.M., Raine C.S. and Kay W.J. 1972. Observations on viral demyelinating encephalomyelitis: canine distemper. *Lab. Invest.*, **26**, 589-599.

Wisniewski H.M., Oppenheimer D. and McDonald W.I. 1976. Relation between myelination and function in MS and EAE (Abst.). *J. Neuropath. Exp. Neurol.*, **35**, 327.

Wisniewski H.M., Brosnan C.F. and Bloom B.R. 1980. Bystander and antibody-dependent cell-mediated demyelination. In *Suppression of Experimental Allergic Encephalomyelitis and Multiple Sclerosis*, ed. by A.N. Davison and M.L. Cuzner, Academic Press, London, pp 45-55.

Wolman M. 1960. The grape-like bodies of the central nervous system. *Confina Neurologica*, **20**, 36-44.

Woodroofe M.N., Bellamy A.S., Feldmann M., Davison A.N. and Cuzner M.L. 1986. Immunocytochemical characterisation of the immune reaction in the CNS in multiple sclerosis. *J. Neurol. Sci.*, **74**, 135-152.

Wright G. Payling 1961. The metabolism of myelin. *Proc. Roy. Soc. Med.*, **54**, 26-30.

Wright, H. Payling, Thompson R.H.S. and Zilkha K.J. 1965. Platelet adhesiveness in multiple sclerosis. *Lancet*, **ii** 1109-1110.

Wright D.G., Laureno R. and Victor M. 1979. Pontine an extra pontine myelinoclasis. *Brain*, **102**, 361-385.

Yakovlev P. and Lecours A.R. 1967. The myelinogenetic cycles of regional maturation of the brain. In *Regional Development of the Brain in Early Life*, ed. by Minkowski A. Blackwell, Oxford, pp 3-70.

Yanagisawa K., Duncan I.D., Hammang J.P., and Quarle R.H. 1986. Myelin deficient rat: analysis of myelin proteins. *J. Neurochem.*, **47**, 1901-1907.

Ziegler E. 1886. A *Textbook of Pathological Anatomy and Pathogenesis*. Macmillan, London, Section 9-12, pp 280-284.

Zimmerman A.W., Matthieu J-M., Quarles R.H., Brady R.O. and Hsu J.M. 1976. Hypomyelination in copper-deficient rats. *Arch. Neurol.*, **33**, 111-119.

Zimmerman H.M. and Netsky M.G. 1950. The patholog of multiple sclerosis. *Res. Publ. Assoc. Res. Nerv. Ment. Dis.*, **28**, 271-312.

Index

Figures in **bold** refer to illustrations; other figures refer to page numbers.